T0263816

# Genitourinary Pathology

*Editor*

MICHELLE S. HIRSCH

# SURGICAL PATHOLOGY CLINICS

www.surgpath.theclinics.com

*Consulting Editor*
JOHN R. GOLDBLUM

December 2015 • Volume 8 • Number 4

**ELSEVIER**

1600 John F. Kennedy Boulevard • Suite 1800 • Philadelphia, Pennsylvania, 19103-2899

http://www.theclinics.com

**SURGICAL PATHOLOGY CLINICS Volume 8, Number 4**
**December 2015 ISSN 1875-9181, ISBN-13: 978-0-323-39587-8**

Editor: Lauren Boyle
Developmental Editor: Donald Mumford

*Surgical Pathology Clinics* (ISSN 1875-9181) is published quarterly by Elsevier Inc., 360 Park Avenue South, New York, NY 10010. Months of issue are March, June, September, and December. Business and Editorial Office: Elsevier Inc., 1600 John F. Kennedy Blvd., Ste. 1800, Philadelphia, PA 19103-2899. Accounting and Circulation Offices: Elsevier Inc., 3251 Riverport Lane, Maryland Heights, MO 63043. Periodicals postage paid at New York, NY and at additional mailing offices. Subscription prices are $200.00 per year (US individuals), $233.00 per year (US institutions), $100.00 per year (US students/residents), $250.00 per year (Canadian individuals), $266.00 per year (Canadian Institutions), $250.00 per year (foreign individuals), $266.00 per year (foreign institutions), and $120.00 per year (international & Canadian students/residents). Foreign air speed delivery is included in all *Clinics'* subscription prices. All prices are subject to change without notice. **POSTMASTER:** Send address changes to *Surgical Pathology Clinics*, Elsevier, 3251 Riverport Lane, Maryland Heights, MO 63043. **Customer Service: 1-800-654-2452 (US). From outside the United States, call 1-314-447-8871. Fax: 1-314-447-8029. E-mail:** JournalsCustomerServiceusa@elsevier.com **(for print support)** and JournalsOnlineSupport-usa@elsevier.com **(for online support)**.

*Reprints.* For copies of 100 or more, of articles in this publication, please contact the Commercial Reprints Department, Elsevier Inc., 360 Park Avenue South, New York, NY 10010-1710. Tel. 212-633-3874; Fax: 212-633-3820; E-mail: reprints@elsevier.com.

*Surgical Pathology Clinics of North America* is covered in *MEDLINE/PubMed (Index Medicus)*.

# Contributors

## CONSULTING EDITOR

**JOHN R. GOLDBLUM, MD**
Chairman, Department of Anatomic Pathology,
Professor of Pathology; Cleveland Clinic Lerner
College of Medicine, Cleveland Clinic,
Cleveland, Ohio

## EDITOR

**MICHELLE S. HIRSCH, MD, PhD**
Chief, Genitourinary Pathology Division, Staff
Pathologist, Department of Pathology,
Brigham and Women's Hospital, Associate
Professor, Harvard Medical School, Boston,
Massachusetts

## AUTHORS

**ADEBOWALE J. ADENIRAN, MD**
Associate Professor, Department of Pathology,
Yale University School of Medicine, New
Haven, Connecticut

**LAURENCE ALBIGES, MD, PhD**
Dana-Farber Cancer Institute, Harvard Medical
School, Boston, Massachusetts

**MAHUL B. AMIN, MD**
Professor, Medical Director and Chairman,
Department of Pathology and Laboratory
Medicine, Cedars-Sinai Medical Center, Los
Angeles, California

**JAVIER A. ARIAS-STELLA III, MD**
Department of Pathology and Laboratory
Medicine, Henry Ford Health System, Detroit,
Michigan

**JUSTINE A. BARLETTA, MD**
Assistant Professor, Department of Pathology,
Brigham and Women's Hospital, Harvard
Medical School, Boston, Massachusetts

**CLAIR BEARD, MD**
Associate Professor, Department of Radiation
Oncology, Brigham and Women's Hospital,
Harvard Medical School, Boston,
Massachusetts

**JOAQUIM BELLMUNT, MD, PhD**
Associate Professor of Medicine, Lank Center
for Genitourinary Oncology, Dana-Farber
Cancer Institute, Harvard Medical School,
Boston, Massachusetts

**BRANDON BERNARD, MD**
Lank Center for Genitourinary Oncology,
Dana-Farber Cancer Institute, Harvard
Medical School, Boston, Massachusetts

**DANIEL M. BERNEY, FRCPath**
Orchid Tissue Laboratory, St. Bartholomew's
Hospital, Barts Cancer Institute, Queen Mary
University of London, London, United Kingdom

**TONI K. CHOUEIRI, MD**
Dana-Farber Cancer Institute; Brigham and
Women's Hospital, Harvard Medical School,
Boston, Massachusetts

**PAOLA DAL CIN, PhD**
Professor, Department of Pathology, Center for
Advanced Molecular Diagnostics, Brigham and
Women's Hospital, Harvard Medical School,
Boston, Massachusetts

**MUKUL DIVATIA, MD**
Department of Pathology and Laboratory
Medicine, Cedars-Sinai Medical Center, Los
Angeles, California

**AYMEN ELFIKY, MD, MA, MPH, MSc**
Attending Physician, Lank Center for
Genitourinary Oncology, Dana-Farber
Cancer Institute/Brigham and Women's
Hospital, Harvard Medical School,
Massachusetts

**ANDRÉ P. FAY, MD**
Dana-Farber Cancer Institute, Harvard Medical
School, Boston, Massachusetts

**DONNA E. HANSEL, MD, PhD**
Chief, Division of Anatomic Pathology,
Department of Pathology, University of
California, San Diego, La Jolla, California

**LAUREN C. HARSHMAN, MD**
Assistant Professor of Medicine, Lank
Center for Genitourinary Oncology,
Dana-Farber Cancer Institute, Harvard
Medical School, Boston, Massachusetts

**MICHELLE S. HIRSCH, MD, PhD**
Chief, Genitourinary Pathology Division,
Staff Pathologist, Associate Professor,
Department of Pathology, Brigham
and Women's Hospital, Harvard
Medical School, Boston, Massachusetts

**BROOKE E. HOWITT, MD**
Department of Pathology, Brigham and
Women's Hospital, Harvard Medical School,
Boston, Massachusetts

**PETER A. HUMPHREY, MD, PhD**
Professor of Pathology, Director of
Genitourinary Pathology, Department
of Pathology, Yale University School of
Medicine, New Haven, Connecticut

**MARINA D. KAYMAKCALAN, PharmD**
Dana-Farber Cancer Institute, Harvard Medical
School, Boston, Massachusetts

**RANA R. McKAY, MD**
Dana-Farber Cancer Institute; Brigham and
Women's Hospital, Harvard Medical School,
Boston, Massachusetts

**ROHIT MEHRA, MD**
Department of Pathology, University of
Michigan Hospital and Health Systems, Ann
Arbor, Michigan

**GEORGE J. NETTO, MD**
Director of Surgical Pathology Molecular
Diagnostics; Professor of Pathology,
Oncology, and Urology, Johns Hopkins
University, Baltimore, Maryland

**ANDRE PINTO, MD**
Surgical Pathology Fellow, Department of
Pathology, Brigham and Women's Hospital,
Harvard Medical School, Boston,
Massachusetts

**MARK POMERANTZ, MD**
Department of Medical Oncology, Dana-Farber
Cancer Institute, Harvard Medical School,
Boston, Massachusetts

**MARK A. PRESTON, MD, MPH**
Instructor in Surgery, Division of Urology,
Brigham and Women's Hospital, Harvard
Medical School, Boston, Massachusetts

**SABINA SIGNORETTI, MD**
Associate Professor, Department of Pathology,
Brigham and Women's Hospital, Harvard
Medical School, Boston, Massachusetts

**STEVEN C. SMITH, MD**
Department of Pathology and Laboratory
Medicine, Cedars-Sinai Medical Center, Los
Angeles, California

**JAMES P. SOLOMON, MD, PhD**
Resident, Department of Pathology, University
of California, San Diego, La Jolla, California

**CHRISTOPHER J. SWEENEY, MBBS**
Lank Center for Genitourinary Oncology, Dana-
Farber Cancer Institute, Harvard Medical
School, Boston, Massachusetts

**SEAN R. WILLIAMSON, MD**
Senior Staff Pathologist, Department of
Pathology and Laboratory Medicine, Henry
Ford Health System; Josephine Ford Cancer
Institute, Henry Ford Health System; Clinical
Assistant Professor of Pathology, Wayne State
University School of Medicine, Detroit,
Michigan

# Contents

**Morphologic Updates in Prostate Pathology** 539

Adebowale J. Adeniran and Peter A. Humphrey

> In the past several years, modifications have been made to the original Gleason sys-
> tem with resultant therapeutic and prognostic implications. Several morphologic
> variants of prostatic adenocarcinoma have also been described. Prostate pathology
> has also evolved over the years with the discovery and utility of new immunohisto-
> chemical stains. The topics discussed in this update include the Gleason grading
> system, prognostic grade grouping, variants of prostatic adenocarcinoma, and the
> application of immunohistochemistry to prostate pathology.

**Molecular Updates in Prostate Cancer** 561

George J. Netto

> A wide array of molecular markers and genomic signatures, reviewed in this article,
> may soon be used as adjuncts to currently established screening strategies, prog-
> nostic parameters, and early detection markers. Markers of genetic susceptibility
> to PCA, recurrent epigenetic and genetic alterations, including *ETS* gene fusions,
> *PTEN* alterations, and urine-based early detection marker *PCA3*, are discussed.
> Impact of recent genome-wide assessment on our understanding of key pathways
> of PCA development and progression and their potential clinical implications are
> highlighted.

**Active Surveillance: Pathologic and Clinical Variables Associated with Outcome** 581

Mark Pomerantz

> Over the past 10 years, active surveillance has emerged as a primary management
> option for men diagnosed with low-risk prostate cancer. Given the morbidity asso-
> ciated with curative treatment, active surveillance maintains quality of life for men
> whose disease may never become symptomatic. In order to confidently and safely
> offer this approach to as many patients as possible, improved metrics are needed to
> fully assess risk. While pathologic and clinical variables currently help determine
> whether active surveillance is a reasonable approach, emerging biomarkers and im-
> aging technologies demonstrate promise for more precise identification of ideal
> candidates.

**Adult Renal Cell Carcinoma: A Review of Established Entities from Morphology to Molecular Genetics** 587

Michelle S. Hirsch, Sabina Signoretti, and Paola Dal Cin

> According to the current World Health Organization (WHO), renal cell carcinomas
> (RCCs) that primarily affect adults are classified into 8 major subtypes. Additional
> emerging entities in renal neoplasia have also been recently recognized and these
> are discussed in further detail by Mehra et al (Emerging Entities in Renal Neoplasia.
> Surgical Pathology Clinics, 2015, Volume 8, Issue 4). In most cases, the diagnosis of

a RCC subtype can be based on morphologic criteria, but in some circumstances the use of ancillary studies can aid in the diagnosis. This review discusses the morphologic, genetic, and molecular findings in RCCs previously recognized by the WHO, and provides clues to distinction from each other and some of the newer subtypes of RCC. As prognosis and therapeutic options vary for the different subtypes of RCC, accurate pathologic distinction is critical for patient care.

This article reviews emerging entities in renal epithelial neoplasia, including tubulocystic carcinoma, clear-cell-papillary renal cell carcinoma (RCC), thyroid-like follicular RCC, ALK-related RCC, translocation RCC, acquired cystic disease-related RCC, succinate dehydrogenase-deficient RCC, and hereditary leiomyomatosis-RCC syndrome-associated RCC. Many of these rarer subtypes of RCC were recently studied in more depth and are included in the upcoming version of the World Health Organization classification of tumors. Emphasis is placed on common gross and morphologic features, differential diagnoses, use of ancillary studies for making accurate diagnoses, molecular alterations, and predicted biologic behavior based on previous studies.

Renal cell carcinoma (RCC) is a heterogeneous disease. A rigorous diagnostic assessment by a pathologist with close communication with the clinician provides more accurate prognostication and informed treatment decisions. In the localized setting, an accurate prognostic assessment directs patients to potential adjuvant clinical trials. For patients with advanced disease, the pathologic assessment may have a direct impact on the systemic therapy algorithm. Additionally, it provides the basis for continuous efforts in biomarker development. In rare histologic subtypes, the interaction between clinicians and pathologists provides an opportunity to offer patients specific clinical trials. Molecular characterization platforms may identify targets for therapeutic intervention.

Bladder cancer is the fourth most common cancer in men, and is associated with significant morbidity and mortality. Pathologic evaluation of urothelial cancers relies predominantly on histomorphologic features but can be aided in a small subset of cases by immunohistochemical analyses. Distinction of papillary versus flat lesions, low-grade versus high-grade cytology, and histologic variants and the presence or absence of invasive tumor is important for proper clinical management. Advances in the molecular alterations associated with the various subtypes of urothelial carcinoma have been made but such studies are ongoing.

In 2014, more than 74,000 new cases and 15,000 deaths from bladder cancer were estimated to occur. The most reliable prognostic factors for survival are pathologic stage and histologic grade. Accordingly, a good understanding of the pathologic features of these cancers is essential to guide optimal clinical treatment, which requires a multidisciplinary team of pathologists, urologists, radiation oncologists, and medical oncologists. This review highlights several clinical scenarios in which detailed pathologic evaluation and accurate reporting impact clinical management.

This article reviews the most frequently encountered tumor of the testis; pure and mixed malignant testicular germ cell tumors (TGCT), with emphasis on adult (post-pubertal) TGCTs and their differential diagnoses. We additionally review TGCT in the postchemotherapy setting, and findings to be integrated into the surgical pathology report, including staging of testicular tumors and other problematic issues. The clinical features, gross pathologic findings, key histologic features, common differential diagnoses, the use of immunohistochemistry, and molecular alterations in TGCTs are discussed.

Testicular germ cell tumors (GCTs) include seminoma and nonseminoma. Chance of cure is excellent for clinical stage I disease regardless of whether adjuvant treatment or a surveillance strategy with treatment only for those who relapse is used. Risk of recurrence is greater in nonseminoma with evidence of lymphovascular invasion, but most can be salvaged with chemotherapy and survival rates remain high. This article outlines key pathologic and clinical considerations in clinical stage I seminoma, non-seminoma, advanced disease, and assessment of cancer of unknown primary as a potential GCT.

Although most adrenal tumors are not diagnostic dilemmas, there are cases that are challenging. This may be due to the tissue provided, for example fragmented tissue received in the setting of morcellation, or it may be due to inherently challenging histology, such as in cases with equivocal features of malignancy. Additionally, much has been learned about the molecular alterations of adrenal tumors, especially pheochromocytomas. Many of these alterations represent germline mutations with significant clinical implications for patients and their families. The aim of this review is to provide an overview of the most common adrenal tumors in adults so that pathologists can tackle these interesting tumors.

Within the category of orphan diseases and rare malignancies, adrenocortical carcinoma (ACC) represents an aggressive entity with high mortality and morbidity. While localized tumors which are diagnosed early can be cured with surgical intervention, there are prognostic factors which predict for micrometastases and consequent recurrent and advanced disease. In such cases, mitotane and cytotoxic chemotherapy have been utilized with a modest degree of benefit. The poor prognosis of recurrent and advanced ACC has underscored the interest in nuanced characterization of ACC cases to guide the personalized use of immunotherapeutic and novel targeted therapies.

Javier A. Arias-Stella III and Sean R. Williamson

The genitourinary tract is a common site for new cancer diagnosis, particularly for men. Therefore, cancer-containing specimens are very common in surgical pathology practice. However, many benign neoplasms and nonneoplastic, reactive, and inflammatory processes in the genitourinary tract may mimic or cause differential diagnostic challenges with malignancies. Emerging clinicopathologic, immunohistochemical, and molecular characteristics have shed light on the pathogenesis and differential diagnosis of these lesions. This review addresses differential diagnostic challenges related to benign genitourinary tract lesions in the kidney, urinary bladder, prostate, and testis, with emphasis on recent advances in knowledge and areas most common in diagnostic practice.

# SURGICAL PATHOLOGY CLINICS

THE CLINICS ARE AVAILABLE ONLINE!
Access your subscription at:
www.theclinics.com

# Preface

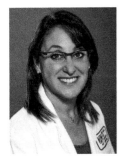

Michelle S. Hirsch, MD, PhD
*Editor*

An Update of Genitourinary Pathology from Morphology to Molecular Genetics with an Emphasis on Clinicopathologic Correlation.

It has been an honor and a pleasure to act as Special Editor for this issue of *Surgical Pathology Clinics*, which places an emphasis on pathology of the genitourinary (GU) tract. It has been approximately six years since the last GU issue of *Surgical Pathology Clinics* was published, and since that time, there have been many significant advances in all areas of GU pathology including morphology and biomarker analysis, genetic and molecular alterations, and clinical treatment. Accordingly, my approach to the current GU issue of *Surgical Pathology Clinics* was to address these updates in the prostate, kidney, bladder, testis, and adrenal gland. In most of the articles, updates in morphology and the molecular basis of disease are addressed concurrently. However, as there have been so many advances in both of these areas for prostatic adenocarcinoma, I felt it was best to separate morphology (including the recent changes made to Gleason grading) from molecular alterations. Similarly, with our improved ability to more precisely subtype kidney tumors, I felt it was important to define those that are well established and those more recently added to the World Health Organization (WHO) Classification of Kidney Tumors in separate articles. Although fewer in frequency, changes made by the WHO in urothelial and testicular pathology are also summarized in their respective articles. Inclusion of the adrenal gland was done intentionally as GU pathologists may encounter such specimens, and adrenal gland neoplasms may subsequently be treated by a urologic medical oncologist. The final pathology article in this issue discusses nonneoplastic lesions in the GU organs, as clearly their distinction from malignancy is clinically relevant. Last, I would like to point out the unique and innovative approach to this GU issue of *Surgical Pathology Clinics*, which included small clinical reviews, written by expert urologic medical oncologists, that discuss the clinicopathologic correlation in regards to all 5 corresponding organ systems. The intent was for this complete collection of reviews to provide clinically significant information for the pathologist so that we can better understand why we make certain diagnoses, as well as pathologically significant information for the clinician including recent changes to nomenclature and reporting. Overall, it is my hope that this comprehensive GU issue of *Surgical Pathology Clinics* will provide a contemporary update for pathologists and clinicians at various levels of experience in regards to the diagnostic workup, differential diagnosis, pathophysiology, and clinical significance of neoplastic and nonneoplastic lesion of the GU tract.

Michelle S. Hirsch, MD, PhD
Harvard Medical School
Brigham and Women's Hospital
Department of Pathology
75 Francis Street, Amory-1
Boston, MA 02115, USA

E-mail address:
mhirsch1@partners.org

*Surgical Pathology 8 (2015) xi*
http://dx.doi.org/10.1016/j.path.2015.10.005
1875-9181/15/$ – see front matter © 2015 Published by Elsevier Inc.

# Morphologic Updates in Prostate Pathology

Adebowale J. Adeniran, MD*, Peter A. Humphrey, MD, PhD

## KEYWORDS

• Prostatic adenocarcinoma • Gleason system • Active surveillance • Immunohistochemistry

## ABSTRACT

In the past several years, modifications have been made to the original Gleason system with resultant therapeutic and prognostic implications. Several morphologic variants of prostatic adenocarcinoma have also been described. Prostate pathology has also evolved over the years with the discovery and utility of new immunohistochemical stains. The topics discussed in this update include the Gleason grading system, prognostic grade grouping, variants of prostatic adenocarcinoma, and the application of immunohistochemistry to prostate pathology.

## OVERVIEW: UPDATE ON THE GLEASON GRADING SYSTEM

Since the original Gleason grading system[1] was derived, so much has changed in the area of prostate pathology, with the discovery and utility of serum prostate-specific antigen (PSA), immunohistochemical stains, 18-gauge core needle biopsies, and improved surgical techniques. In 2005, the International Society of Urologic Pathology (ISUP) reviewed and made changes to the original Gleason grading system[2] and these changes have had a profound impact on contemporary pathology and urology practices worldwide.[3–10] A second modification to the Gleason diagram entailed placement of cribriform adenocarcinomas into pattern 4 (Fig. 1).[8] Conventional and modified Gleason grading both correlate with age, serum PSA, and cancer involvement in needle biopsies. It has been shown that the stage distribution of modified Gleason grades of radical prostatectomy (RP) specimens differs from that of conventional Gleason grades, but a good correlation exists between grade and primary tumor (pT) stage.[5,10] Some of issues concerning the various Gleason grades/patterns are as follows.

## GLEASON GRADE 1

Gleason grade 1 glands consist of a circumscribed nodule of closely packed but distinct, uniform, medium-sized acinar structures, which are round to oval and usually larger than glands seen in pattern 3. It is recommended that Gleason score of 1 + 1 = 2 should not be assigned to prostatic adenocarcinoma, regardless of the specimen, with rare exceptions. A majority of cases in this group are actually adenosis (atypical adenomatous hyperplasia).[2,9,11–13]

## GLEASON GRADE 2

The glands in the Gleason grade 2 group are fairly circumscribed but may have minimal infiltration at the edge. These glands are more loosely arranged than those seen in pattern 1. This pattern is characteristic of transition zone cancers, so should rarely be seen in needle biopsy sampling that typically targets the peripheral zone. This fact along with poor reproducibility has led to the recommendation that a diagnosis of Gleason score 2 + 2 = 4 should be made "rarely, if ever" in needle biopsy.[2,14,15] A majority of the cases assigned a Gleason score of 4 on core needle biopsies have a higher Gleason score on corresponding prostatectomies.

## GLEASON GRADE 3

The glands in the Gleason grade 3 category are typically smaller than those seen in pattern 1 or

Department of Pathology, Yale University School of Medicine, 310 Cedar Street, LH 108, New Haven, CT 06520, USA

* Corresponding author.

*E-mail address:* adebowale.adeniran@yale.edu

Surgical Pathology 8 (2015) 539–560

http://dx.doi.org/10.1016/j.path.2015.08.002

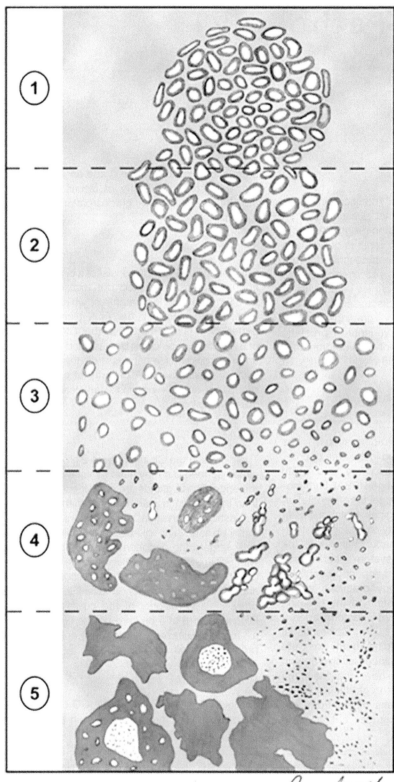

*Fig. 1.* Gleason grading diagram: 2010 modification of ISUP 2005 modified scheme. (*From* Epstein JI. An update of the Gleason grading system. J Urol 2010;183: 433–40; with permission.) Note that a new ISUP modification of this diagram will be published (Epstein JI, Egevad L, Amin MB, et al. The 2014 international society of urological pathology [ISUP] Consensus Conference on Gleason grading of prostatic carcinoma: Definition of grading patterns and proposal for a new grading system. Am J Surg Pathol 2015, in press).

2. They usually present as discrete glandular units with marked variation in size and shape and they are characterized by infiltration in and among benign glands. The consensus among urologic pathologists now is that invasive cribriform glands and glands with glomeruloid architecture more accurately reflect Gleason pattern 4 and hence should not be diagnosed as Gleason pattern 3.[7,8,16] Pitfalls in grading of pattern 3 include overgrading of pattern 3 as pattern 4 with crowded pattern 3 glands (Fig. 2), atrophic pattern 3B, tangentially sectioned glands, branching glands, crush artifact, and glands with perineural invasion.[17]

## GLEASON GRADE 4

The glands in the Gleason grade 4 category are characterized by fused microacinar glands, cribriform glands (Fig. 3), ill-defined glands with poorly formed glandular lumina (Fig. 4), and glands with glomeruloid pattern. In the past, the hypernephromatoid adenocarcinoma was viewed as pattern 4 but it is vanishingly rare.[18] It is now clear that invasive cribriform adenocarcinoma is more aggressive than grade 3[19–22] and should be included in pattern 4, as indicated by the second modification of the Gleason system (see Fig. 1).[8] Ill-defined glands with poorly formed glandular lumina are now also considered as pattern 4 when a tangential section of pattern 3 glands cannot account for the histology. Diagnosis of poorly formed glands remains a significant challenge, with reproducibility an issue.

## GLEASON GRADE 5

In pattern 5, there is essentially no glandular differentiation, with tumor consisting of solid sheets, cords, or single cells. The presence of comedonecrosis surrounded by papillary, cribriform, or solid masses, also falls into the pattern 5 category. Small solid nests (Fig. 5), linear arrays (Fig. 6), and solid cylinders should also be considered grade

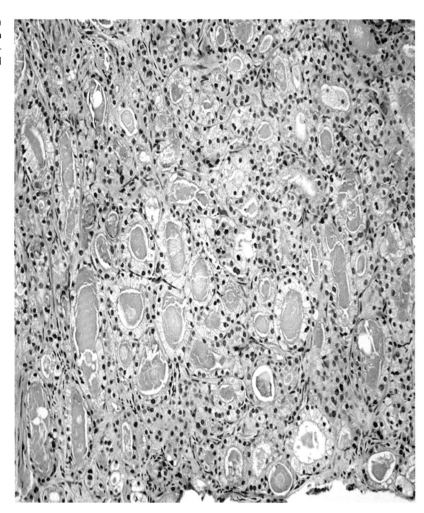

*Fig. 2.* Crowded Gleason grade 3 adenocarcinoma of the prostate (hematoxylin-eosin, original magnification ×200).

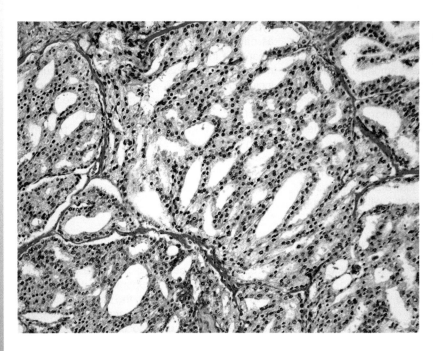

Fig. 3. Cribriform Gleason grade 4 adenocarcinoma of the prostate (hematoxylin-eosin, original magnification ×200).

5.[18] One pitfall is that the presence of signet ring-like cells is indicative of pattern 5 and these should be distinguished from clear vacuoles, which are typically seen in pattern 4 tumors, but which can also be found in pattern 3 glands. Grade 5 is readily underdiagnosed, particularly when it is not the primary pattern.[23] A challenge for the future for diagnosis of pattern 5 is the determination of how many single cells are needed to assign pattern 5 (Fig. 7). This is currently unsettled.

## PROGNOSTIC GLEASON GRADE GROUPS

Based on the clinical outcome and excellent prognosis for patients with low Gleason scores, 5

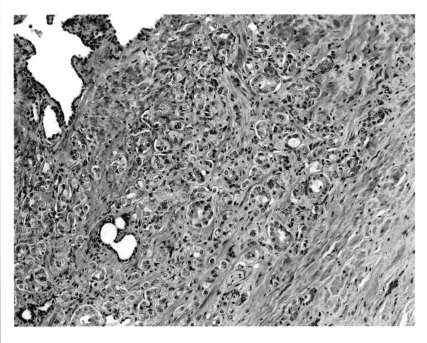

Fig. 4. Poorly formed glands of Gleason grade 4 adenocarcinoma of the prostate (hematoxylin-eosin, original magnification ×100).

*Fig. 5.* Small solid nests of Gleason grade 5 adenocarcinoma of the prostate (hematoxylin-eosin, original magnification ×200).

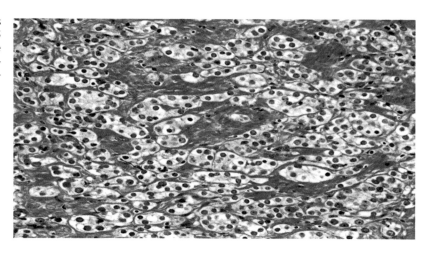

prognostic groups have been proposed, and these accurately reflect tumor behavior and prognosis in prostate cancer.[24] Additionally, by defining Gleason score 6 carcinoma as group 1 of 5, rather than 6 of 10 using the Gleason system, physicians and patients can appreciate the indolent and low-risk nature of this common score, where it is in the lowest-risk grade group (1/5) rather than considered intermediate (6/10) in the Gleason system. The 5 prognostic groups are defined as follows:

Grade group 1 (Gleason score 2–6)
Grade group 2 (Gleason score 3 + 4 = 7)
Grade group 3 (Gleason score 4 + 3 = 7)
Grade group 4 (Gleason score 4 + 4 = 8)
Grade group 5 (Gleason score 9–10)

Several studies have shown that in the modified Gleason system, Gleason score 6 has an excellent prognosis.[24–26] In 1 of the studies, Gleason score 6 tumor was associated with an extremely low risk of progression after RP.[25] In that study, 94.6% and 96.6% of patients with pure Gleason 6 cancer at biopsy and RP, respectively, were biochemically free of tumor 5 years after RP. Additionally, in a multi-institutional study of more than 14,000 RP cases of modified Gleason score 6, there was not a single patient with lymph node

*Fig. 6.* Linear array growth pattern of Gleason grade 5 adenocarcinoma of the prostate (hematoxylin-eosin, original magnification ×200).

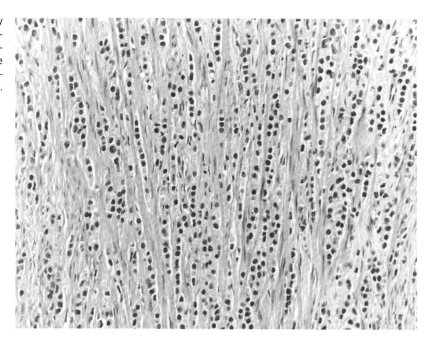

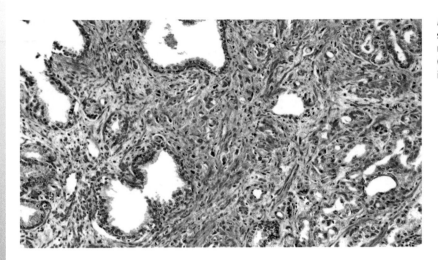

*Fig. 7.* Single cell Gleason grade 5 adenocarcinoma of the prostate (hematoxylin-eosin, original magnification ×40).

metastasis.[27] Best evidence using various parameters, such as competing risk analyses, surgical series, nonrandomized cohort studies, and randomized trials, has shown similar outcomes for patients with Gleason score 2 to 6 tumors treated or not in the PSA era.[28–32] An analysis of these data shows that using a time frame of 10 to 15 years, less than 3% of men diagnosed with Gleason score less than or equal to 6 and classified as low risk (based on a PSA <10 ng/mL and stage ≤pT2a) die as a result of prostate cancer whether treated or not. This calls into question the rationale for treating patients with Gleason score 6 tumors who otherwise have a life expectancy of less than 10 to 15 years. This has also led to questions as to whether or not tumors in this category should be labeled as cancer.[24,26,33] Esserman and colleagues[34] proposed the reclassification of cancers without metastatic potential as indolent lesions of epithelial origin. Tumors in this category continue to be labeled as cancer because it is generally believed that they share cytologic and molecular alterations associated with higher Gleason patterns (including loss of basal cell layer, up-regulation of alpha-methylacyl-CoA racemase [AMACR], glutathione S-transferase hypermethylation and down-regulation, and TMPRSS2-ERG gene fusions),[35] and they have the ability for extraprostatic extension and perineural invasion. Renaming Gleason score 6 tumors as noncancer could also result in missed opportunity for cure because a Gleason score 6 tumor may reflect the presence of a higher-grade tumor or a more extensive disease that was not sampled as well as possibility of progression to a higher-grade tumor in a small percent of patients. This rate of progression is unknown but presumably it increases with time.[36] Of particular concern to pathologists and urologists is that renaming Gleason score 6 tumors as noncancer would result in medical liability.[37]

The difference between Gleason score 3 + 4 and 4 + 3 has been extensively investigated and a majority of the studies demonstrate worse pathologic stage and biochemical recurrence rates for Gleason score 4 + 3 compared with 3 + 4.[38–42] Using the modified Gleason system, Gleason score 7 has been separated into 2 prognostic groups. This is based on the evidence that Gleason score 3 + 4 has a favorable prognosis and an estimated 5-year biochemical recurrence-free survival (BFS) rates of 82.7% and 88.1% after biopsy and RP, respectively.[25]

Gleason score 4 + 3 tumors have been demonstrated to behave more similarly to tumors with Gleason 8 score than they do to those with Gleason score 3 + 4 = 7. They have BFS rates of 65.1% and 69.7% for biopsy and RP, respectively.[25]

The prognosis worsens considerably with Gleason score 8 tumors but not to the level of Gleason scores 9 to 10. In the literature, Gleason scores 8 to 10 have traditionally been grouped together as 1 grade category and some have considered Gleason score 8 as having the same prognosis as Gleason score 9 to 10.[25,43] A recent study showed that Gleason 9 to 10 tumors have almost twice the risk of progression when compared with tumors with Gleason score 8. The estimated 5-year BFS rates are 63.1% and 67.1% after biopsy and RP, respectively, in Gleason score 8 tumors whereas they are 34.5% and 34.5% after biopsy and RP, respectively, in Gleason score 9 to 10 tumors.[25] There are also studies in the radiation literature that allude to the worse prognosis for Gleason score 9 to 10 tumors compared with Gleason score 8.[44] So, the separation of Gleason score 8 (prognostic grade group 4) from Gleason score 9 to 10 (prognostic grade group 5) is a new way of thinking about and approaching high-grade prostate cancer.

## GLEASON SCORE AND ACTIVE SURVEILLANCE

Active surveillance is an important management strategy for decreasing the prostate cancer over-treatment rate, thereby decreasing patient morbidity and the harm of universal PSA-based prostate cancer screening.[45,46] The basic concept underlying active surveillance is that Gleason score 6 prostate cancer is an indolent disease and does not pose a significant mortality threat to patients.[47] Because a small percentage of these patients harbor high-grade cancer that potentially poses a significant threat and also the small proportion that dedifferentiates over time, ongoing follow-up is needed to identify the patients with a higher risk for progression in whom treatment is warranted. Many studies have suggested that active surveillance is associated with prostate cancer mortality similar to that under immediate treatment.[48–50] The 2011 National Institutes of Health consensus conference on active surveillance concluded that active surveillance has emerged as a viable option that should be offered to patients with low-risk cancer.[51] There are many different sets of clinical and pathologic criteria that have been used for enrollment into active surveillance programs. One common set of criteria that is widely accepted includes Gleason score 6 or less on biopsy, no more than 2 positive cores, no involvement of more than 50% of a core, PSA density less than 0.15, and unilateral cancer.[45,47,52,53] In some studies, absolute PSA value is used instead of PSA density.[54–58]

There is a group of patients with intermediate risk disease who may be candidates for active surveillance. These patients typically have predominantly Gleason pattern 3 cancer with a small component of pattern 4. Patients who are in this category and have a PSA of less than 10 have a natural history of disease and rate of progression that are comparable to Gleason score 6.[59–61] Given the increased risk of disease progression with Gleason pattern 4, it has been suggested that this approach be restricted to patients over age 65.[56]

## GLEASON GRADE OF TUMOR AT THE MARGIN AS AN INDEPENDENT PREDICTOR OF PROGNOSIS

Approximately 11% to 37% of patients with RP have a positive surgical margin.[62–65] Only 30% to 35% of these patients with positive margins eventually develop biochemical recurrence.[62,63,65] Patients with positive surgical margins have a 2-fold increase in the risk of biochemical recurrence compared with those with a negative surgical margin.[62,63,65] Various pathologic parameters, such as location and extent of positive margins, have been proposed as possible prognostic factors in patients with margin-positive prostate cancer. A positive surgical margin involving the bladder neck or posterolateral surface of the prostate has been reported as having a more significant adverse impact on prognosis than an involved apical or anterior margin.[66–69]

Cao and colleagues[70] reported an association between Gleason score of the tumor at the margin and biochemical recurrence in a cohort with a median follow-up of 32 months. On both univariate and multivariate analysis, the Gleason score of the tumor at the margin was a strong and statistically significant predictive factor for biochemical recurrence. These results suggest that the Gleason score of the tumor at the margin could be reported in addition to the Gleason score of the main tumor for radical prostatectomy. Other studies have confirmed that the Gleason grade of the carcinoma at a positive surgical margin is an independent predictor of biochemical recurrence.[71–73] Savdie and colleagues[71] concluded that the 5-year actual BFS was significantly lower for patients with Gleason pattern 4 or 5 carcinoma at the margin than for patients with Gleason grade 3 at the margin or clear margins. Assessment of Gleason grade at the margin may aid the optimum selection of patients for adjuvant radiotherapy after radical prostatectomy.

## UPDATE ON VARIANTS OF PROSTATIC ADENOCARCINOMA

Most prostatic adenocarcinoma cases are typical/conventional/usual acinar-type adenocarcinoma. Although less common, there are also many variants of prostatic adenocarcinoma that are of diagnostic and/or prognostic and therapeutic significance. This component of the review focuses on 2 broad classes of variants: the deceptively benign-appearing variants of typical acinar adenocarcinoma and emerging variants of prostatic adenocarcinoma.

## DECEPTIVELY BENIGN-APPEARING VARIANTS OF TYPICAL ACINAR ADENOCARCINOMA

### Foamy Gland Adenocarcinoma

Foamy gland adenocarcinoma is a variant of acinar adenocarcinoma, which is characterized by abundant foamy cytoplasm and often by pyknotic nuclei with minimal atypia.[74–77] Because of the minimal nuclear atypia seen in this variant, foamy gland adenocarcinoma may be deceptively benign appearing (**Fig. 8**) and accounts for a large percentage of prostatic carcinoma cases misdiagnosed as benign on needle biopsy.[78] The mean age of patients with foamy gland adenocarcinoma is 62 years, which is similar to that for nonfoamy usual acinar adenocarcinoma.[74] Foamy glands can be found admixed with usual acinar adenocarcinoma in 17% of cases on needle biopsy[78] and 15% to 23% of RP cases.[74] In needle biopsies, however, the carcinoma may be pure foamy gland.[75]

Microscopically, the glands are crowded or infiltrative. High-grade growth patterns, in order of frequency of detection, include cribriform, fused/poorly formed glands, cords/single cells, and solid sheets.[75,79] The typical cytologic features of acinar adenocarcinoma, such as nuclear enlargement and prominent nucleoli, are frequently absent, making this variant more difficult to diagnose, especially on needle biopsy.[20,80,81] Another study, however, found that, in prostatectomy specimens, a substantial percentage of foamy gland carcinomas harbor prominent nucleoli.[74] The usual Gleason grade for foamy gland adenocarcinoma has often been described as 3 + 3 = 6.[8,78,79,82] Other studies have shown, however, that Gleason score 7 represents the most common score and that a majority of the cases with foamy gland carcinoma

have a component of high Gleason grade 4 or 5 carcinoma.[74,79] The discrepancy may be due to different clinical populations. Biochemical failure in foamy gland carcinoma is significantly associated with preoperative PSA level, Gleason score, percentage of total carcinoma (foamy and nonfoamy components combined), and percentage of foamy gland tumor.[74] These are the same factors that are important for nonfoamy usual acinar adenocarcinomas in predicting outcome after radical prostatectomy.[20] The presence of foamy glands does not seem to impart a prognostic difference. In a series of consecutive RP cases, progression after RP was not significantly different between the foamy gland and nonfoamy gland cases.[74]

## Prostatic Adenocarcinoma with Atrophic Features (Atrophic Pattern Adenocarcinoma)

Atrophic adenocarcinoma of the prostate represents a diagnostic pitfall and it is important to distinguish this entity from benign acinar atrophy to avoid underdiagnosis of carcinoma.[83,84] Atrophy in malignant acini can be seen sporadically or after hormonal or radiation treatment. The incidence of atrophic adenocarcinoma in the absence of hormonal or radiation treatment is 2% in needle biopsy cases[83] and 16% in RP cases.[85] The average age of patients is 60 years (range, 50–76 years).[83] Useful diagnostic features include infiltrative architecture (**Fig. 9**) with individual small atrophic glands situated between larger glands;

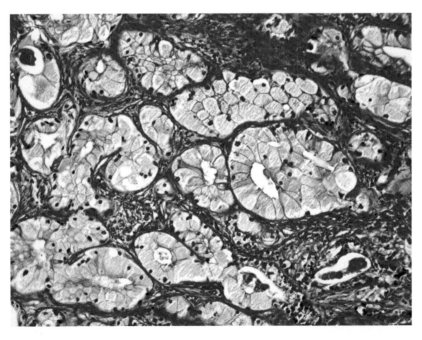

Fig. 8. Foamy gland adenocarcinoma of the prostate (hematoxylin-eosin, original magnification ×200).

*Fig. 9.* Atrophic pattern adenocarcinoma (*left*) adjacent to benign atrophy (*right*) (hematoxylin-eosin, original magnification ×40).

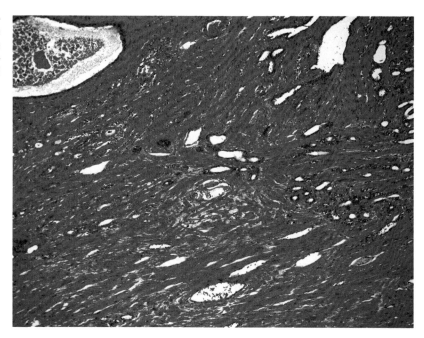

the concomitant presence of conventional, less atrophic carcinoma; and greater cytologic atypia (such as enlarged nuclei and macronucleoli) than is seen in benign atrophy.[75,84,85] The cells usually have cytoplasmic volume loss and this gives the tumor a typical basophilic appearance. The luminal contents of acini also provide a clue to the malignant nature of this lesion. Most cases contain intraluminal proteinaceous secretions and blue mucin.[83] The diagnosis of atrophic adenocarcinoma should be made with caution in needle biopsy specimens. Most atrophic adenocarcinomas are Gleason grade 3. This variant does not seem to have a different prognosis from usual acinar adenocarcinoma because adenocarcinoma of the prostate with and without atrophic features does not differ in Gleason grade or pathologic stage.[85]

## Pseudohyperplastic Adenocarcinoma

Pseudohyperplastic adenocarcinoma is a variant of acinar adenocarcinoma that may be misdiagnosed as usual epithelial hyperplasia. The incidence of pseudohyperplastic prostatic adenocarcinoma in biopsy specimen is 2% to 2.2%.[86,87] In a consecutive series of 202 radical prostatectomies, the incidence was 11%.[86] The difference in the incidence rates between biopsy and prostatectomy specimens may be attributed to the fact that some cases are found in the transition zone, which is not commonly sampled by needle biopsy. Pseudohyperplastic carcinoma is common in

prostate cancer patients with a germline mutation in the homeobox transcription factor *HOXB13 G84E* gene, which predisposes to prostate cancer.[88]

Microscopically, the architectural patterns seen in pseudohyperplastic adenocarcinoma include papillary infoldings, luminal undulations, and branching and cystic dilatation, with or without papillary projections (**Fig. 10**). The malignant epithelial cells resemble hyperplastic cells in cell shape, cytoplasmic quality, and location of nuclei. The cells are almost always columnar, the cytoplasm is pale-staining to almost granular, and the nuclei are basally oriented.[75,86,89,90] It has been suggested that nuclear atypia, including macronucleoli and complete absence of basal cells, are present in most cases.[75] Pure pseudohyperplastic adenocarcinoma is rare. It is usually in direct continuity with well to moderately differentiated adenocarcinoma. Gleason pattern 3 is recommended for this variant. Prognosis is not certain but pathologic stages of carcinoma with or without hyperplastic changes are not significantly different.[86]

## Microcystic Adenocarcinoma

Cystic change or glandular dilatation within the spectrum of atrophic and pseusohyperplastic patterns with a flat luminal lining layer is typically referred to as microcystic adenocarcinoma (**Fig. 11**).[91] The incidence of microcystic adenocarcinoma in prostatectomy specimens is 11%.

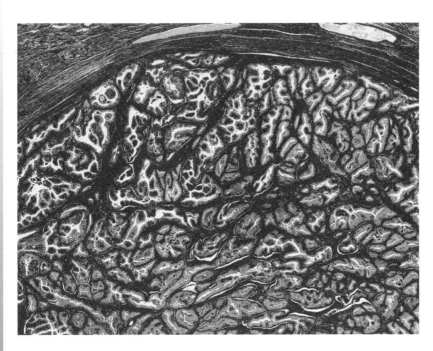

*Fig. 10.* Pseudohyperplastic adenocarcinoma of the prostate (hematoxylin-eosin, original magnification ×40).

The incidence is higher if focusing specifically on pseudohyperplastic (32%) and atrophic (22%) pattern adenocarcinomas.[85,86] The Gleason grade of microcystic adenocarcinoma is best considered pattern 3, similar to pseudohyperplastic and atrophic pattern adenocarcinoma.[91]

## EMERGING VARIANTS OF PROSTATIC ADENOCARCINOMA

### *Pleomorphic Giant Cell Adenocarcinoma*

Pleomorphic giant cell adenocarcinoma is an extremely rare, highly aggressive variant of

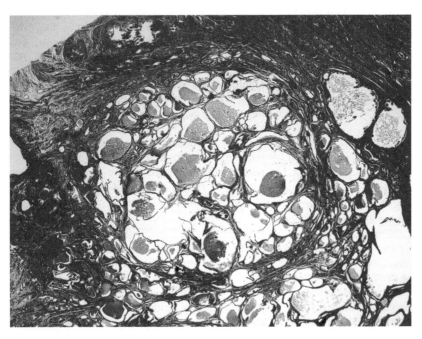

*Fig. 11.* Microcystic adenocarcinoma of the prostate (hematoxylin-eosin, original magnification ×20).

adenocarcinoma, which is characterized by the presence of giant pleomorphic nuclei.[92,93] Fewer than 10 cases have been reported in the literature. In the largest series of 6 cases, mean patient age was 65.8 years (range, 59–76).[92] Histologically, the tumor is characterized by the presence of aggregates or sheets of mononucleated and multinucleated giant, bizarre, anaplastic cells with abundant cytoplasm. The tumor cells lack cohesiveness and extensive necrosis is usually present. In addition to the pleomorphic giant cell component, multiple histologic components coexist with the tumor, the most notable of which is Gleason score 9 conventional adenocarcinoma. Based on the limited number of cases in the literature, this entity portends a particularly aggressive clinical course.

## Prostatic Intraepithelial Neoplasia–like Adenocarcinoma

Prostatic intraepithelial neoplasia (PIN)-like adenocarcinoma is an unusual variant of prostatic adenocarcinoma that bears a close resemblance to gland architecture seen in high-grade PIN (HGPIN) (Fig. 12). It accounts for 1.3% of prostatic adenocarcinomas.[94] The mean age of patients at presentation is 68 years, which is similar to the mean age in usual prostatic adenocarcinoma.[95] Histologically, this variant of prostatic adenocarcinoma has pseudostratified cuboidal or columnar epithelium in contrast to the typically single-cell lining layer of cuboidal epithelium of small acinar prostatic adenocarcinoma.

The main differential diagnosis of PIN-like adenocarcinoma is high-grade PIN. Distinguishing between the 2 might not be critical if areas of usual prostatic adenocarcinoma are present elsewhere in the biopsy material. PIN-like adenocarcinoma can be comprised of either acinar (see Fig. 12) or ductal cells. PIN-like ductal adenocarcinoma is distinct from HGPIN by the higher prevalence of flat epithelium, more crowded glands, and, often, large dilated glands. PIN-like adenocarcinoma may have less cytologic atypia than HGPIN. Whereas HGPIN by definition requires the presence of prominent nucleoli, PIN-like ductal adenocarcinoma often had tall-pseudostratified epithelium in the absence of visible nucleoli.[95] In difficult cases, the identification of basal cells in hematoxylin-eosin sections or by basal cell marker positivity in immunohistochemistry points toward a diagnosis of HGPIN, whereas lack of basal cells and the presence of glandular crowding point toward a diagnosis of prostatic adenocarcinoma. PIN-like ductal adenocarcinoma seems to behave less aggressively than conventional ductal adenocarcinoma.[94]

## Proposed Morphologic Classification of Prostate Carcinoma with Neuroendocrine Differentiation

The amount of neuroendocrine differentiation of prostate adenocarcinoma increases with disease progression and in response to androgen deprivation therapy.[96,97] Emerging clinical and molecular data from prostate cancers treated by

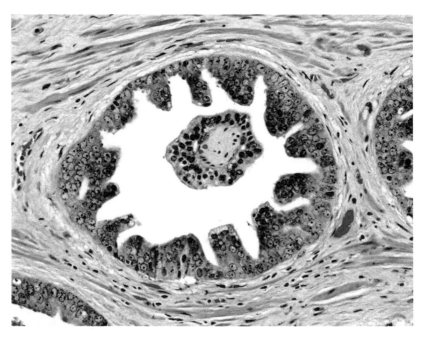

*Fig. 12.* PIN-like adenocarcinoma, with invasion around small nerve twig in center (hematoxylin-eosin, original magnification ×200).

contemporary androgen deprivation therapies have demonstrated the need to refine the diagnostic terminology to encompass the full spectrum of neuroendocrine differentiation. To address this, the Prostate Cancer Foundation working committee on the molecular biology and pathologic classification of neuroendocrine classification in prostate cancer proposed the classification of neuroendocrine prostate carcinoma as follows: usual prostate adenocarcinoma with neuroendocrine differentiation, adenocarcinoma with Paneth cell neuroendocrine differentiation, carcinoid tumor, small cell carcinoma, large cell neuroendocrine carcinoma and mixed neuroendocrine carcinoma–acinar carcinoma.[98]

## Usual Prostate Adenocarcinoma with Neuroendocrine Differentiation

Usual prostate adenocarcinoma with neuroendocrine differentiation is characterized morphologically by usual acinar or ductal adenocarcinoma in which neuroendocrine differentiation is demonstrated by immunohistochemistry alone. It is uncertain whether neuroendocrine differentiation in usual adenocarcinoma has any prognostic significance, because there are conflicting data from several studies[99–103]; hence, the routine use of immunohistochemistry in an otherwise morphologically typical primary adenocarcinoma of the prostate is not recommended.[98]

## Adenocarcinoma with Paneth Cell–like Neuroendocrine Differentiation

The distinctive morphologic feature of adenocarcinoma with Paneth cell–like neuroendocrine differentiation is the presence of usual prostatic adenocarcinoma with varying proportions of cells with eosinophilic granular cytoplasm that are positive for neuroendocrine markers and negative for lysozyme, making them distinct from true Paneth cells of the small intestine.[98,104–106] Electron microscopy studies reveal dense core neurosecretory granules within the cytoplasm of Paneth cell–like cells.[106] The Paneth cells can be seen as either patchy isolated cells or diffusely involving glands or nests (Fig. 13).[105,107] They may be present in well-formed glands of Gleason pattern 3 as well as in cords of cells with bland cytology, which ordinarily would be assigned Gleason pattern 5 on strict application of the Gleason grading system. This, however, may represent overgrading because, based on the limited data available, this entity is generally believed to have a favorable prognosis.[107]

## Carcinoid Tumor

Carcinoid tumor is a well-differentiated neuroendocrine tumor of the prostate, which shows the classic morphology of carcinoid tumor seen at other sites (Fig. 14). True carcinoid tumors of the prostate are extremely rare and for this diagnosis to be made, the tumor must not be closely

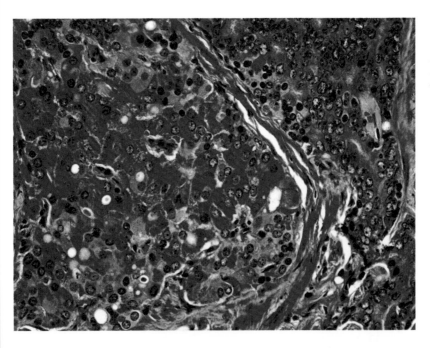

Fig. 13. Paneth cell–like neuroendocrine differentiation in prostatic carcinoma (hematoxylin-eosin, original magnification ×400).

*Fig. 14.* Carcinoid tumor of the prostate (hematoxylin-eosin, original magnification ×100). (*Courtesy of* Dr John Srigley, Mississauga, Ontario.)

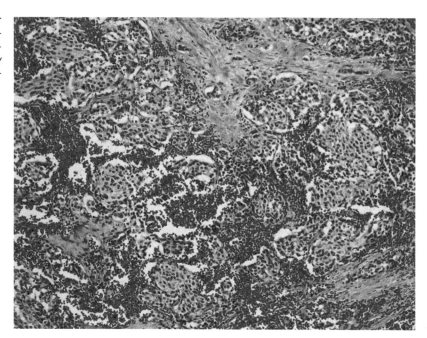

associated with concomitant usual prostatic adenocarcinoma, must express neuroendocrine markers and not express PSA, and must arise in the prostatic parenchyma as opposed to the urethra or extension from the bladder.[98,108,109] When this diagnosis is made in young patients, multiple endocrine neoplasia IIB syndrome must be excluded.[110,111] Although the data are limited, prostatic carcinoid seems to have a favorable prognosis even in cases with locally advanced disease.[98]

## Small Cell Carcinoma

This high-grade tumor, small cell carcinoma, is defined by characteristic nuclear features, including nuclear molding, lack of prominent nucleoli, high nuclear-to-cytoplasmic ratio, high mitotic rate, apoptotic bodies, and crush artifact (**Fig. 15**). Geographic necrosis may be frequent in resection specimens. Morphologic variations may include intermediate cell type with more open chromatin and visible small nucleoli.[112] Up to half of small cell carcinomas have a history of usual prostatic adenocarcinoma, followed by hormonal and/or radiation treatment. Historically, pure small cell carcinoma was seen at initial diagnosis in approximately 50% to 60% of cases.[112] Because of the rarity of small cell carcinoma of the prostate, metastasis from other sites and local extension from the bladder must be excluded. Expression of thyroid transcription factor (TTF)-1 has been demonstrated in greater than 50% of prostatic small cell carcinoma, hence the limitation in its utility for differentiating primary prostatic small cell carcinoma from a metastasis from the lung.[112,113] Demonstration of the *TMPRSS2-ERG* gene rearrangement by fluorescence in situ hybridization is specific for prostatic small cell carcinoma in the differential diagnosis with small cell carcinomas originating at other anatomic sites, such as urinary bladder or lung.[114] The sensitivity is, however, not high, at 48%. Despite the emergence of more-aggressive treatment modalities, the prognosis of men with prostatic small cell carcinoma remains dismal.[115]

## Large Cell Neuroendocrine Carcinoma

Large cell neuroendocrine carcinoma is an extremely rare, aggressive, high-grade tumor with neuroendocrine differentiation. The histologic features are identical to those of large cell carcinoma in the lung. Tumor consists of large nests with peripheral palisading and geographic necrosis. Tumor generally shows prominent nucleoli, vesicular clumpy chromatin, and fair amount of cytoplasm, features that are reminiscent of non–small cell carcinoma. Neuroendocrine differentiation is confirmed by the expression of at least 1 neuroendocrine marker. A significant proportion of the cases reported in the literature had a history of adenocarcinoma treated with hormonal therapy.[116] Prognosis is dismal, with death from metastatic disease at an average of 7 months.[116]

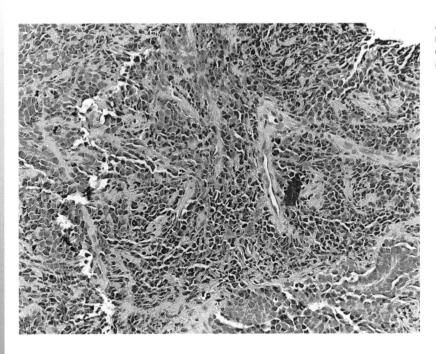

*Fig. 15.* Small cell carcinoma of the prostate (hematoxylin-eosin, original magnification ×200).

## Mixed Neuroendocrine Carcinoma–Acinar Carcinoma

Mixed neuroendocrine carcimona–acinar carcinoma is a biphasic tumor with distinct, recognizable, admixed components of neuroendocrine carcinoma and usual conventional adenocarcinoma. Most cases that are encountered in clinical practice are mixed small cell carcinoma–acinar carcinoma.[98] Gleason score is assigned to the conventional adenocarcinoma component if untreated. It is recommended that the percentage and grade of the acinar component be provided at histologic diagnosis, because this information might be valuable for individual case management.

## Update on Immunohistochemistry in Prostate Cancer

Immunohistochemical stains have been used over the years in cases in which morphology alone was insufficient for a definitive diagnosis of prostate cancer. Immunohistochemistry has also been of tremendous help in the diagnosis of benign mimickers of prostatic adenocarcinoma as well as in the confirmation of the diagnosis of deceptively benign prostatic adenocarcinomas and minimal (limited) adenocarcinoma.[117] The markers that are most widely used are the enzyme AMACR (also known as racemase or p504S), which is overexpressed in neoplastic prostatic epithelial cells and basal cell markers (p63 and high-molecular-

weight cytokeratins [HMWCKs], as detected by antibody 34betaE12, also known as CK903), or antibodies directed against CK5/6, which are typically negative in prostatic adenocarcinoma.[118–130] These antibodies can be used in double (basal cell markers) or triple (AMACR, p63, and 34betaE12) cocktails (**Fig. 16**). There are caveats in the interpretation of both AMACR and basal cell marker immunostains.[117] Basal cell stains must be interpreted with caution because some benign glands can lack basal cells[117] and because there are some rare cases of acinar adenocarcinoma that stain positively for HMWCKs and less so with p63 in a non–basal cell distribution. Rare acinar adenocarcinomas can show aberrant diffuse expression of p63.[131–133] These p63-expressing prostatic adenocarcinomas seem molecularly distinct from usual-type prostatic adenocarcinoma.[134] A majority (80% to 100%) of prostate cancers are positive for AMACR by immunohistochemistry. Atrophic pattern, pseudohyperplastic, and hormonally treated prostatic adenocarcinomas can show less frequent AMACR staining.[117] Initial work indicated a diminished frequency of AMACR staining in foamy gland carcinoma but a recent investigation revealed that AMACR is a highly sensitive marker for this variant.[78] Also, benign mimickers of prostatic adenocarcinoma, such as partial atrophy, nephrogenic adenoma, and adenosis, can exhibit AMACR overexpression.[117] A recently proposed addition to the panel of diagnostic markers

*Fig. 16.* Triple-stain immunohistochemistry with red stain indicating AMACR overexpression and brown stain indicating basal cells, as detected by 34betaE12 and p63 antibodies (original magnification ×100).

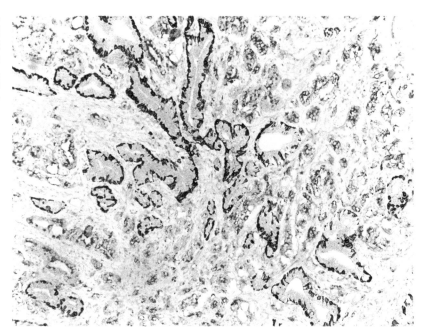

is ERG. The recently discovered *TMPRSS2-ERG* gene fusion has been identified as a highly specific alteration in prostate cancer and monoclonal anti-ERG antibodies are now available.[135–138] Although ERG protein overexpression is specific for neoplastic prostatic epithelium, it is not sensitive (at approximately 40%) and for minimal adenocarcinoma diagnosis ERG immunohistochemistry only rarely provides added value beyond AMACR and basal cell marker immunostains.[139] ERG immunostaining could potentially be useful in the diagnosis of the AMACR-positive cases of atrophy or adenosis, because ERG is negative in these benign mimickers of prostate cancer.[140,141]

For the work-up of small foci of atypical glands suspicious for adenocarcinoma, ISUP recommends HMWCK, p63, or a combination of the 2 with AMACR either in a double or triple cocktail. There is no justification to perform AMACR and basal cell staining in the setting of obvious carcinoma or obvious benign glands. In the work-up of atypical foci with definite cancer in other parts, IHC is justified only if subsequent therapy is affected or when active surveillance is an option.[142]

The distinction between poorly differentiated prostatic adenocarcinoma and poorly differentiated urothelial carcinoma can sometimes be difficult but is critical because the 2 are treated differently. Although PSA and prostate-specific acid phosphatase are useful in identifying prostate lineage, their sensitivity decreases because the

tumor becomes less differentiated. In such a scenario, newer prostate lineage markers, such as prostein (P501S) (**Fig. 17**), prostate-specific membrane antigen, NKX3.1, and androgen receptor, could be of added utility.[143–145] These prostate lineage markers are combined with urothelial lineage markers, such as HMWCKs, p63, uroplakins, thrombomodulin, and GATA-3.[144,146–153] The ISUP recommendation is to use PSA as a first test to identify prostatic adenocarcinoma and GATA-3 to identify urothelial carcinoma. If GATA-3 is not available, then HMWCKs and p63 can be used. If the tumor is equivocal or negative for PSA and negative for p63 and HMWCKs, then staining for P501S, NKX3.1, and GATA-3 should be performed.[142] CK7 and CK20 are of limited utility in this differential because they may both be positive in a subset of prostatic adenocarcinoma.[154,155]

The diagnosis of small cell carcinoma of the prostate can be made based on morphology in most cases. In cases in which morphology is equivocal, a combination of prostate markers, neuroendocrine markers, and TTF-1 and ki-67 can be used.[112,113] The small cell carcinoma component is positive for 1 or more neuroendocrine markers. Of the commonly used neuroendocrine markers, synaptophysin has the best combination of sensitivity and specificity. CD56 is the most sensitive but least specific, whereas chromogranin is the most specific but is often negative or only shows rare positive cells.[142] Expression of

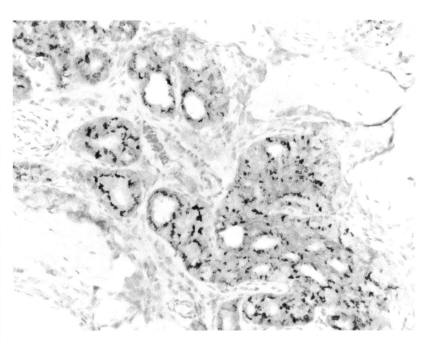

*Fig. 17.* Prostein expression in adenocarcinoma of the prostate, with characteristic granular, perinuclear staining (original magnification ×200).

TTF-1 is a common occurrence in prostatic small cell carcinoma, so its utility for differentiating primary prostatic small cell carcinoma from a metastasis from the lung is limited.[112,113]

Colorectal adenocarcinoma may directly invade the prostate. Usually this does not present a diagnostic dilemma because there is almost always a prior diagnosis. In cases of primary presentation as metastasis to the prostate, it may be confused with one of the patterns of prostatic ductal adenocarcinomas. If there is a difficulty in differentiating colorectal adenocarcinoma from prostatic adenocarcinoma, it is recommended that the usual prostate markers be done in addition to CDX-2, villin, and β-catenin.[142,156–158]

Xanthomas and nonspecific granulomatous prostatitis are 2 entities that can mimic high-grade prostatic carcinoma. Both are usually positive for CD68 while negative for keratins and prostate specific markers.[159,160]

Currently there are no prognostic immunohistochemistry markers that are recommended to be routinely performed on biopsy and resection specimens.[142]

## REFERENCES

1. Mellinger GT, Gleason D, Bailar J 3rd. The histology and prognosis of prostatic cancer. J Urol 1967;97: 331–7.
2. Epstein JI, Allsbrook WC Jr, Amin MB, et al, ISUP Grading Committee. The 2005 International Society of Urological Pathology (ISUP) consensus conference on gleason grading of prostatic carcinoma. Am J Surg Pathol 2005;29:1228–42.
3. Helpap B, Egevad L. The significance of modified Gleason grading of prostatic carcinoma in biopsy and radical prostatectomy specimens. Virchows Arch 2006;449:622–7.
4. Billis A, Guimaraes MS, Freitas LL, et al. The impact of the 2005 international society of urological pathology consensus conference on standard Gleason grading of prostatic carcinoma in needle biopsies. J Urol 2008;180:548–52.
5. Helpap B, Egevad L. Correlation of modified Gleason grading of prostate carcinoma with age, serum prostate specific antigen and tumor extent in needle biopsy specimens. Anal Quant Cytol Histol 2008;30:133–8.
6. Uemura H, Hoshino K, Sasaki T, et al. Usefulness of the 2005 International Society of Urologic Pathology Gleason grading system in prostate biopsy and radical prostatectomy specimens. BJU Int 2009;103:1190–4.
7. Zareba P, Zhang J, Yilmaz A, et al. The impact of the 2005 International Society of Urological Pathology (ISUP) consensus on Gleason grading in contemporary practice. Histopathology 2009;55:384–91.
8. Epstein JI. An update of the Gleason grading system. J Urol 2010;183:433–40.
9. Osunkoya AO. Update on prostate pathology. Pathology 2012;44:391–406.
10. Helpap B, Egevad L. Correlation of modified Gleason grading with pT stage of prostatic carcinoma after radical prostatectomy. Anal Quant Cytol Histol 2008;30:1–7.

11. Young RH, Clement PB. Sclerosing adenosis of the prostate. Arch Pathol Lab Med 1987;111:363–6.
12. Jones EC, Clement PB, Young RH. Sclerosing adenosis of the prostate gland. A clinicopathological and immunohistochemical study of 11 cases. Am J Surg Pathol 1991;15:1171–80.
13. Gaudin PB, Epstein JI. Adenosis of the prostate. Histologic features in transurethral resection specimens. Am J Surg Pathol 1994;18:863–70.
14. Shah RB. Current perspectives on the Gleason grading of prostate cancer. Arch Pathol Lab Med 2009;133:1810–6.
15. Epstein JI. Gleason score 2-4 adenocarcinoma of the prostate on needle biopsy: a diagnosis that should not be made. Am J Surg Pathol 2000;24: 477–8.
16. Helpap B, Egevad L. Modified Gleason grading. An updated review. Histol Histopathol 2009;24: 661–6.
17. Epstein JI. The Gleason grading system: a complete guide for pathologists and clinicians. Philadelphia: Wolters Kluwer; 2013.
18. Gottipati S, Warncke J, Vollmer R, et al. Usual and unusual histologic patterns of high Gleason score 8 to 10 adenocarcinoma of the prostate in needle biopsy tissue. Am J Surg Pathol 2012;36:900–7.
19. Kweldam CF, Wildhagen MF, Steyerberg EW, et al. Cribriform growth is highly predictive for postoperative metastasis and disease-specific death in Gleason score 7 prostate cancer. Mod Pathol 2015;28(3):457–64.
20. Epstein JI, Cubilla AL, Humphrey PA. Acinar (usual) adenocarcinoma of the prostate (Chapter 4). In: Tumors of the prostate gland, seminal vesicles, penis and scrotum. AFIP atlas of tumor pathology, Fascicle 14, Series 4. Washington, DC: American Registry of Pathology; 2011. p. 77–238.
21. Dong F, Yang P, Wang C, et al. Architectural heterogeneity and cribriform pattern predict adverse clinical outcome for Gleason grade 4 prostatic adenocarcinoma. Am J Surg Pathol 2013;37:1855–6.
22. Iczkowski KA, Torkko KC, Kotnis GR, et al. Digital quantification of five high-grade prostate cancer patterns, including the cribriform pattern, and their association with adverse outcome. Am J Clin Pathol 2011;136:98–107.
23. Fajardo DA, Miyamoto H, Miller JS, et al. Identification of Gleason pattern 5 on prostatic needle core biopsy: frequency of underdiagnosis and relation to morphology. Am J Surg Pathol 2011;35:1706–11.
24. Carter HB, Partin AW, Walsh PC, et al. Gleason score 6 adenocarcinoma: should it be labeled as cancer? J Clin Oncol 2012;30:4294–6.
25. Pierorazio PM, Walsh PC, Partin AW, et al. Prognostic Gleason grade grouping: data based on the modified Gleason scoring system. BJU Int 2013;111:753–60.
26. Berman DM, Epstein JI. When is prostate cancer really cancer? Urol Clin North Am 2014;41:339–46.
27. Ross HM, Kryvenko ON, Cowan JE, et al. Do adenocarcinomas of the prostate with Gleason score (GS) $\leq 6$ have the potential to metastasize to lymph nodes? Am J Surg Pathol 2012;36:1346–52.
28. Parker C, Muston D, Melia J, et al. A model of the natural history of screen-detected prostate cancer, and the effect of radical treatment on overall survival. Br J Cancer 2006;94:1361–8.
29. Stattin P, Holmberg E, Johansson JE, et al, National Prostate Cancer Register (NPCR) of Sweden. Outcomes in localized prostate cancer: National Prostate Cancer Register of Sweden follow-up study. J Natl Cancer Inst 2010;102:950–8.
30. Shappley WV 3rd, Kenfield SA, Kasperzyk JL, et al. Prospective study of determinants and outcomes of deferred treatment or watchful waiting among men with prostate cancer in a nationwide cohort. J Clin Oncol 2009;27:4980–5.
31. Eggener SE, Scardino PT, Walsh PC, et al. Predicting 15-year prostate cancer specific mortality after radical prostatectomy. J Urol 2011;185:869–75.
32. Wilt TJ, Brawer MK, Barry MJ, et al. The prostate cancer intervention versus observation trial: VA/NCI/AHRQ cooperative studies program #407 (PIVOT): design and baseline results of a randomized controlled trial comparing radical prostatectomy to watchful waiting for men with clinically localized prostate cancer. Contemp Clin Trials 2009;30:81–7.
33. Nickel JC, Speakman M. Should we really consider Gleason 6 prostate cancer? BJU Int 2012;109: 645–6.
34. Esserman LJ, Thompson IM, Reid B, et al. Addressing overdiagnosis and overtreatment in cancer: a prescription for change. Lancet Oncol 2014;15:e234–42.
35. Netto GJ, Cheng L. Emerging critical role of molecular testing in diagnostic genitourinary pathology. Arch Pathol Lab Med 2012;136:372–90.
36. Sheridan TB, Carter HB, Wang W, et al. Change in prostate cancer grade over time in men followed expectantly for stage T1c disease. J Urol 2008; 179:901–4.
37. Dunn IB, Kirk D. Legal pitfalls in the diagnosis of prostate cancer. BJU Int 2000;86:304–7.
38. Burdick MJ, Reddy CA, Ulchaker J, et al. Comparison of biochemical relapse-free survival between primary Gleason score 3 and primary Gleason score 4 for biopsy Gleason score 7 prostate cancer. Int J Radiat Oncol Biol Phys 2009;73:1439–45.
39. Chan TY, Partin AW, Walsh PC, et al. Prognostic significance of Gleason score 3+4 versus Gleason score 4+3 tumor at radical prostatectomy. Urology 2000;56:823–7.

40. Kang DE, Fitzsimons NJ, Presti JC Jr, et al, SEARCH Database Study Group. Risk stratification of men with Gleason score 7 to 10 tumors by primary and secondary Gleason score: results from the SEARCH database. Urology 2007;70:277–82.

41. Koontz BF, Tsivian M, Mouraviev V, et al. Impact of primary Gleason grade on risk stratification for Gleason score 7 prostate cancers. Int J Radiat Oncol Biol Phys 2012;82:200–3.

42. Makarov DV, Sanderson H, Partin AW, et al. Gleason score 7 prostate cancer on needle biopsy: is the prognostic difference in Gleason scores 4 + 3 and 3 + 4 independent of the number of involved cores? J Urol 2002;167:2440–2.

43. Stenmark MH, Blas K, Halverson S, et al. Continued benefit to androgen deprivation therapy for prostate cancer patients treated with dose-escalated radiation therapy across multiple definitions of high-risk disease. Int J Radiat Oncol Biol Phys 2011;81:e335–44.

44. Sabolch A, Feng FY, Daignault-Newton S, et al. Gleason pattern 5 is the greatest risk factor for clinical failure and death from prostate cancer after dose-escalated radiation therapy and hormonal ablation. Int J Radiat Oncol Biol Phys 2011;81:e351–60.

45. Reese AC, Landis P, Han M, et al. Expanded criteria to identify men eligible for active surveillance of low risk prostate cancer at Johns Hopkins: a preliminary analysis. J Urol 2013;190:2033–8.

46. Xia J, Trock BJ, Cooperberg MR, et al. Prostate cancer mortality following active surveillance versus immediate radical prostatectomy. Clin Cancer Res 2012;18:5471–8.

47. Klotz L. Active surveillance: patient selection. Curr Opin Urol 2013;23:239–44.

48. van den Bergh RC, Steyerberg EW, Khatami A, et al, Swedish and Dutch sections of the European Randomized Study of Screening for Prostate Cancer. Is delayed radical prostatectomy in men with low-risk screen-detected prostate cancer associated with a higher risk of unfavorable outcomes? Cancer 2010;116:1281–90.

49. Hayes JH, Ollendorf DA, Pearson SD, et al. Active surveillance compared with initial treatment for men with low-risk prostate cancer: a decision analysis. JAMA 2010;304:2373–80.

50. Warlick C, Trock BJ, Landis P, et al. Delayed versus immediate surgical intervention and prostate cancer outcome. J Natl Cancer Inst 2006;98:355–7.

51. Ganz PA, Barry JM, Burke W, et al. WNIH State-of-the-Science Conference Statement: role of active surveillance in the management of men with localized prostate cancer. NIH Consens State Sci Statements 2011;28:1–27.

52. Epstein JI, Walsh PC, Carmichael M, et al. Pathologic and clinical findings to predict tumor extent of nonpalpable (stage T1c) prostate cancer. JAMA 1994;271:368–74.

53. Kryvenko ON, Carter HB, Trock BJ, et al. Biopsy criteria for determining appropriateness for active surveillance in the modern era. Urology 2014;83:869–74.

54. Berglund RK, Masterson TA, Vora KC, et al. Pathological upgrading and up staging with immediate repeat biopsy in patients eligible for active surveillance. J Urol 2008;180:1964–7.

55. Dall'Era MA, Konety BR, Cowan JE, et al. Active surveillance for the management of prostate cancer in a contemporary cohort. Cancer 2008;112:2664–70.

56. Klotz L, Zhang L, Lam A, et al. Clinical results of long-term follow-up of a large, active surveillance cohort with localized prostate cancer. Clin Oncol 2010;28:126–31.

57. Soloway MS, Soloway CT, Williams S, et al. Active surveillance; a reasonable management alternative for patients with prostate cancer: the Miami experience. BJU Int 2008;101:165–9.

58. van As NJ, Norman AR, Thomas K, et al. Predicting the probability of deferred radical treatment for localised prostate cancer managed by active surveillance. Eur Urol 2008;54:1297–305.

59. Choo R, Klotz L, Danjoux C, et al. Feasibility study: watchful waiting for localized low to intermediate grade prostate carcinoma with selective delayed intervention based on prostate specific antigen, histological and/or clinical progression. J Urol 2002;167:1664–9.

60. Cooperberg MR, Carroll PR, Klotz L. Active surveillance for prostate cancer: progress and promise. J Clin Oncol 2011;29:3669–76.

61. Bul M, van den Bergh RC, Zhu X, et al. Outcomes of initially expectantly managed patients with low or intermediate risk screen-detected localized prostate cancer. BJU Int 2012;110:1672–7.

62. Kausik SJ, Blute ML, Sebo TJ, et al. Prognostic significance of positive surgical margins in patients with extraprostatic carcinoma after radical prostatectomy. Cancer 2002;95:1215–9.

63. Swindle P, Eastham JA, Ohori M, et al. Do margins matter? The prognostic significance of positive surgical margins in radical prostatectomy specimens. J Urol 2005;174:903–7.

64. Boorjian SA, Karnes RJ, Crispen PL, et al. The impact of positive surgical margins on mortality following radical prostatectomy during the prostate specific antigen era. J Urol 2010;183:1003–9.

65. Wright JL, Dalkin BL, True LD, et al. Positive surgical margins at radical prostatectomy predict prostate cancer specific mortality. J Urol 2010;183:2213–8.

66. Eastham JA, Kuroiwa K, Ohori M, et al. Prognostic significance of location of positive margins in

radical prostatectomy specimens. Urology 2007; 70:965–9.

67. Blute ML, Bergstralh EJ, Iocca A, et al. Use of Gleason score, prostate specific antigen, seminal vesicle and margin status to predict biochemical failure after radical prostatectomy. J Urol 2001; 165:119–25.

68. Obek C, Sadek S, Lai S, et al. Positive surgical margins with radical retropubic prostatectomy: anatomic site-specific pathologic analysis and impact on prognosis. Urology 1999;54:682–8.

69. Poulos CK, Koch MO, Eble JN, et al. Bladder neck invasion is an independent predictor of prostate-specific antigen recurrence. Cancer 2004;101: 1563–8.

70. Cao D, Kibel AS, Gao F, et al. The Gleason score of tumor at the margin in radical prostatectomy is predictive of biochemical recurrence. Am J Surg Pathol 2010;34(7):994–1001.

71. Savdie R, Horvath LG, Benito RP, et al. High Gleason grade carcinoma at a positive surgical margin predicts biochemical failure after radical prostatectomy and may guide adjuvant radiotherapy. BJU Int 2012;109:1794–800.

72. Viers BR, Sukov WR, Gettman MT, et al. Primary Gleason grade 4 at the positive margin is associated with metastasis and death among patients with Gleason 7 prostate cancer undergoing radical prostatectomy. Eur Urol 2014;66(6):1116–24.

73. Brimo F, Partin AW, Epstein JI. Tumor grade at margins of resection in radical prostatectomy specimens is an independent predictor of prognosis. Urology 2010;76:1206–9.

74. Hudson J, Cao D, Vollmer R, et al. Foamy gland adenocarcinoma of the prostate: incidence, Gleason grade, and early clinical outcome. Hum Pathol 2012;43:974–9.

75. Humphrey PA. Histological variants of prostatic carcinoma and their significance. Histopathology 2012;60:59–74.

76. Humphrey PA. Variants of prostatic carcinoma. Prostate pathology. Chicago: ASCP Press; 2003. p. 390–429.

77. Humphrey PA. Unusual prostatic neoplasms. Prostate pathology. Chicago: ASCP Press; 2003. p. 430–55.

78. Warrick JI, Humphrey PA. Foamy gland carcinoma of the prostate in needle biopsy: incidence, Gleason grade, and comparative α-methylacyl-CoA racemase vs. ERG expression. Am J Surg Pathol 2013;37:1709–14.

79. Zhao J, Epstein JI. High-grade foamy gland prostatic adenocarcinoma on biopsy or transurethral resection: a morphologic study of 55 cases. Am J Surg Pathol 2009;33:583–90.

80. Arista-Nasr J, Martinez-Benitez B, Camorlinga-Tagle N, et al. Foamy gland microcarcinoma in needle prostatic biopsy. Ann Diagn Pathol 2008; 12:349–55.

81. Wolters T, van der Kwast TH, Vissers CJ, et al. False-negative prostate needle biopsies: frequency, histopathologic features, and follow-up. Am J Surg Pathol 2010;34:35–43.

82. Nelson RS, Epstein JI. Prostatic carcinoma with abundant xanthomatous cytoplasm. Foamy gland carcinoma. Am J Surg Pathol 1996;20:419–26.

83. Egan AJ, Lopez-Beltran A, Bostwick DG. Prostatic adenocarcinoma with atrophic features: malignancy mimicking a benign process. Am J Surg Pathol 1997;21:931–5.

84. Cina SJ, Epstein JI. Adenocarcinoma of the prostate with atrophic features. Am J Surg Pathol 1997;21:289–95.

85. Kaleem Z, Swanson PE, Vollmer RT, et al. Prostatic adenocarcinoma with atrophic features: a study of 202 consecutive completely embedded radical prostatectomy specimens. Am J Clin Pathol 1998; 109:695–703.

86. Humphrey PA, Kaleem Z, Swanson PE, et al. Pseudohyperplastic prostatic adenocarcinoma. Am J Surg Pathol 1998;22:1239–46.

87. Arista-Nasr J, Cortés E, Pichardo R. Low grade adenocarcinoma simulating benign glandular lesions in needle prostatic biopsy. Rev Invest Clin 1997;49:37–40.

88. Smith SC, Palanisamy N, Zuhlke KA, et al. HOXB13 G84E-related familial prostate cancers: a clinical, histologic, and molecular survey. Am J Surg Pathol 2014;38:615–26.

89. Levi AW, Epstein JI. Pseudohyperplastic prostatic adenocarcinoma on needle biopsy and simple prostatectomy. Am J Surg Pathol 2000;24:1039–46.

90. Arista-Nasr J, Martinez-Benitez B, Fernandez-Amador JA, et al. Pseudohyperplastic prostatic carcinoma in simple prostatectomy. Ann Diagn Pathol 2011;15:170–4.

91. Yaskiv O, Cao D, Humphrey PA. Microcystic adenocarcinoma of the prostate: a variant of pseudohyperplastic and atrophic patterns. Am J Surg Pathol 2010;34:556–61.

92. Parwani AV, Herawi M, Epstein JI. Pleomorphic giant cell adenocarcinoma of the prostate: report of 6 cases. Am J Surg Pathol 2006;30:1254–9.

93. Lopez-Beltran A, Eble JN, Bostwick DG. Pleomorphic giant cell carcinoma of the prostate. Arch Pathol Lab Med 2005;129:683–5.

94. Hameed O, Humphrey PA. Stratified epithelium in prostatic adenocarcinoma: a mimic of high-grade prostatic intraepithelial neoplasia. Mod Pathol 2006;19:899–906.

95. Tavora F, Epstein JI. High-grade prostatic intraepithelial neoplasialike ductal adenocarcinoma of the prostate: a clinicopathologic study of 28 cases. Am J Surg Pathol 2008;32:1060–7.

96. Hirano D, Okada Y, Minei S, et al. Neuroendocrine differentiation in hormone refractory prostate cancer following androgen deprivation therapy. Eur Urol 2004;45:586–92.

97. Berruti A, Mosca A, Porpiglia F, et al. Chromogranin A expression in patients with hormone naïve prostate cancer predicts the development of hormone refractory disease. J Urol 2007;178:838–43.

98. Epstein JI, Amin MB, Beltran H, et al. Proposed morphologic classification of prostate cancer with neuroendocrine differentiation. Am J Surg Pathol 2014;38:756–67.

99. Berruti A, Mosca A, Tucci M, et al. Independent prognostic role of circulating chromogranin A in prostate cancer patients with hormone-refractory disease. Endocr Relat Cancer 2005;12:109–17.

100. Bostwick DG, Qian J, Pacelli A, et al. Neuroendocrine expression in node positive prostate cancer: correlation with systemic progression and patient survival. J Urol 2002;168:1204–11.

101. Theodorescu D, Broder SR, Boyd JC, et al. Cathepsin D and chromogranin A as predictors of long term disease specific survival after radical prostatectomy for localized carcinoma of the prostate. Cancer 1997;80:2109–19.

102. Shariff AH, Ather MH. Neuroendocrine differentiation in prostate cancer. Urology 2006;68:2–8.

103. Ishida E, Nakamura M, Shimada K, et al. Immunohistochemical analysis of neuroendocrine differentiation in prostate cancer. Pathobiology 2009;76: 30–8.

104. Heinrich E, Trojan L, Friedrich D, et al. Neuroendocrine tumor cells in prostate cancer: evaluation of the neurosecretory products serotonin, bombesin, and gastrin - impact on angiogenesis and clinical follow-up. Prostate 2011;71:1752–8.

105. Adlakha H, Bostwick DG. Paneth cell-like change in prostatic adenocarcinoma represents neuroendocrine differentiation: report of 30 cases. Hum Pathol 1994;25:135–9.

106. di Sant' Agnese PA. Divergent neuroendocrine differentiation in prostatic carcinoma. Semin Diagn Pathol 2000;17:149–61.

107. So JS, Gordetsky J, Epstein JI. Variant of prostatic adenocarcinoma with Paneth cell-like neuroendocrine differentiation readily misdiagnosed as Gleason pattern 5. Hum Pathol 2014;45(12): 2388–93.

108. Freschi M, Colombo R, Naspro R, et al. Primary and pure neuroendocrine tumor of the prostate. Eur Urol 2004;45:166–9.

109. Giordano S, Tolonen T, Tolonen T, et al. A pure primary low-grade neuroendocrine carcinoma (carcinoid tumor) of the prostate. Int Urol Nephrol 2010; 42:683–7.

110. Goulet-Salmon B, Berthe E, Franc S, et al. Prostatic neuroendocrine tumor in multiple endocrine neoplasia Type 2B. J Endocrinol Invest 2004;27: 570–3.

111. Whelan T, Gatfield CT, Robertson S, et al. Primary carcinoid of the prostate in conjunction with multiple endocrine neoplasia IIb in a child. J Urol 1995;153:1080–2.

112. Wang W, Epstein JI. Small cell carcinoma of the prostate. A morphologic and immunohistochemical study of 95 cases. Am J Surg Pathol 2008;32: 65–71.

113. Yao JL, Madeb R, Bourne P, et al. Small cell carcinoma of the prostate: an immunohistochemical study. Am J Surg Pathol 2006;30:705–12.

114. Schelling LA, Williamson SR, Zhang S, et al. Frequent TMPRSS2-ERG rearrangement in prostatic small cell carcinoma detected by fluorescence in situ hybridization: the superiority of fluorescence in situ hybridization over ERG immunohistochemistry. Hum Pathol 2013;44:2227–33.

115. Nadal R, Schweizer M, Kryvenko ON, et al. Small cell carcinoma of the prostate. Nat Rev Urol 2014; 11:213–9.

116. Evans AJ, Humphrey PA, Belani J, et al. Large cell neuroendocrine carcinoma of prostate: a clinicopathologic summary of 7 cases of a rare manifestation of advanced prostate cancer. Am J Surg Pathol 2006;30:684–93.

117. Hameed O, Humphrey PA. Immunohistochemistry in diagnostic surgical pathology of the prostate. Semin Diagn Pathol 2005;22:88–104.

118. Stein BS, Vangore S, Petersen RO, et al. Immunoperoxidase localization of prostate-specific antigen. Am J Surg Pathol 1982;6:553–7.

119. Epstein JI. PSA and PAP as immunohistochemical markers in prostate cancer. Urol Clin North Am 1993;20:757–70.

120. Wright GL Jr, Haley C, Beckett ML, et al. Expression of prostate-specific membrane antigen in normal, benign, and malignant prostate tissues. Urol Oncol 1995;1:18–28.

121. Green R, Epstein JI. Use of intervening unstained slides for immunohistochemical stains for high molecular weight cytokeratin on prostate needle biopsies. Am J Surg Pathol 1999;23:567–70.

122. Parsons JK, Gage WR, Nelson WG, et al. p63 protein expression is rare in prostate adenocarcinoma: implications for cancer diagnosis and carcinogenesis. Urology 2001;58:619–24.

123. Luo J, Zha S, Gage WR, et al. Alpha-methylacyl-CoA racemase: a new molecular marker for prostate cancer. Cancer Res 2002;62:2220–6.

124. Shah RB, Zhou M, LeBlanc M, et al. Comparison of the basal cell-specific markers, 34betaE12 and p63, in the diagnosis of prostate cancer. Am J Surg Pathol 2002;26:1161–8.

125. Rubin MA, Zhou M, Dhanasekaran SM, et al. alpha-Methylacyl coenzyme A racemase as a tissue

biomarker for prostate cancer. JAMA 2002;287: 1662–70.

126. Zhou M, Chinnaiyan AM, Kleer CG, et al. Alpha-Methylacyl-CoA racemase: a novel tumor marker over-expressed in several human cancers and their precursor lesions. Am J Surg Pathol 2002;26: 926–31.

127. Sanderson SO, Sebo TJ, Murphy LM, et al. An analysis of the p63/alpha-methylacyl coenzyme A racemase immunohistochemical cocktail stain in prostate needle biopsy specimens and tissue microarrays. Am J Clin Pathol 2004;121:220–5.

128. Farinola MA, Epstein JI. Utility of immunohistochemistry for alpha-methylacyl-CoA racemase in distinguishing atrophic prostate cancer from benign atrophy. Hum Pathol 2004;35:1272–8.

129. Sheridan T, Herawi M, Epstein JI, et al. The role of P501S and PSA in the diagnosis of metastatic adenocarcinoma of the prostate. Am J Surg Pathol 2007;31:1351–5.

130. Trpkov K, Bartczak-McKay J, Yilmaz A. Usefulness of cytokeratin 5/6 and AMACR applied as double sequential immunostains for diagnostic assessment of problematic prostate specimens. Am J Clin Pathol 2009;132:211–20.

131. Oliai BR, Kahane H, Epstein JI. Can basal cells be seen in adenocarcinoma of the prostate?: an immunohistochemical study using high molecular weight cytokeratin (clone 34betaE12) antibody. Am J Surg Pathol 2002;26:1151–60.

132. Ali TZ, Epstein JI. False positive labeling of prostate cancer with high molecular weight cytokeratin: p63 a more specific immunomarker for basal cells. Am J Surg Pathol 2008;32:1890–5.

133. Osunkoya AO, Hansel DE, Sun X, et al. Aberrant diffuse expression of p63 in adenocarcinoma of the prostate on needle biopsy and radical prostatectomy: report of 21 cases. Am J Surg Pathol 2008;32:461–7.

134. Tan HL, Haffner MC, Esopi DM, et al. Prostate adenocarcinomas aberrantly expressing p63 are molecularly distinct from usual-type prostatic adenocarcinomas. Mod Pathol 2015;28(3):446–56.

135. Tomlins SA, Rhodes DR, Perner S, et al. Recurrent fusion of TMPRSS2 and ETS transcription factor genes in prostate cancer. Science 2005;310: 644–8.

136. Clark JP, Cooper CS. ETS gene fusions in prostate cancer. Nat Rev Urol 2009;6:429–39.

137. Park K, Tomlins SA, Mudaliar KM, et al. Antibody-based detection of ERG rearrangement-positive prostate cancer. Neoplasia 2010;12:590–8.

138. He H, Magi-Galluzzi C, Li J, et al. The diagnostic utility of novel immunohistochemical marker ERG in the workup of prostate biopsies with 'atypical glands suspicious for cancer'. Am J Surg Pathol 2011;35:608–14.

139. Andrews C, Humphrey PA. Utility of ERG versus AMACR expression in diagnosis of minimal adenocarcinoma of the prostate in needle biopsy tissue. Am J Surg Pathol 2014;38:1007–12.

140. Cheng L, Davidson DD, Maclennan GT, et al. Atypical adenomatous hyperplasia of prostate lacks TMPRSS2-ERG gene fusion. Am J Surg Pathol 2013;37:1550–4.

141. Green WM, Hicks JL, De Marzo A, et al. Immunohistochemical evaluation of TMPRSS2-ERG gene fusion in adenosis of the prostate. Hum Pathol 2013;44:1895–901.

142. Epstein JI, Egevad L, Humphrey PA, et al, Members of the ISUP Immunohistochemistry in Diagnostic Urologic Pathology Group. Best practices recommendations in the application of immunohistochemistry in the prostate: report from the International Society of Urologic Pathology consensus conference. Am J Surg Pathol 2014;38:e6–19.

143. Downes MR, Torlakovic EE, Aldaoud N, et al. Diagnostic utility of androgen receptor expression in discriminating poorly differentiated urothelial and prostate carcinoma. J Clin Pathol 2013;66:779–86.

144. Chuang AY, DeMarzo AM, Veltri RW, et al. Immunohistochemical differentiation of high-grade prostate carcinoma from urothelial carcinoma. Am J Surg Pathol 2007;31:1246–55.

145. Miyamoto H, Yao JL, Chaux A, et al. Expression of androgen and oestrogen receptors and its prognostic significance in urothelial neoplasm of the urinary bladder. BJU Int 2012;109:1716–26.

146. Varma M, Morgan M, Amin MB, et al. High molecular weight cytokeratin antibody (clone 34betaE12): a sensitive marker for differentiation of high-grade invasive urothelial carcinoma from prostate cancer. Histopathology 2003;42:167–72.

147. Huang HY, Shariat SF, Sun TT, et al. Persistent uroplakin expression in advanced urothelial carcinomas: implications in urothelial tumor progression and clinical outcome. Hum Pathol 2007;38:1703–13.

148. Kaufmann O, Volmerig J, Dietel M. Uroplakin III is a highly specific and moderately sensitive immunohistochemical marker for primary and metastatic urothelial carcinomas. Am J Clin Pathol 2000;113: 683–7.

149. Ordonez NG. Thrombomodulin expression in transitional cell carcinoma. Am J Clin Pathol 1998; 110:385–90.

150. Higgins JP, Kaygusuz G, Wang L, et al. Placental S100 (S100P) and GATA3: markers for transitional epithelium and urothelial carcinoma discovered by complementary DNA microarray. Am J Surg Pathol 2007;31:673–80.

151. Liu H, Shi J, Wilkerson ML, et al. Immunohistochemical evaluation of GATA3 expression in tumors and normal tissues: a useful immunomarker for

breast and urothelial carcinomas. Am J Clin Pathol 2012;138:57–64.

152. Miettinen M, McCue PA, Sarlomo-Rikala M, et al. GATA3: a multispecific but potentially useful marker in surgical pathology: a systematic analysis of 2500 epithelial and nonepithelial tumors. Am J Surg Pathol 2014;38:13–22.

153. Chang A, Amin A, Gabrielson E, et al. Utility of GATA3 immunohistochemistry in differentiating urothelial carcinoma from prostate adenocarcinoma and squamous cell carcinomas of the uterine cervix, anus, and lung. Am J Surg Pathol 2012;36:1472–6.

154. Genega EM, Hutchinson B, Reuter VE, et al. Immunophenotype of high-grade prostatic adenocarcinoma and urothelial carcinoma. Mod Pathol 2000; 13:1186–91.

155. Mhawech P, Uchida T, Pelte MF. Immunohistochemical profile of high-grade urothelial bladder carcinoma and prostate adenocarcinoma. Hum Pathol 2002;33:1136–40.

156. Osunkoya AO, Netto GJ, Epstein JI. Colorectal adenocarcinoma involving the prostate: report of 9 cases. Hum Pathol 2007;38:1836–41.

157. Owens CL, Epstein JI, Netto GJ. Distinguishing prostatic from colorectal adenocarcinoma on biopsy samples: the role of morphology and immunohistochemistry. Arch Pathol Lab Med 2007;131: 599–603.

158. Contreras HR, Ledezma RA, Vergara J, et al. The expression of syndecan-1 and -2 is associated with Gleason score and epithelial-mesenchymal transition markers, E-cadherin and beta-catenin, in prostate cancer. Urol Oncol 2010;28:534–40.

159. Oppenheimer JR, Kahane H, Epstein JI. Granulomatous prostatitis on needle biopsy. Arch Pathol Lab Med 1997;121:724–9.

160. Chuang AY, Epstein JI. Xanthoma of the prostate: a mimicker of high-grade prostate adenocarcinoma. Am J Surg Pathol 2007;31:1225–30.

# Molecular Updates in Prostate Cancer

George J. Netto, MD

## KEYWORDS

- Prostate cancer • PCA3 • Carcinogenesis • Genomic classification

## ABSTRACT

A wide array of molecular markers and genomic signatures, reviewed in this article, may soon be used as adjuncts to currently established screening strategies, prognostic parameters, and early detection markers. Markers of genetic susceptibility to PCA, recurrent epigenetic and genetic alterations, including *ETS* gene fusions, *PTEN* alterations, and urine-based early detection marker *PCA3*, are discussed. Impact of recent genome-wide assessment on our understanding of key pathways of PCA development and progression and their potential clinical implications are highlighted.

## OVERVIEW

Deciphering the molecular pathways of prostate cancer (PCA) development has facilitated the pursuit of molecular biomarkers that would soon help refine early detection strategy, accurately predict outcome, and serve as potential targets of therapy.[1–3] Such efforts have gained an unprecedented momentum from the staggering amount of information that has been brought to light evaluating datasets of genomic, transcriptomic, and proteomic analyses using sophisticated bioinformatics tools.[4–6] Furthermore, genomic studies have been instrumental in identifying germline (host) markers of genetic susceptibility associated with risk of developing early and aggressive disease. The latter will in turn help refine the current "one-size-fits-all" screening strategy.

The recent debate questioning whether current serum prostate-specific antigen (PSA)-based screening strategies are potentially leading to "overtreatment" of at least a subset of patients with PCA[7–10] has further emphasized the need to identify molecular markers of biologically "significant" PCA that would merit "definitive" therapy.

Currently used clinicopathologic algorithms and National Comprehensive Cancer Network guidelines that define "insignificant" very low risk (http://www.nccn.org/professionals/physician_gls/f_guidelines.asp) PCA are in dire need of being buttressed by molecular signature(s) that will enhance confidence in accurately assigning the right patients to such approach while vigilantly monitoring using molecular imaging tools and signatures of molecular biologic progression in tissue samples.

## CARCINOGENESIS AND GENETIC SUSCEPTIBILITY

The variation in PCA incidence among geographic populations has long pointed to differences in ethnic genetic determinants as well as environmental causes as significant etiologic factors. Although higher incidence of the disease in African American individuals compared with Asian American individuals is likely genetically based,[11] the alteration in risk on migration in a given ethnic group strongly suggests environmental and lifestyle factors as additional contributing determinants of risk.[1,2,12–14]

### ENVIRONMENTAL FACTORS

Lifestyle and dietary habits have long been linked to PCA risk.[15–17] Accumulating evidence points to glandular epithelial cell injury by dietary carcinogens, estrogens, or oxidants as a trigger for a chronic inflammatory milieu that set the stage for cancer development.[12,13,17,18] Pinpointing the exact culprit environmental carcinogen(s) has proven to be a difficult endeavor; however, epidemiologic dietary association data and animal model studies[19,20] have strongly supported dietary intake of red meats and animal fats as risk factors. Cooking with high temperature and char-broiling

Johns Hopkins University, Baltimore, Maryland, USA
*E-mail address:* gnetto1@jhmi.edu

Surgical Pathology 8 (2015) 561–580
http://dx.doi.org/10.1016/j.path.2015.08.003
1875-9181/15/$ – see front matter © 2015 Elsevier Inc. All rights reserved.

of red meat result in the formation of heterocyclic aromatic amine (eg, 2-amino-1-methyl-6-phenyli-midazopyrine) and polycyclic aromatic hydrocarbon carcinogens, some of which have been linked to disease pathogenesis in animal models.[21–23] Other cited environmental risk factors include exposures to sex steroid hormones and infectious agents. Animal data link estrogen to prostate epithelial cell damage and inflammation potentially though induction of autoimmunity.[24,25] Likewise, sexually transmitted infections (eg, trichomonas, chlamydia, and gonorrhea) have been cited as potential initiators of predisposing chronic inflammation of the prostate (Fig. 1).[26–29] Epithelial damage and ensuing inflammation is the common pathogenic link between environmental "carcinogens" and PCA development. Faced with persistent oxidative stress, the epithelial cells mount a genome damage defense and cell survival response by initially inducing their expression of $\alpha$ and $\pi$ class glutathione S-transferases, cyclooxygenase-2, and other mediators.[15,30–32] Ultimately, this is followed by epigenetic silencing of hundreds of genes, including the crucial caretaker gene GSTP1 that persists throughout subsequent cancer progression phases. Proliferative inflammatory atrophy (PIA) has been forwarded by some as the earliest histologic manifestation of the injury response exhibiting increased epithelial proliferation and inflammation. That view is supported by the fact that PIA shares many of the somatic genetic and epigenetic alterations that are exhibited by prostatic intraepithelial neoplasm (PIN) and PCA.[33–35]

## GENETIC SUSCEPTIBILITY

PCA has increasingly been recognized as one of the most heritable cancer types driven by numerous common and few rare inherited germline genetic variants of risk (Figs. 2 and 3). Family pedigree and twin studies have consistently supported genetic predisposition as a risk factor for PCA.[11,36,37] Men with a first-degree relative diagnosed with PCA are at twice the risk (more than fourfold if diagnosed before age 60).[38,39]

Early linkage analysis studies suggested various inheritance models (eg, dominant, X-linked) and numerous chromosomal loci of association that failed to be consistently validated.[38,40–47] Evidence supporting the initial suggestion that inflammatory and infection response gene loci (ELAC2, RANSEL, and MSR1) are associated with risk have not been consistently replicated.[48–51] In the largest linkage study performed by the international consortium of PCA genetics, only one locus (22q) stood out.[52] Subsequent studies also pointed to 8q24[53–55] as a region harboring genetic risk variants. The detection of far more common germline genetic variants with only low to moderate penetrance had to await the advent of Genome-Wide Association Studies (GWAS). GWAS that are able to assess millions of single nucleotide polymorphisms (SNPs) in a given individual for disease risk association were first used to assess PCA risk variants in 2006.[56] To date, at least 92 SNPs associated with PCA risk (Table 1) have been established by such studies (A catalog of published genome-wide

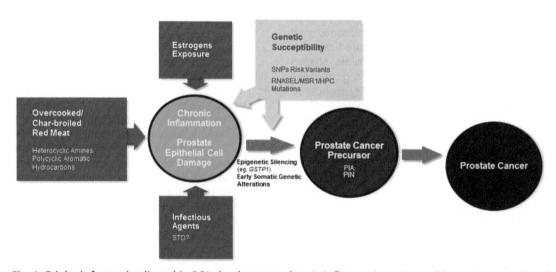

Fig. 1. Etiologic factors implicated in PCA development: chronic inflammation triggered by environmental and lifestyle exposures leads to persistent prostate epithelial cell damage. Inherited genetic predisposition also plays a determining factor in promoting oncogenesis.

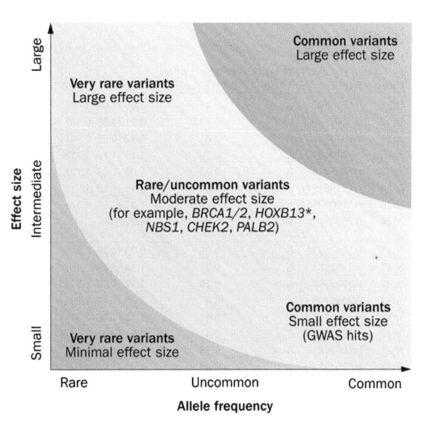

Fig. 2. Mixed model of common and rare genetic variants with different effect size determining genetic risk of PCA. (*Adapted from* Eeles R, Goh C, Castro E, et al. The genetic epidemiology of prostate cancer and its clinical implications. Nat Rev Urol 2014;11: 18–31; with permission.)

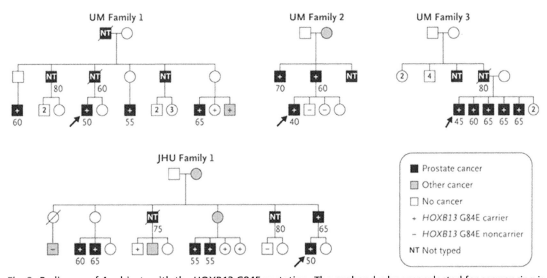

Fig. 3. Pedigrees of 4 subjects with the HOXB13 G84E mutation. The proband who was selected for sequencing is indicated by the arrow in each pedigree. Squares indicate male sex, and circles indicate female sex. Ages of subjects are shown under the symbols. A slash through the symbol indicates that the subject is deceased. Two subjects in 2 families, family 1 from the University of Michigan PCA Genetics Project (UM) and family 1 from Johns Hopkins University (JHU), who were inferred to be obligate carriers of the HOXB13 G84E mutation, died of PCA. (*Adapted from* Xu J, Lange EM, Lu L, et al. HOXB13 is a susceptibility gene for prostate cancer: results from the international consortium for prostate cancer genetics (ICPCG). Hum Genet 2013;132:5–14.)

*Table 1*
Common prostate cancer genetic susceptibility loci from here to 29 performed GWAS studies

| Locus | SNP | Effect (Risk) Allele | Effect Allele Frequency | Per Allele OR (95% CI)/Beta | Nearby Genes |
|---|---|---|---|---|---|
| 1q21 | rs1218582 | G | 0.45 | 1.06 (1.03–1.09) | KCNN3 |
| 1q32 | rs4245739 | C | 0.25 | 0.91 (0.88–0.95) | MDM4, PIK3C2B |
| 2p11 | rs10187424 | G | 0.41 | 0.92 (0.89–0.94) | GGCX/VAMP8 |
| 2p15 | rs721048 | A | 0.19 | 1.15 (1.10–1.21) | EHBP1 |
| 2p21 | rs1465618 | A | 0.23 | 1.08 (1.03–1.12) | THADA |
| 2p24 | rs13385191 | G | 0.56 | 1.15 (1.10–1.21) | C2orf43 |
| 2p25 | rs11902236 | A | 0.27 | 1.07 (1.03–1.10) | TAF1B:GRHL1 |
| 2q24 | rs7582141 | T | 0.04 | 0.37 (NR) | TANC1, BTF3L4P2, GSTM3P2 |
| 2q31 | rs12621278 | G | 0.06 | 0.75 (0.70–0.80) | ITGA6 |
| 2q37 | rs2292884 | G | 0.25 | 1.14 (1.09–1.19) | MLPH |
| 2q37 | rs3771570 | A | 0.15 | 1.12 (1.08–1.17) | FARP2 |
| 3p11 | rs2055109 | C | 0.9 | 1.20 (1.13–1.29) | Unknown |
| 3p12 | rs2660753 | T | 0.11 | 1.18 (1.06–1.31) | Unknown |
| 3q13 | rs7611694 | C | 0.41 | 0.91 (0.88–0.93) | SIDT1 |
| 3q21 | rs10934853 | A | 0.28 | 1.12 (1.08–1.16) | EEFSEC |
| 3q23 | rs6763931 | T | 0.45 | 1.04 (1.01–1.07) | ZBTB38 |
| 3q26 | rs10936632 | C | 0.48 | 0.90 (0.88–0.93) | CLDN11/SKIL |
| 4q13 | rs1894292 | A | 0.48 | 0.91 (0.89–0.94) | AFM, RASSF6 |
| 4q22 | rs17021918 | T | 0.34 | 0.90 (0.87–0.93) | PDLIM5 |
| 4q22 | rs12500426 | A | 0.46 | 1.08 (1.05–1.12) | PDLIM5 |
| 4q24 | rs7679673 | A | 0.45 | 0.91 (0.88–0.94) | TET2 |
| 5p12 | rs2121875 | G | 0.34 | 1.05 (1.02–1.08) | FGF10 |
| 5p15 | rs2242652 | A | 0.19 | 0.87 (0.84–0.90) | TERT |
| 5p15 | rs12653946 | T | 0.44 | 1.26 (1.20–1.33) | IRX4 |
| 5q35 | rs6869841 | A | 0.21 | 1.07 (1.04–1.11) | FAM44B (BOD1) |
| 6p21 | rs130067 | G | 0.21 | 1.05 (1.02–1.09) | CCHCR1 |
| 6p21 | rs1983891 | T | 0.41 | 1.15 (1.09–1.21) | FOXP4 |
| 6p21 | rs3096702 | A | 0.4 | 1.07 (1.04–1.10) | NOTCH4 |
| 6p21 | rs2273669 | G | 0.15 | 1.07 (1.03–1.11) | ARMC2, SESN1 |
| 6q22 | rs339331 | T | 0.63 | 1.22 (1.15–1.28) | RFX6 |
| 6q25 | rs9364554 | T | 0.29 | 1.17 (1.08–1.26) | SLC22A3 |
| 6q25 | rs1933488 | G | 0.41 | 0.89 (0.87–0.92) | RSG17 |
| 7p15 | rs10486567 | G | 0.77 | 0.74 (0.66–0.83) | JAZF1 |
| 7p21 | rs12155172 | A | 0.23 | 1.11 (1.07–1.15) | SP8 |
| 7q21 | rs6465657 | C | 0.46 | 1.12 (1.05–1.20) | LMTK2 |
| 8p21 | rs2928679 | T | 0.42 | 1.05 (1.01–1.09) | SLC25A37 |
| 8p21 | rs1512268 | A | 0.45 | 1.18 (1.14–1.22) | NKX3.1 |
| 8p21 | rs11135910 | A | 0.16 | 1.11 (1.07–1.16) | EBF2 |
| 8q24 | rs1447295 | A | 0.13 | 1.62 (NR) | Unknown |
| 8q24 | rs6983267 | G | 0.5 | 1.26 (1.13–1.41) | Unknown |
| 8q24 | rs16901979 | A | 0.09 | 1.79 (1.36–2.34) | Unknown |
| 8q24 | rs10086908 | C | 0.3 | 0.87 (0.81–0.94) | Unknown |
| 8q24 | rs12543663 | C | 0.31 | 1.08 (1.00–1.16) | Unknown |

(continued on next page)

**Table 1**
*(continued)*

| Locus | SNP | Effect (Risk) Allele | Effect Allele Frequency | Per Allele OR (95% CI)/Beta | Nearby Genes |
|-------|-----|------|------|------|------|
| 8q24 | rs620861 | T | 0.39 | 0.90 (0.84–0.96) | Unknown |
| 8q24 | rs6983267 | G | NR | 0.29 (0.22–0.36) unit increase | SRRM1P1, POU5F1B |
| 8q24 | rs1447295 | A | NR | 0.51 (0.40–0.63) unit increase | MYC |
| 8q24 | rs12682344 | G | NR | 0.67 (0.48–0.86) unit increase | SRRM1P1, POU5F1B |
| 8q24 | rs6983267 | G | NR | 1.36 (NR) | NR |
| 8q24 | rs10505477 | A | 0.49 | 1.39 (1.28–1.50) | MYC |
| 9q31 | rs817826 | C | 0.08 | 1.41 (1.29–1.54) | RAD23B–KLF4 |
| 9q33 | rs1571801 | A | 0.25 | 1.27 (1.10–1.48) | DAB21P |
| 10q11 | rs10993994 | T | 0.4 | 1.25 (1.17–1.34) | MSMB |
| 10q11 | rs10993994 | T | NR | 0.40 (0.33–0.47) unit increase | MSMB |
| 10q11 | rs10993994 | T | 0.42 | 1.32 (1.21–1.43) | MSMB |
| 10q24 | rs3850699 | G | 0.29 | 0.91 (0.89–0.94) | TRIM8 |
| 10q26 | rs4962416 | C | 0.27 | 1.20 (1.07–1.34) | CTBP2 |
| 10q26 | rs2252004 | G | 0.77 | 1.16 (1.10–1.22) | Unknown |
| 11p15 | rs7127900 | A | 0.2 | 1.22 (1.17–1.27) | Unknown |
| 11p15 | rs7127900 | A | NR | 1.4 (NR) | NR |
| 11p15 | rs7126629 | C | 0.21 | 1.44 (1.31–1.57) | TH |
| 11q12 | rs1938781 | C | 0.3 | 1.16 (1.11–1.21) | FAM111A |
| 11q13 | rs7931342 | T | 0.49 | 0.84 (0.79–0.90) | Unknown |
| 11q13 | rs7931342 | G | NR | 1.30 (NR) | NR |
| 11q13 | rs11228583 | T | 0.52 | 1.33 (1.22–1.44) | MYEOV |
| 11q22 | rs11568818 | G | 0.44 | 0.91 (0.88–0.94) | MMP7 |
| 12q13 | rs10875943 | C | 0.31 | 1.07 (1.04–1.10) | TUBA1C/PRPH |
| 12q13 | rs902774 | A | 0.15 | 1.17 (1.11–1.24) | KRT8 |
| 12q24 | rs1270884 | A | 0.49 | 1.07 (1.04–1.10) | TBX5 |
| 13q22 | rs9600079 | T | 0.38 | 1.18 (1.12–1.24) | Unknown |
| 14q22 | rs8008270 | A | 0.18 | 0.89 (0.86–0.93) | FERMT2 |
| 14q24 | rs7141529 | G | 0.5 | 1.09 (1.06–1.12) | RAD51L1 |
| 17p13 | rs684232 | G | 0.36 | 1.10 (1.07–1.14) | VPS53, FAM57A |
| 17q12 | rs4430796 | A | 0.49 | 1.22 (1.15–1.30) | HNF1B |
| 17q12 | rs11649743 | G | 0.8 | 1.28 (1.07–1.52) | HNF1B |
| 17q12 | rs2005705 | G | 0.56 | 1.35 (1.23–1.47) | TCF2 |
| 17q21 | rs7210100 | G | 0.05 | 1.51 (1.35–1.69) | ZNF652 |
| 17q21 | rs11650494 | A | 0.08 | 1.15 (1.09–1.22) | SPOP, HOXB13 |
| 17q24 | rs1859962 | G | 0.46 | 1.20 (1.14–1.27) | Unknown |
| 17q24 | rs4793529 | T | NR | 0.28 (0.20–0.35) unit increase | CALM2P1, SOX9 |
| 18q23 | rs7241993 | A | 0.3 | 0.92 (0.89–0.95) | SALL3 |
| 19q13 | rs2735839 | A | 0.15 | 0.83 (0.75–0.91) | KLK2/KLK3 |
| 19q13 | rs8102476 | C | 0.54 | 1.12 (1.08–1.15) | Unknown |
| 19q13 | rs11672691 | A | 0.76 | 1.12 (1.03–1.21) | Unknown |
| 19q13 | rs103294 | C | 0.24 | 1.28 (1.21–1.36) | LILRA3 |
| 19q13 | rs17632542 | T | NR | 0.73 (0.60–0.86) unit increase | KLK3 |
| 19q13 | rs17632542 | T | 0.92 | 1.85 (1.61–2.09) | KLK3 |
| 20q13 | rs2427345 | A | 0.37 | 0.94 (0.91–0.97) | GATAS, CABLES2 |

*(continued on next page)*

**Table 1**
*(continued)*

| Locus | SNP | Effect (Risk) Allele | Effect Allele Frequency | Per Allele OR (95% CI)/Beta | Nearby Genes |
|-------|-----|----------------------|--------------------------|------------------------------|--------------|
| 20q13 | rs6062509 | C | 0.3 | 0.89 (0.66–0.92) | ZGPAT |
| 22q13 | rs5759167 | T | 0.47 | 0.86 (0.83–0.88) | BIL/TTLL1 |
| Xp11 | rs5945619 | C | 0.36 | 1.19 (1.07–1.31) | NUDT11 |
| Xp22 | rs2405942 | G | 0.21 | 0.88 (0.83–0.92) | SHROOM2 |
| Xq12 | rs5919432 | G | 0.19 | 0.94 (0.89–0.98) | AR |

*Abbreviations:* A, adenine; C, cytosine; CI, confidence interval; G, guanine; GWAS, genome-wide association studies; NR, not reported; OR, odds ratio; SNP, single nucleotide polymorphism; T, thymine.

*From* Hindorff LA, MacArthur J, Morales J, et al. A catalog of published genome-wide association studies. Available at: www.genome.gov/gwastudies.

association studies. Available at: www.genome. gov/gwastudies). These SNPs may account for up to one-third of PCA familial risk. Of note are regions such as the 8q24 region[57,58] containing SNPs exerting a modifier effect on the neighboring *MYC* oncogene, a recognized player in PCA pathogenesis.[54] Other SNP variants are located on chromosome 19 q13 that harbor kallikreins *KLK2* and *KLK3* (*PSA*) genes.[59,60] Although each susceptibility SNP allele individually carries only a small risk, multiplicatively, a subject SNP profile can be deduced from risk algorithm models that will identify individuals in the upper 1% risk tier with an approximately fivefold the risk of the general population.[61,62] Evidently such approach could soon prove instrumental in refining the best groups of men to target for screening and prevention strategies that can address the current concerns of overdiagnosis and overtreatment of PCA.[8,9]

Rare but strongly penetrant germline variants (>5% frequencies) are not detectable by current SNP array-based GWAS. Their detection requires exhaustive direct sequencing of many case versus control subjects that only recently became possible with the advent of next-generation sequencing (NGS) technologies. Albeit rare and therefore accounts for only a minute fraction of PCA incidence, such rare variants impart a high risk in carrier subjects for early onset (fivefold to sevenfold) and at times more aggressive PCA. Among these, germline mutations in *BRCA 2* tumor suppressor gene[63] and *HOXB13* (*G84E*)[64,65] have the most established evidence of association with hereditary PCA. A 5% germline carrier frequency for *HOXB13* (*G84E*) mutation was shown in families of PCA of mostly European descent.[65] The Breast Cancer Linkage Consortium study revealed that men with the *BRCA2* germline mutation are at fivefold the risk for PCA (sevenfold the risk of early disease).[66] Of the 6 molecular studies,

32 (73%, 95% confidence interval [CI] 57%–85%) of 44 PCA tumors in carriers were mismatch repair gene (MMR) deficient, which equates to carriers having a 3.67-fold increased risk of PCA (95% CI 2.32–6.67). The evidence from molecular and risk studies supports increased susceptibility for PCA in Lynch syndrome. A recent meta-analysis of 12 risk studies showed a 2.28-fold (95% CI 1.37–3.19) increased risk of PCA for all men from MMR mutation-carrying families. In one of the largest studies in MMR mutation carriers, the relative risk was greatest for MSH2 carriers (5.8, 95% CI 2.6–20.9). PCA was the first or only diagnosed tumor in 37% of carriers.[67–69]

Evidence for *BRCA1*[70] and other DNA repair genes, such as *PALB2, CHECK2, BRIP1,* and *NBS1,* is less robust at this time.[71–74] Several multinational consortia (PCA Association Group to Investigate Cancer Associated Alterations in the Genome, online: http://practical.ccge. medschl.cam.ac.uk/; International Consortium for PCA Genetics, online: http://www.icpcg.org/? q=content/about-icpcg; Elucidating Loci Involved in PCA Susceptibility, online: http://epi.grants. cancer.gov/gameon/personnel.html#ellipse) are currently investigating the important clinical impact of genetic susceptibility to PCA so as to address the potential screening, risk management guidelines, functional and treatment implications of the growing list of identified germline genetic variants.

## EPIGENETIC ALTERATIONS

As mentioned previously, changes in DNA methylation marks, accompanied by epigenetic gene silencing, are the earliest somatic changes of PCA development.[35] Novel genome-wide, high-throughput strategies for detection of specific DNA sequences carrying 5-meC, offer promising opportunities for potential clinical tests for PCA screening, detection (eg, GSTP1, APC, PTGS2, MDR1, and RASSF1a), diagnosis, staging, and risk stratification (eg, *PTGS2*).[45]

Hypermethylation of glutathione S-transferase-π (*GSTP1*) transcriptional regulatory sequences has been consistently detected in more than 90% of PCAs. *GSTP1* encodes an enzyme responsible for detoxifying electrophiles and oxidants, thus shielding the cell from genome damage. As indicated previously, loss of *GSTP1* expression is an early event in the initiation of prostatic carcinogenesis as evidenced by the presence of *GSTP1* methylation in 5% to 10% of PIA and in more than 70% of high-grade PIN lesions.[33,34]

More than 40 additional genes also have been found to be altered by epigenetic hypermethylation.[75] That CpG island hypermethylation is found at an extremely high frequency in PCA tissues and is not found in the normal tissues clearly presents opportunity for noninvasive detection. In a recent study,[76] our group evaluated the extent of promoter methylation of 9 candidate genes (*AIM1, APC, CCND2, GPX3, GSTP1, MCAM, RARbeta2, SSBP2,* and *TIMP3*) by quantitative fluorogenic methylation-specific polymerase chain reaction. Higher extent of *GSTP1* promoter methylation was independently associated with

the risk of recurrence in patients with early PCA. The finding suggests the extent of *GSTP1* promoter methylation as a potential marker of biochemical recurrence marker.

CpG island hypermethylation changes occur early and nearly universally in PCA and are closely maintained throughout disease.[45] In contrast, DNA hypomethylation changes appear to occur late during PCA progression. Importantly, incremental global loss of CpG methylation is associated with progression from primary to hormone-naïve metastatic lesions to castration-resistant prostate cancer (CRPC). Furthermore, hypomethylation signatures appear to be heterogeneous across different metastatic deposits within the same subject. The latter fact carries significant implication for therapeutic strategies targeting genes that are overexpressed as a result of hypomethylation of their promoters (eg, cancer testis antigen genes).[77,78]

## GENETIC SOMATIC MOLECULAR ALTERATIONS

Delineation of pathogenetic pathways (**Fig. 4**) and key driver molecular alterations (**Table 2**) involved

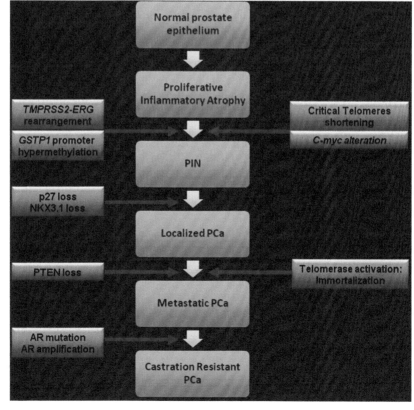

*Fig. 4.* Somatic genetic alterations involved in the pathogenetic steps of Prostate Carcinoma progression. (*From* Netto GJ, Cheng L. Emerging critical role of molecular testing in diagnostic genitourinary pathology. Arch Pathol Lab Med 2012;136(4):372–90; with permission.)

*Table 2*
Genetic and epigenetic alterations in prostate cancer (PCA)

| Gene and Gene Type | Location | Notes |
|---|---|---|
| **Tumor-suppressor genes** | | |
| CDKN1B | 12p13.1–p12 | Encodes cyclin-dependent kinase inhibitor p27. One allele is frequently deleted in primary PCA. |
| NKX3.1 | 8p21.2 | Encodes prostate-restricted homeobox protein that can suppress the growth of prostate epithelial cells. One allele is frequently deleted in primary PCA. |
| PTEN | 10q23.31 | Encodes phosphatase and tensin homologue, suppresses cell proliferation and increases apoptosis. One allele is frequently lost in primary PCA tumors. Mutations are found more frequently in metastatic PCA. |
| TP53 | 17p13.1 | Mutations are uncommon early, but occur in about 50% of advanced or castrate-resistant PCA. |
| **Oncogenes** | | |
| MYC | 8q24 | Transcription factor, regulates genes involved in cell proliferation, senescence, apoptosis, and cell metabolism. mRNA levels increased in all stages. Low-level amplification of the MYC locus is common in advanced PCA. |
| ERG | 21q22.3 | Fusion transcripts with the 5′ portion of androgen-regulated gene (TMPRSS22) arise from deletion or chromosomal rearrangements commonly found in PCA. |
| ETV1–4 | 7p21.3, 19q13.12, 1q21,-q23, 17q21.31 | Encodes ETS-like transcription factors 1–4, which are proposed to be new oncogenes for PCA. Fusion transcripts with the 5′ portion of androgen-regulated gene (TMPRSS22) arise from chromosomal rearrangements commonly found in all disease stages. |
| AR | Xq11–12 | Encodes the androgen receptor. Protein is expressed in most PCA. Locus is amplified or mutated in advanced and castrate-resistant PCA. |
| Activation of the enzyme telomerase | | Maintains telomere function and contributes to cell immortalization. Activated in most PCA, mechanism of activation may be through MYC activation. |
| **Caretaker genes** | | |
| GSTP1 | 11q13 | Encodes the enzyme that catalyses the conjugation of reduced glutathione to electrophilic substrates. Functions to detoxify carcinogens. Inactivated >90% of PCA by somatic hypermethylation of the CpG island within the upstream regulatory region. |
| Telomere dysfunction | Chromosome termini | Contributes to chromosomal instability. Shortened telomeres are found in more than 90% of prostatic intraepithelial neoplasia (PIN) lesions and PCA lesions. |

*(continued on next page)*

| Table 2 (continued) | | |
|---|---|---|
| **Gene and Gene Type** | **Location** | **Notes** |
| Centrosome abnormalities | N/A | Contributes to chromosomal instability. Centrosomes are structurally and numerically abnormal in most PCA. |
| Other somatic changes | | |
| PTGS2, APC, MDR1, EDNRB, RASSF1α, RARβ2 | Various | The hypermethylation of CpG islands within upstream regulatory regions occurs in most primary tumors and metastatic lesions. The functional significance of these changes is not yet known. |

*Adapted from* Netto GJ. Clinical applications of recent molecular advances in urologic malignancies: No longer chasing a "mirage"? Adv Anat Pathol 2013;20:175–203, with permission; and De Marzo AM, Platz EA, Sutcliffe S, et al. Inflammation in prostate carcinogenesis. Nat Rev Cancer 2007;7:256–69.

in PCA development has provided a roadmap for the evaluation of an exhaustive list of biomarkers for their potential role in predicting disease outcome and as therapeutic targets.[1,2,12,35,79–81] They include markers of proliferation index (ki67),[82–85] tumor suppression genes (eg, p53, p21, p27, NKX3.1, PTEN, retinoblastoma gene), oncogenes (eg, Bcl2, c-myc, EZH2, and HER2/neu), adhesion molecules (CD44, E-Cadherin), PI3K/akt/mTOR pathway members,[86] apoptosis regulators (eg, survivin and transforming growth factor β 1), androgen receptor status,[87] and prostate tissue lineage-specific markers (PSA, PSAP, and prostate-specific membrane antigen).

## ETS GENE FUSIONS

In 2005, Tomlins and colleagues[88,89] identified a recurrent chromosomal rearrangement in more than one-half of their analyzed PCA cases. The rearrangements lead to fusion of the androgen-responsive promoter elements of the *TMPRSS2* gene (21q22) to 1 of 3 members of the ETS transcription factors family members *ERG, ETV1,* and *ETV4* located at chromosomes 21q22, 7p21, and 17q21, respectively. Although the prognostic role of assessing *TMPRSS2-ETS* rearrangements in PCA tissue samples, as a standalone marker, was subsequently not substantiated in well-designed large cohort studies,[90,91] the discovery had great implications in terms of furthering our understanding of PCA pathogenesis and provided a new marker for molecular diagnosis in PCA.[92–96] Furthermore, as shown later in this article, recent genome-wide studies have repointed to the prognostic significance of *TMPRSS2-ERG* fusion status as part of genomic signatures that could stratify disease aggressiveness. The potential diagnostic and prognostic role of detecting

*TMPRSS2-ERG* fusion in postprostate massage urine samples is also very promising.[97–99]

Recently, commercial anti-ERG monoclonal antibodies became available that make it possible to use immunohistochemistry (IHC) for evaluating ERG protein expression as a surrogate approach to detecting *TMPRSS2-ERG* fusion by fluorescence in situ hybridization. Park and colleagues[100] and Chaux and colleagues[101] have demonstrated a strong correlation between ERG overexpression by IHC and *ERG* fusion status with more than 86% sensitivity and specificity rates. ERG IHC may offer an accurate, simpler, and less costly alternative for evaluation of *ERG* fusion status in PCA on needle biopsy and radical prostatectomy samples. IHC ERG staining also may have utility in assessing small atypical foci on needle biopsy in combination with other immunomarkers, such as Racemase, p63, and phosphatase and tensin homologue (PTEN).

## PTEN AND PI3K/MAMMALIAN TARGET OF RAPAMYCIN PATHWAY

The PI3K/mTOR (mammalian target of rapamycin) pathway plays an important role in cell growth, proliferation, and oncogenesis in PCA.[102–104] *PTEN* is a master negative regulator of the pathway. Several well-designed retrospective studies have revealed that loss of *PTEN* tumor suppressor gene activity, and the ensuing mTOR pathway activation, is associated with poor prognosis in PCA. In a large nested cases control tissue microarray Chaux and colleagues[105] showed loss of PTEN immunoexpression to be an independent predictor of biochemical recurrence (BCR). Lotan and colleagues[106] also demonstrated the prognostic role of assessing PTEN alteration in a surgical cohort of high-risk patients with PCA where its loss was also predictive of decreased time to metastatic spread.

In the largest study (more than 4750 cases) on PTEN in PCA to date, Krohn and colleagues[107] demonstrated that biallelic *PTEN* inactivation, by either homozygous deletion or deletion of one allele and mutation of the other, occurs in most PTEN-defective cancers and characterizes a particularly aggressive subset of metastatic and hormone-refractory PCA. *PTEN* deletions were present in 20% of PCA (8% heterozygous and 12% homozygous). *PTEN* deletions were associated with early BCR, advanced tumor stage, high Gleason grade, presence of lymph node metastasis, hormone-refractory disease, presence of *ERG* gene fusion, and nuclear p53 accumulation. The prognostic impact of *PTEN* deletion was seen in both *ERG* fusion-positive and *ERG* fusion-negative tumors (**Fig. 5**).[107]

The mTOR pathway is also a potential target of therapy in PCA. Several rapamycin analogs are currently being assessed as potential therapeutic agents for PCA.[104,108,109] We have previously reported the results of a pilot study evaluating the pharmacodynamic efficacy of neoadjuvant rapamycin therapy in PCA.[108] Using IHC analysis, we found a significant decrease in Phos-S6 protein, the main downstream effector of mTOR pathway, in patients receiving neoadjuvant mTOR inhibitor agent.[108]

## OTHER TUMOR SUPPRESSOR GENES AND ONCOGENES

Among tumor suppressor genes, the role of p53 expression in predicting prognosis in prostate carcinoma has been extensively studied. Brewster and colleagues[110] found p53 expression and Gleason score in needle biopsy to be independent predictors of biochemical relapse after radical prostatectomy. Many retrospective studies evaluating prostatectomy specimens found p53 to be of prognostic significance independent of grade, stage, and margin status.[111–113] As discussed later in this article, more recent genome-wide studies seem to support the prognostic role of p53 alterations.[114] Likewise, most retrospective studies of another tumor suppressor gene, p27, a cell cycle inhibitor, also have supported a correlation with progression after prostatectomy, although less robust evidence exists for the prognostic role of p21,[115] a downstream mediator of p53, and

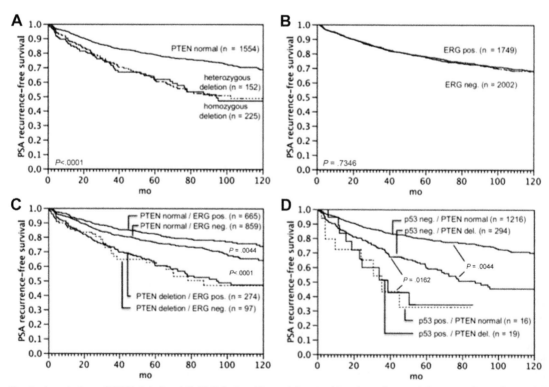

**Fig. 5.** Association of PTEN deletion (*A*), ERG fusion (*B*), and the combination of PTEN deletion and ERG fusion (*C*) or nuclear p53 accumulation with BCR in PCA (*D*). del., deletion; neg., negative; pos., positive. (*Adapted from* Lotan TL, Gurel B, Sutcliffe S, et al. PTEN protein loss by immunostaining: analytical validation and prognostic indicator for a high risk surgical cohort of prostate cancer patients. Clin Cancer Res 2011;17:6563–73; with permission.)

transcription factors such as NKX3.1.[116,117] A preponderance of evidence supports a prognostic role for Bcl2[110,112] and myc oncogenes[118] as potential adjuncts to histologic prognostic parameters. In the absence of prospective randomized data, none of the later markers have transitioned into clinical use.

## GENOMIC SIGNATURES

Early on, in sentinel gene expression profiling (cDNA microarrays), Lapointe and colleagues[5] were able to identify 3 subclasses of PCA based on their distinct patterns of gene expression. The same group subsequently used array-based comparative genomic hybridization[119] to identify recurrent copy number genetic alterations (CNA) that corresponded to 3 prognostically distinct groups: (1) deletions at 5q21 and 6q15 group associated with favorable outcome group, (2) a 8p21 (NKX3-1) and 21q22 (resulting in TMPRSS2-ERG fusion) deletion group, and (3) 8q24 (MYC) and 16p13 gains, and loss at 10q23 (PTEN) and 16q23 groups correlating with metastatic disease and aggressive outcome.

More recent genome-wide characterizing of the PCA transcriptome and genome has further identified chromosomal rearrangements and copy number gains and losses, including ETS gene family fusions, PTEN loss, and androgen receptor (AR) amplification, which drive PCA development and progression to lethal, metastatic castration-resistant PCA. Assessing DNA copy number, mRNA expression, and focused exon resequencing, Taylor and colleagues[120] using DNA CNA data, defined clusters of low-risk and high-risk disease beyond what is achieved by Gleason score. Six clusters of PCA tumors are identified by unsupervised hierarchical clustering with distinct risk for BCR. Markert and colleagues[114] evaluated mRNA microarray signature profiles in a large Swedish watchful-waiting cohort of patients with PCA and found mRNA "stemlike signatures" in combination with p53 and PTEN inactivation to be associated with very poor survival outcome. TMPRSS2-ERG fusion group had intermediate survival outcome compared with the remaining groups with more favorable outcome. The findings were validated in an independent clinical cohort at Memorial Sloan-Kettering Cancer Center.

Berger and colleagues[121] are credited with a monumental report of whole genome sequencing (WGS) in PCA. Their analysis of the entire genome of 7 PCA tissue samples from warm autopsy brought to light the occurrence of complex chains of balanced (that is, "copy-neutral") rearrangements within or adjacent to known cancer genes that on average includes 90 rearrangements per genome. This process of complex rearrangements, termed chromoplexy, was further confirmed in a subsequent larger WGS study by the same investigators performed on 57 PCA samples.[122] Distinctive patterns of chromoplexy appear to take place in (ETS$^{neg}$ CHD1$^{del}$) tumors compared with those that are (ETS$^{pos}$ CHD1$^{wt}$) (Fig. 6). Tumors with a deletion of CHD1 demonstrated an excess of intrachromosomal chained rearrangements and gene deletions clustered in 1 or 2 chromosome(s) with breakpoints concentrated in GC-poor nonexpressed DNA sites. In contrast, in ETS$^{pos}$ tumors, many single chromopexy events joined DNA from dispersed regions of 6 or more chromosomes. In the latter group, the chain rearrangements primarily involved breakpoints enriched near open (actively transcribed) chromatin, AR, and ERG DNA binding sites. The latter suggests a link between chromatin and transcriptional regulation and the genesis of genomic aberrations. Among the genes that are most frequently disrupted by the rearrangements are adhesion molecule gene CADM2 and not surprisingly PTEN and MAGI2, a gene that encodes for PTEN interacting protein.

WGS analysis has helped to further define the chronology of oncogenic events in PCA progression. Genome-wide germline SNP coverage permitted the identification of DNA alterations that arose after a founder clone is established. As illustrated in Fig. 7, a suggested consensus path of PCA tumor evolution may begin with loss of NKX3-1, FOXP1, or TMPRSS2–ERG fusion. The path then proceeds with loss of CDKN1B, CHD1, and TP53 and then leads to loss of PTEN as a progression-related gate event.[122]

Finally, a better understanding of the mutational landscape of CRPC is also emerging with the aid of genomics. Whole-exome sequencing analyses, as the one performed by Grasso and colleagues[123] in 50 lethal metastatic CRPCs, has defined recurrent mutations in genes encoding proteins that physically interact with AR. These included ERG gene fusion product, FOXA1, MLL2, UTX (also known as KDM6A), and ASXL1. The findings shed light on the mechanistic alterations in AR signaling in CRPC and thus present new opportunities for targets of novel therapies in lethal PCA.

## EMERGING CLINICAL GENOMIC MOLECULAR CLASSIFIER ASSAYS

As discussed previously, genomic studies suggest that PCAs develop via a limited number of alternative preferred genetic pathways. The resultant

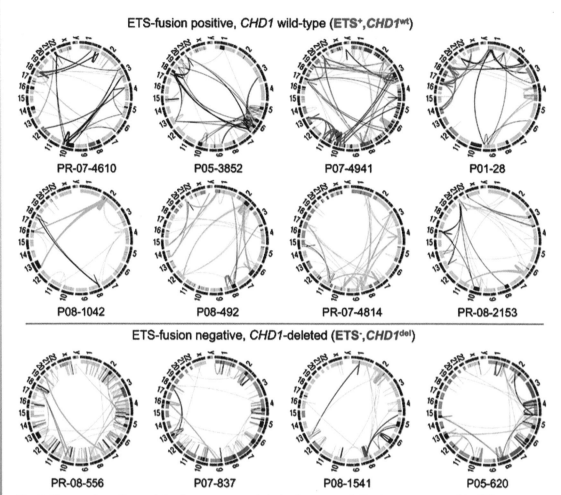

**ETS-fusion positive, *CHD1* wild-type (ETS⁺,*CHD1*ʷᵗ)**

PR-07-4610          P05-3852          P07-4941          P01-28

P08-1042          P08-492          PR-07-4814          PR-08-2153

**ETS-fusion negative, *CHD1*-deleted (ETS⁻,*CHD1*ᵈᵉˡ)**

PR-08-556          P07-837          P08-1541          P05-620

*Fig. 6.* Chromoplexy. Circos plots of rearrangement chains in representative tumors, grouped by ETS rearrangements and CHD1 disruption status. Rearrangements in the same chain are depicted in one color. Rearrangements in gray were not assigned to a chain. The inner ring shows copy number gain and loss in red and blue, respectively. Note that rearrangement chains in ETS-positive tumors contain a greater proportion of interchromosomal fusions than chains in ETS-negative tumors. (*Adapted from* Taylor BS, Schultz N, Hieronymus H, et al. Integrative genomic profiling of human prostate cancer. Cancer Cell 2010;18:11–22.)

molecular genetic subtypes provide a new framework for investigating PCA biology and ultimately stratification of disease outcome and clinical heterogeneity of the disease.

Transitioning the previously described findings to the clinical arena will no doubt be accelerated by the increased implementation of genomic and NGS technologies in commercial and hospital-based clinical molecular diagnostic laboratories. Only a few examples of burgeoning "genomic molecular classifiers" are discussed in this article without implying any endorsement for their utilization (Table 3). Although the role of some of these assays has been supported by initial studies, additional prospective validation studies are accumulating to justify their future implementation as standard of care. Decipher genomic classifier[124,125] is one example of such assays offered by GenomeDx (San Diego, CA). Ross and colleagues[125] demonstrated that the Decipher genomic classifier outperformed clinicopathologic variables (Gleason grade, PSA doubling time, and time to BCR) in predicting metastatic progression in a cohort of 85 patients with radical prostatectomy from our institution. In another study, both Decipher genomic classifier and CAPRA-S (Cancer of the Prostate Risk Assessment post-Surgical score) were significant independent predictors of cancer-specific mortality in a high-risk prostatectomy cohort. If prospectively validated, these would support the integration of genomic and clinical classifiers for identification of postprostatectomy patients who may benefit from early adjuvant therapeutic intervention following BCR.[126]

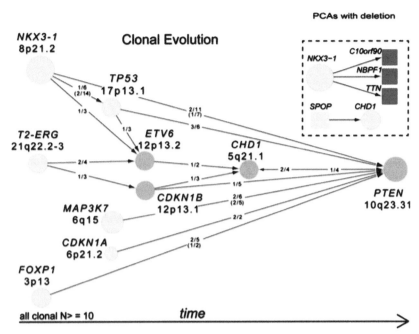

*Fig. 7.* Clonality and evolution of PCA. Patterns of tumor evolution were inferred on the basis of clonality estimates. Arrows indicate the direction of clonal-subclonal hierarchy between genes that are deleted in the same sample in multiple cases. Deleted genes are represented by circles with size and color intensity reflecting the frequency of overall deletions and subclonal deletions, respectively. Ratios along the arrows indicate the number of samples demonstrating directionality of the hierarchy out of samples with deletion of both genes. (*Adapted from* Taylor BS, Schultz N, Hieronymus H, et al. Integrative genomic profiling of human prostate cancer. Cancer Cell 2010;18:11–22.)

The Oncotype DX prostate cancer assay (Genomic Health, Redwood City, CA) is a multigene reverse transcriptase polymerase chain reaction (RT-PCR) expression assay that was developed for use in formalin-fixed paraffin-embedded (FFPE) prostate needle biopsies. The assay evaluates the expression of 12 cancer genes representing several pathways implicated in prostate tumorigenesis. These include the androgen pathway (*AZGP1, KLK2, SRD5A2,* and *FAM13C*), cellular organization (*FLNC, GSN, TPM2,* and *GSTM2*), proliferation (*TPX2*), and stromal response (*BGN, COL1A1,* and *SFRP4*). The expression of 5 "reference" genes is simultaneously assessed to control for sources of preanalytical and analytical variability as well as allow for variable RNA inputs. The calculated Genomic Prostate Score has been shown to predict adverse PCA pathology beyond conventional clinical/pathologic factors in 2 recently completed clinical validation studies.[127,128]

**Table 3**
**Prognostic commercial genomic classifier assays**

| Genomic Assay | Manufacturer | Sample | Comment |
|---|---|---|---|
| Prolaris | Myriad Genetics | FFPE prostatectomy tissue | *CCP score:* Expression of 31 cell-cycle genes; quantitative RT-PCR |
| Oncotype DX | Genomic Health | FFPE needle Bx tissue | *GPS:* Expression of 12 genes; (androgen pathway, cellular organization, cell proliferation and stromal response) Risk assessment before treatment intervention |
| Decipher | GenomeDx | FFPE prostatectomy tissue | *GC:* Expression of 22 genes Calculate risk for metastasis post RP |

*Abbreviations:* Bx, Biopsy; CCP, cell-cycle progression; FFPE, formalin-fixed paraffin-embedded; GC, genomic classifier; GPS, genomic predictor score; RP, radical prostatectomy; RT-PCR, reverse transcriptase polymerase chain reaction.

A third commercial molecular risk classifier assay, termed Prolaris, has been advanced by Myriad Genetics (Salt Lake City, UT).[129,130] In this assay, the expression of 31 genes involved in cell-cycle progression (CCP) is evaluated with quantitative RT-PCR on RNA extracted from radical prostatectomy (RP) FFPE tumor samples. A CCP score is assigned based on the average expression of the CCP genes normalized to 15 housekeeper genes. The signature was initially assessed in an RP cohort of patients from the United States and a separate British cohort of conservatively managed patients diagnosed by Trans-urethral resection of prostate (TRUP).[129] The primary endpoint was time to BCR in the RP cohort and time to death from disease in the TURP cohort. On multivariate analyses, CCP score and initial serum PSA were the best predictors of BCR after RP, whereas CCP score was the best predictor of time to death from PCA (hazard ratio [HR] 2.57). The prognostic significance of CCP score was subsequently validated in a study by Cooperberg and colleagues.[130] The CCP score was assessed, in 413 patients treated with RP for localized disease, for prognostic utility beyond that achieved by standard postoperative risk assessment (CAPRA-S score). The HR of BCR for each unit increase in CCP score was 2.1. The CCP score was also able to substratify patients with low clinical risk as defined by CAPRA-S $\leq 2$. Combining the CCP and CAPRA-S improved the concordance index for both the overall cohort and low-risk subset and outperformed both individual scores on decision curve analysis.[130]

Metamark Genetics Inc (Cambridge, MA) has developed an automated, quantitative protein-based multiplex imaging platform designated Pro-Mark. Metamark's automated proteomics imaging platform is applied to standard FFPE tissue biopsy sections. The tissue sections are subjected to multiplex immunofluorescent staining with monoclonal antibodies, as well as 4',6-diamidino-2-phenylindole, by using a proprietary assay format that enables the quantitative biomarker measurements in the tumor epithelium regions only. Awaiting prospective validation studies, the assay could be of value in predicting indolent disease (organ confined, Gleason grade 3 = 3 or 3 + 4) in patients with positive biopsies that would hence be potential active surveillance candidates.

## EMERGING EARLY DETECTION MARKERS AND TARGETS OF THERAPY

PCA detection markers that can be applied to blood, urine, or prostatic secretion fluid (ejaculate or prostate massage fluids) have been the focus of active recent research. Examples include gene promoter hypermethylation profile assays[75,131–133] and DD3 (differential display code 3), also known as PCA3 in urine or prostatic secretions.

DD3 is a noncoding RNA that was initially identified by Bussemakers and colleagues[134] as one of the most specific markers of PCA. The PCA3 gene is located on chromosome 9q21.2. Quantitative real-time RT-PCR assay detecting PCA3 can be applied to blood, urine, or prostatic fluid.[135] Evaluation of PCA3 in urine samples, obtained following an "attentive" prostate massage, using transcription-mediated amplification technology, has shown to be superior to serum PSA in prediction biopsy outcome with sensitivity and specificity approximating 70% and 80%, respectively, and a negative predictive value of 90%[136–139]; it is currently approved by the Food and Drug Administration and offered by commercial laboratories in the United States.

Multiplex urine assays, including PCA3, TMPRSS2-ERG, SPINK1, and GOLPH2, are also under evaluation with recent data suggesting an improved performance of such assays compared with PCA3 alone.[140] PCA3 may also have a role in predicting the risk for higher Gleason score and larger tumor volume on radical retropubic prostatectomy. If confirmed, the latter could be of great value in defining candidates for active surveillance.[141–144] As part of the multi-institutional Canary Prostate Active Surveillance Study (PASS), PCA3 and TMPRSS2-ERG fusion were analyzed in urine samples prospectively collected at study entry. Both PCA3 and TMPRSS2-ERG scores were significantly associated with higher volume disease and presence of high-grade disease.[145] Encouraging data from the REDUCE trial support a role for PCA3 in postattentive prostate massage urine sample to predict the incidence of PCA in needle biopsies obtained following an initial negative biopsy.

In a different approach to early detection, assays that can be applied to negative biopsy tissue samples that may help predict the presence of non-sampled "occult" PCA is also gaining interest. Such approach will help alleviate the morbidity associated with repeat biopsies. ConfirmMDx is an epigenetic assay developed by MDxHealth (Irvine, CA) that assesses the methylation status of 3 genes, GSTP1, APC, and RASSF1, with a multiplexed methylation-specific PCR technique. A positive methylation result for any of the tested markers in any of the negative cores signify a positive test that will imply a higher risk of harboring "occult" PCA. Recently, the results of an international multi-institutional study involving 498 patients with initial negative prostate biopsies, followed by positive (cases) or negative (controls) repeat biopsy within 30 months were reported. The epigenetic assay had an impressive negative predictive value of 90% (95% confidence interval 87–93) and predicted incidence of PCA independently from clinicopathologic variables (odds ratio 3.17).[146]

Finally, several markers are being investigated as potential targets of therapy for PCA. Among heavily investigated agents are those directed toward tyrosine kinase receptors (eg, *EGFR*), angiogenesis targets (eg, *VEGF*), and *PI3K/akt/mTOR* mammalian target of rapamycin.[109,147–151]

## REFERENCES

1. DeMarzo AM, Nelson WG, Isaacs WB, et al. Pathological and molecular aspects of prostate cancer. Lancet 2003;361:955–64.
2. Nelson WG, De Marzo AM, Isaacs WB. Prostate cancer. N Engl J Med 2003;349:366–81.
3. Netto GJ. Clinical applications of recent molecular advances in urologic malignancies: no longer chasing a "mirage"? Adv Anat Pathol 2013;20:175–203.
4. Prowatke I, Devens F, Benner A, et al. Expression analysis of imbalanced genes in prostate carcinoma using tissue microarrays. Br J Cancer 2007;96:82–8.
5. Lapointe J, Li C, Higgins JP, et al. Gene expression profiling identifies clinically relevant subtypes of prostate cancer. Proc Natl Acad Sci U S A 2004;101:811–6.
6. Tomlins SA, Mehra R, Rhodes DR, et al. Integrative molecular concept modeling of prostate cancer progression. Nat Genet 2007;39:41–51.
7. Andriole GL, Crawford ED, Grubb RL 3rd, et al. Mortality results from a randomized prostate-cancer screening trial. N Engl J Med 2009;360:1310–9.
8. Andriole GL, Crawford ED, Grubb RL 3rd, et al. Prostate cancer screening in the randomized prostate, lung, colorectal, and ovarian cancer screening trial: mortality results after 13 years of follow-up. J Natl Cancer Inst 2012;104:125–32.
9. Schroder FH, Hugosson J, Roobol MJ, et al. Prostate-cancer mortality at 11 years of follow-up. N Engl J Med 2012;366:981–90.
10. Schroder FH, Hugosson J, Roobol MJ, et al. Screening and prostate-cancer mortality in a randomized European study. N Engl J Med 2009;360:1320–8.
11. Zeigler-Johnson CM, Rennert H, Mittal RD, et al. Evaluation of prostate cancer characteristics in four populations worldwide. Can J Urol 2008;15:4056–64.
12. De Marzo AM, Platz EA, Sutcliffe S, et al. Inflammation in prostate carcinogenesis. Nat Rev Cancer 2007;7:256–69.
13. Sfanos KS, Hempel HA, De Marzo AM. The role of inflammation in prostate cancer. Adv Exp Med Biol 2014;816:153–81.
14. Lee J, Demissie K, Lu SE, et al. Cancer incidence among Korean-American immigrants in the United States and native Koreans in South Korea. Cancer Control 2007;14:78–85.
15. Nelson WG, Demarzo AM, Yegnasubramanian S. The diet as a cause of human prostate cancer. Cancer Treat Res 2014;159:51–68.
16. Nelson WG, DeWeese TL, DeMarzo AM. The diet, prostate inflammation, and the development of prostate cancer. Cancer Metastasis Rev 2002;21:3–16.
17. Coffey DS. Similarities of prostate and breast cancer: evolution, diet, and estrogens. Urology 2001;57:31–8.
18. Sfanos KS, Wilson BA, De Marzo AM, et al. Acute inflammatory proteins constitute the organic matrix of prostatic corpora amylacea and calculi in men with prostate cancer. Proc Natl Acad Sci U S A 2009;106:3443–8.
19. Nakai Y, Nonomura N. Inflammation and prostate carcinogenesis. Int J Urol 2013;20:150–60.
20. Nakai Y, Nelson WG, De Marzo AM. The dietary charred meat carcinogen 2-amino-1-methyl-6-phenylimidazo[4,5-b]pyridine acts as both a tumor initiator and promoter in the rat ventral prostate. Cancer Res 2007;67:1378–84.
21. Giovannucci E, Stampfer MJ, Colditz G, et al. Relationship of diet to risk of colorectal adenoma in men. J Natl Cancer Inst 1992;84:91–8.
22. Knize MG, Salmon CP, Mehta SS, et al. Analysis of cooked muscle meats for heterocyclic aromatic amine carcinogens. Mutat Res 1997;376:129–34.
23. Wakabayashi K, Totsuka Y, Fukutome K, et al. Human exposure to mutagenic/carcinogenic heterocyclic amines and comutagenic beta-carbolines. Mutat Res 1997;376:253–9.
24. Stoker TE, Robinette CL, Cooper RL. Perinatal exposure to estrogenic compounds and the subsequent effects on the prostate of the adult rat: evaluation of inflammation in the ventral and lateral lobes. Reprod Toxicol 1999;13:463–72.
25. Seethalakshmi L, Bala RS, Malhotra RK, et al. 17 beta-estradiol induced prostatitis in the rat is an autoimmune disease. J Urol 1996;156:1838–42.
26. Sutcliffe S, Platz EA. Inflammation and prostate cancer: a focus on infections. Curr Urol Rep 2008;9:243–9.
27. Sutcliffe S, Neace C, Magnuson NS, et al. Trichomonosis, a common curable STI, and prostate carcinogenesis–a proposed molecular mechanism. PLoS Pathog 2012;8:e1002801.
28. Elkahwaji JE. The role of inflammatory mediators in the development of prostatic hyperplasia and prostate cancer. Res Rep Urol 2012;5:1–10.

29. Elkahwaji JE, Hauke RJ, Brawner CM. Chronic bacterial inflammation induces prostatic intraepithelial neoplasia in mouse prostate. Br J Cancer 2009; 101:1740–8.

30. van Leenders GJ, Gage WR, Hicks JL, et al. Intermediate cells in human prostate epithelium are enriched in proliferative inflammatory atrophy. Am J Pathol 2003;162:1529–37.

31. Parsons JK, Nelson CP, Gage WR, et al. GSTA1 expression in normal, preneoplastic, and neoplastic human prostate tissue. Prostate 2001;49:30–7.

32. Zha S, Gage WR, Sauvageot J, et al. Cyclooxygenase-2 is up-regulated in proliferative inflammatory atrophy of the prostate, but not in prostate carcinoma. Cancer Res 2001;61:8617–23.

33. Brooks JD, Weinstein M, Lin X, et al. CG island methylation changes near the GSTP1 gene in prostatic intraepithelial neoplasia. Cancer Epidemiol Biomarkers Prev 1998;7:531–6.

34. Nakayama M, Bennett CJ, Hicks JL, et al. Hypermethylation of the human glutathione S-transferase-pi gene (GSTP1) CpG island is present in a subset of proliferative inflammatory atrophy lesions but not in normal or hyperplastic epithelium of the prostate: a detailed study using laser-capture microdissection. Am J Pathol 2003;163:923–33.

35. Nelson WG, De Marzo AM, Yegnasubramanian S. Epigenetic alterations in human prostate cancers. Endocrinology 2009;150:3991–4002.

36. Carter BS, Beaty TH, Steinberg GD, et al. Mendelian inheritance of familial prostate cancer. Proc Natl Acad Sci U S A 1992;89:3367–71.

37. MacInnis RJ, Antoniou AC, Eeles RA, et al. Prostate cancer segregation analyses using 4390 families from UK and Australian population-based studies. Genet Epidemiol 2010;34:42–50.

38. Eeles R, Goh C, Castro E, et al. The genetic epidemiology of prostate cancer and its clinical implications. Nat Rev Urol 2014;11:18–31.

39. Goldgar DE, Easton DF, Cannon-Albright LA, et al. Systematic population-based assessment of cancer risk in first-degree relatives of cancer probands. J Natl Cancer Inst 1994;86:1600–8.

40. Christensen GB, Baffoe-Bonnie AB, George A, et al. Genome-wide linkage analysis of 1,233 prostate cancer pedigrees from the international consortium for prostate cancer genetics using novel sumLINK and sumLOD analyses. Prostate 2010; 70:735–44.

41. Camp NJ, Cannon-Albright LA, Farnham JM, et al. Compelling evidence for a prostate cancer gene at 22q12.3 by the International Consortium for Prostate Cancer Genetics. Hum Mol Genet 2007;16: 1271–8.

42. Camp NJ, Farnham JM, Cannon-Albright LA. Localization of a prostate cancer predisposition gene to an 880-kb region on chromosome 22q12.3 in Utah high-risk pedigrees. Cancer Res 2006;66:10205–12.

43. Tavtigian SV, Simard J, Teng DH, et al. A candidate prostate cancer susceptibility gene at chromosome 17p. Nat Genet 2001;27:172–80.

44. Schleutker J, Baffoe-Bonnie AB, Gillanders E, et al. Genome-wide scan for linkage in Finnish hereditary prostate cancer (HPC) families identifies novel susceptibility loci at 11q14 and 3p25-26. Prostate 2003;57:280–9.

45. Seppala EH, Ikonen T, Autio V, et al. Germ-line alterations in MSR1 gene and prostate cancer risk. Clin Cancer Res 2003;9:5252–6.

46. Xu J, Zheng SL, Komiya A, et al. Germline mutations and sequence variants of the macrophage scavenger receptor 1 gene are associated with prostate cancer risk. Nat Genet 2002;32:321–5.

47. Smith JR, Freije D, Carpten JD, et al. Major susceptibility locus for prostate cancer on chromosome 1 suggested by a genome-wide search. Science 1996;274:1371–4.

48. Xu J, Zheng SL, Hawkins GA, et al. Linkage and association studies of prostate cancer susceptibility: evidence for linkage at 8p22-23. Am J Hum Genet 2001;69:341–50.

49. Maier C, Vesovic Z, Bachmann N, et al. Germline mutations of the MSR1 gene in prostate cancer families from Germany. Hum Mutat 2006;27:98–102.

50. Maier C, Haeusler J, Herkommer K, et al. Mutation screening and association study of RNASEL as a prostate cancer susceptibility gene. Br J Cancer 2005;92:1159–64.

51. Meitz JC, Edwards SM, Easton DF, et al. HPC2/ELAC2 polymorphisms and prostate cancer risk: analysis by age of onset of disease. Br J Cancer 2002;87:905–8.

52. Xu J, Dimitrov L, Chang BL, et al. A combined genomewide linkage scan of 1,233 families for prostate cancer-susceptibility genes conducted by the international consortium for prostate cancer genetics. Am J Hum Genet 2005;77:219–29.

53. Lu L, Cancel-Tassin G, Valeri A, et al. Chromosomes 4 and 8 implicated in a genome wide SNP linkage scan of 762 prostate cancer families collected by the ICPCG. Prostate 2012;72:410–26.

54. Ahmadiyeh N, Pomerantz MM, Grisanzio C, et al. 8q24 prostate, breast, and colon cancer risk loci show tissue-specific long-range interaction with MYC. Proc Natl Acad Sci U S A 2010;107:9742–6.

55. Freedman ML, Haiman CA, Patterson N, et al. Admixture mapping identifies 8q24 as a prostate cancer risk locus in African-American men. Proc Natl Acad Sci U S A 2006;103:14068–73.

56. Schaid DJ, McDonnell SK, Zarfas KE, et al. Pooled genome linkage scan of aggressive prostate cancer: results from the International Consortium for Prostate Cancer Genetics. Hum Genet 2006;120:471–85.

57. Gudmundsson J, Sulem P, Gudbjartsson DF, et al. A study based on whole-genome sequencing yields a rare variant at 8q24 associated with prostate cancer. Nat Genet 2012;44:1326–9.

58. Gudmundsson J, Sulem P, Manolescu A, et al. Genome-wide association study identifies a second prostate cancer susceptibility variant at 8q24. Nat Genet 2007;39:631–7.

59. Cramer SD, Chang BL, Rao A, et al. Association between genetic polymorphisms in the prostate-specific antigen gene promoter and serum prostate-specific antigen levels. J Natl Cancer Inst 2003;95:1044–53.

60. Kote-Jarai Z, Amin Al Olama A, Leongamornlert D, et al. Identification of a novel prostate cancer susceptibility variant in the KLK3 gene transcript. Hum Genet 2011;129:687–94.

61. Kote-Jarai Z, Easton DF, Stanford JL, et al. Multiple novel prostate cancer predisposition loci confirmed by an international study: the PRACTICAL consortium. Cancer Epidemiol Biomarkers Prev 2008;17:2052–61.

62. Eeles RA, Olama AA, Benlloch S, et al. Identification of 23 new prostate cancer susceptibility loci using the iCOGS custom genotyping array. Nat Genet 2013;45:385–91 391.e1–2.

63. Castro E, Goh C, Olmos D, et al. Germline BRCA mutations are associated with higher risk of nodal involvement, distant metastasis, and poor survival outcomes in prostate cancer. J Clin Oncol 2013; 31:1748–57.

64. Ewing CM, Ray AM, Lange EM, et al. Germline mutations in HOXB13 and prostate-cancer risk. N Engl J Med 2012;366:141–9.

65. Xu J, Lange EM, Lu L, et al. HOXB13 is a susceptibility gene for prostate cancer: results from the international consortium for prostate cancer genetics (ICPCG). Hum Genet 2013;132:5–14.

66. Breast Cancer Linkage Consortium. Cancer risks in BRCA2 mutation carriers. J Natl Cancer Inst 1999; 91:1310–6.

67. Ryan S, Jenkins MA, Win AK. Risk of prostate cancer in Lynch syndrome: a systematic review and meta-analysis. Cancer Epidemiol Biomarkers Prev 2014;23:437–49.

68. Raymond VM, Mukherjee B, Wang F, et al. Elevated risk of prostate cancer among men with Lynch syndrome. J Clin Oncol 2013;31:1713–8.

69. Haraldsdottir S, Hampel H, Wei L, et al. Prostate cancer incidence in males with Lynch syndrome. Genet Med 2014;16:553–7.

70. Leongamornlert D, Mahmud N, Tymrakiewicz M, et al. Germline BRCA1 mutations increase prostate cancer risk. Br J Cancer 2012;106:1697–701.

71. Cybulski C, Huzarski T, Gorski B, et al. A novel founder CHEK2 mutation is associated with increased prostate cancer risk. Cancer Res 2004; 64:2677–9.

72. Erkko H, Xia B, Nikkila J, et al. A recurrent mutation in PALB2 in Finnish cancer families. Nature 2007; 446:316–9.

73. Kote-Jarai Z, Jugurnauth S, Mulholland S, et al. A recurrent truncating germline mutation in the BRIP1/FANCJ gene and susceptibility to prostate cancer. Br J Cancer 2009;100:426–30.

74. Cybulski C, Gorski B, Debniak T, et al. NBS1 is a prostate cancer susceptibility gene. Cancer Res 2004;64:1215–9.

75. Bastian PJ, Yegnasubramanian S, Palapattu GS, et al. Molecular biomarker in prostate cancer: the role of CpG island hypermethylation. Eur Urol 2004;46:698–708.

76. Maldonado L, Brait M, Loyo M, et al. GSTP1 promoter methylation is associated with recurrence in early stage prostate cancer. J Urol 2014;192: 1542–8.

77. Yegnasubramanian S, Kowalski J, Gonzalgo ML, et al. Hypermethylation of CpG islands in primary and metastatic human prostate cancer. Cancer Res 2004;64:1975–86.

78. Yegnasubramanian S, Haffner MC, Zhang Y, et al. DNA hypomethylation arises later in prostate cancer progression than CpG island hypermethylation and contributes to metastatic tumor heterogeneity. Cancer Res 2008;68:8954–67.

79. Amin M, Boccon-Gibod L, Egevad L, et al. Prognostic and predictive factors and reporting of prostate carcinoma in prostate needle biopsy specimens. Scand J Urol Nephrol Suppl 2005;216:20–33.

80. De Marzo AM, DeWeese TL, Platz EA, et al. Pathological and molecular mechanisms of prostate carcinogenesis: implications for diagnosis, detection, prevention, and treatment. J Cell Biochem 2004;91:459–77.

81. Srigley JR, Amin M, Boccon-Gibod L, et al. Prognostic and predictive factors in prostate cancer: historical perspectives and recent international consensus initiatives. Scand J Urol Nephrol Suppl 2005;216:8–19.

82. Bettencourt MC, Bauer JJ, Sesterhenn IA, et al. Ki-67 expression is a prognostic marker of prostate cancer recurrence after radical prostatectomy. J Urol 1996;156:1064–8.

83. Cheng L, Pisansky TM, Sebo TJ, et al. Cell proliferation in prostate cancer patients with lymph node metastasis: a marker for progression. Clin Cancer Res 1999;5:2820–3.

84. Stapleton AM, Zbell P, Kattan MW, et al. Assessment of the biologic markers p53, ki-67, and apoptotic index as predictive indicators of prostate carcinoma recurrence after surgery. Cancer 1998; 82:168–75.

85. Vis AN, van Rhijn BW, Noordzij MA, et al. Value of tissue markers p27(kip1), MIB-1, and CD44s for the pre-operative prediction of tumour features in

screen-detected prostate cancer. J Pathol 2002;197: 148–54.

86. Kremer CL, Klein RR, Mendelson J, et al. Expression of mTOR signaling pathway markers in prostate cancer progression. Prostate 2006;66:1203–12.

87. Sanchez D, Rosell D, Honorato B, et al. Androgen receptor mutations are associated with Gleason score in localized prostate cancer. BJU Int 2006; 98:1320–5.

88. Tomlins SA, Rhodes DR, Perner S, et al. Recurrent fusion of TMPRSS2 and ETS transcription factor genes in prostate cancer. Science 2005;310:644–8.

89. Tomlins SA, Mehra R, Rhodes DR, et al. TMPRSS2:ETV4 gene fusions define a third molecular subtype of prostate cancer. Cancer Res 2006; 66:3396–400.

90. Toubaji A, Albadine R, Meeker AK, et al. Increased gene copy number of ERG on chromosome 21 but not TMPRSS2-ERG fusion predicts outcome in prostatic adenocarcinomas. Mod Pathol 2011; 24(11):1511–20.

91. Gopalan A, Leversha MA, Satagopan JM, et al. TMPRSS2-ERG gene fusion is not associated with outcome in patients treated by prostatectomy. Cancer Res 2009;69:1400–6.

92. Demichelis F, Fall K, Perner S, et al. TMPRSS2:ERG gene fusion associated with lethal prostate cancer in a watchful waiting cohort. Oncogene 2007;26: 4596–9.

93. Yoshimoto M, Joshua AM, Cunha IW, et al. Absence of TMPRSS2:ERG fusions and PTEN losses in prostate cancer is associated with a favorable outcome. Mod Pathol 2008;21:1451–60.

94. FitzGerald LM, Agalliu I, Johnson K, et al. Association of TMPRSS2-ERG gene fusion with clinical characteristics and outcomes: results from a population-based study of prostate cancer. BMC Cancer 2008;8:230.

95. Perner S, Mosquera JM, Demichelis F, et al. TMPRSS2-ERG fusion prostate cancer: an early molecular event associated with invasion. Am J Surg Pathol 2007;31:882–8.

96. Netto GJ. TMPRSS2-ERG fusion as a marker of prostatic lineage in small-cell carcinoma. Histopathology 2010;57:633 [author reply: 633–4].

97. Rostad K, Hellwinkel OJ, Haukaas SA, et al. TMPRSS2:ERG fusion transcripts in urine from prostate cancer patients correlate with a less favorable prognosis. APMIS 2009;117:575–82.

98. Rice KR, Chen Y, Ali A, et al. Evaluation of the ETS-related gene mRNA in urine for the detection of prostate cancer. Clin Cancer Res 2010;16: 1572–6.

99. Nguyen PN, Violette P, Chan S, et al. A panel of TMPRSS2:ERG fusion transcript markers for urine-based prostate cancer detection with high specificity and sensitivity. Eur Urol 2011;59:407–14.

100. Park K, Tomlins SA, Mudaliar KM, et al. Antibody-based detection of ERG rearrangement-positive prostate cancer. Neoplasia 2010;12:590–8.

101. Chaux A, Albadine R, Toubaji A, et al. Immunohistochemistry for ERG expression as a surrogate for TMPRSS2-ERG fusion detection in prostatic adenocarcinomas. Am J Surg Pathol 2011;35:1014–20.

102. Bismar TA, Yoshimoto M, Vollmer RT, et al. PTEN genomic deletion is an early event associated with ERG gene rearrangements in prostate cancer. BJU Int 2011;107(3):477–85.

103. Han B, Mehra R, Lonigro RJ, et al. Fluorescence in situ hybridization study shows association of PTEN deletion with ERG rearrangement during prostate cancer progression. Mod Pathol 2009;22:1083–93.

104. Sarker D, Reid AH, Yap TA, et al. Targeting the PI3K/AKT pathway for the treatment of prostate cancer. Clin Cancer Res 2009;15:4799–805.

105. Chaux A, Peskoe SB, Gonzalez-Roibon N, et al. Loss of PTEN expression is associated with increased risk of recurrence after prostatectomy for clinically localized prostate cancer. Mod Pathol 2012;25:1543–9.

106. Lotan TL, Gurel B, Sutcliffe S, et al. PTEN protein loss by immunostaining: analytic validation and prognostic indicator for a high risk surgical cohort of prostate cancer patients. Clin Cancer Res 2011; 17:6563–73.

107. Krohn A, Diedler T, Burkhardt L, et al. Genomic deletion of PTEN is associated with tumor progression and early PSA recurrence in ERG fusion-positive and fusion-negative prostate cancer. Am J Pathol 2012;181:401–12.

108. Armstrong AJ, Netto GJ, Rudek MA, et al. A pharmacodynamic study of rapamycin in men with intermediate- to high-risk localized prostate cancer. Clin Cancer Res 2010;16:3057–66.

109. Zhang Z, Hou X, Shao C, et al. Plk1 inhibition enhances the efficacy of androgen signaling blockade in castration-resistant prostate cancer. Cancer Res 2014;74:6635–47.

110. Brewster SF, Oxley JD, Trivella M, et al. Preoperative p53, bcl-2, CD44 and E-cadherin immunohistochemistry as predictors of biochemical relapse after radical prostatectomy. J Urol 1999;161: 1238–43.

111. Bauer JJ, Sesterhenn IA, Mostofi FK, et al. Elevated levels of apoptosis regulator proteins p53 and bcl-2 are independent prognostic biomarkers in surgically treated clinically localized prostate cancer. J Urol 1996;156:1511–6.

112. Theodorescu D, Broder SR, Boyd JC, et al. p53, bcl-2 and retinoblastoma proteins as long-term prognostic markers in localized carcinoma of the prostate. J Urol 1997;158:131–7.

113. Kuczyk MA, Serth J, Bokemeyer C, et al. The prognostic value of p53 for long-term and

recurrence-free survival following radical prosta-tectomy. Eur J Cancer 1998;34:679–86.

114. Markert EK, Mizuno H, Vazquez A, et al. Molecular classification of prostate cancer using curated expression signatures. Proc Natl Acad Sci U S A 2011;108:21276–81.

115. Lacombe L, Maillette A, Meyer F, et al. Expression of p21 predicts PSA failure in locally advanced prostate cancer treated by prostatectomy. Int J Cancer 2001;95:135–9.

116. Aslan G, Irer B, Tuna B, et al. Analysis of NKX3.1 expression in prostate cancer tissues and correlation with clinicopathologic features. Pathol Res Pract 2006;202:93–8.

117. Bethel CR, Faith D, Li X, et al. Decreased NKX3.1 protein expression in focal prostatic atrophy, prostatic intraepithelial neoplasia, and adenocarcinoma: association with Gleason score and chromosome 8p deletion. Cancer Res 2006;66:10683–90.

118. Gurel B, Iwata T, Koh CM, et al. Nuclear MYC protein overexpression is an early alteration in human prostate carcinogenesis. Mod Pathol 2008;21:1156–67.

119. Lapointe J, Li C, Giacomini CP, et al. Genomic profiling reveals alternative genetic pathways of prostate tumorigenesis. Cancer Res 2007;67:8504–10.

120. Taylor BS, Schultz N, Hieronymus H, et al. Integrative genomic profiling of human prostate cancer. Cancer Cell 2010;18:11–22.

121. Berger MF, Lawrence MS, Demichelis F, et al. The genomic complexity of primary human prostate cancer. Nature 2011;470:214–20.

122. Baca SC, Prandi D, Lawrence MS, et al. Punctuated evolution of prostate cancer genomes. Cell 2013;153:666–77.

123. Grasso CS, Wu YM, Robinson DR, et al. The mutational landscape of lethal castration-resistant prostate cancer. Nature 2012;487:239–43.

124. Karnes RJ, Bergstralh EJ, Davicioni E, et al. Validation of a genomic classifier that predicts metastasis following radical prostatectomy in an at risk patient population. J Urol 2013;190(6):2047–53.

125. Ross AE, Feng FY, Ghadessi M, et al. A genomic classifier predicting metastatic disease progression in men with biochemical recurrence after prostatectomy. Prostate Cancer Prostatic Dis 2014;17(1):64–9.

126. Cooperberg MR, Davicioni E, Crisan A, et al. Combined value of validated clinical and genomic risk stratification tools for predicting prostate cancer mortality in a high-risk prostatectomy cohort. Eur Urol 2015;67(2):326–33.

127. Knezevic D, Goddard AD, Natraj N, et al. Analytical validation of the oncotype DX prostate cancer assay—a clinical RT-PCR assay optimized for prostate needle biopsies. BMC Genomics 2013;14:690.

128. Klein EA, Cooperberg MR, Magi-Galluzzi C, et al. A 17-gene assay to predict prostate cancer aggressiveness in the context of Gleason grade heterogeneity, tumor multifocality, and biopsy undersampling. Eur Urol 2014;66:550–60.

129. Cuzick J, Swanson GP, Fisher G, et al. Prognostic value of an RNA expression signature derived from cell cycle proliferation genes in patients with prostate cancer: a retrospective study. Lancet Oncol 2011;12:245–55.

130. Cooperberg MR, Simko JP, Cowan JE, et al. Validation of a cell-cycle progression gene panel to improve risk stratification in a contemporary prostatectomy cohort. J Clin Oncol 2013;31:1428–34.

131. Bastian PJ, Ellinger J, Wellmann A, et al. Diagnostic and prognostic information in prostate cancer with the help of a small set of hypermethylated gene loci. Clin Cancer Res 2005;11:4097–106.

132. Bastian PJ, Nakayama M, De Marzo AM, et al. GSTP1 CpG island hypermethylation as a molecular marker of prostate cancer. Urologe A 2004;43:573–9.

133. Bastian PJ, Palapattu GS, Lin X, et al. Preoperative serum DNA GSTP1 CpG island hypermethylation and the risk of early prostate-specific antigen recurrence following radical prostatectomy. Clin Cancer Res 2005;11:4037–43.

134. Bussemakers MJ, van Bokhoven A, Verhaegh GW, et al. DD3: a new prostate-specific gene, highly overexpressed in prostate cancer. Cancer Res 1999;59:5975–9.

135. de Kok JB, Verhaegh GW, Roelofs RW, et al. DD3(PCA3), a very sensitive and specific marker to detect prostate tumors. Cancer Res 2002;62:2695–8.

136. Groskopf J, Aubin SM, Deras IL, et al. APTIMA PCA3 molecular urine test: development of a method to aid in the diagnosis of prostate cancer. Clin Chem 2006;52:1089–95.

137. Deras IL, Aubin SM, Blase A, et al. PCA3: a molecular urine assay for predicting prostate biopsy outcome. J Urol 2008;179:1587–92.

138. Haese A, de la Taille A, van Poppel H, et al. Clinical utility of the PCA3 urine assay in European men scheduled for repeat biopsy. Eur Urol 2008;54:1081–8.

139. Sokoll LJ, Ellis W, Lange P, et al. A multicenter evaluation of the PCA3 molecular urine test: preanalytical effects, analytical performance, and diagnostic accuracy. Clin Chim Acta 2008;389:1–6.

140. Laxman B, Morris DS, Yu J, et al. A first-generation multiplex biomarker analysis of urine for the early detection of prostate cancer. Cancer Res 2008;68:645–9.

141. Aubin SM, Reid J, Sarno MJ, et al. PCA3 molecular urine test for predicting repeat prostate biopsy

outcome in populations at risk: validation in the placebo arm of the dutasteride REDUCE trial. J Urol 2010;184:1947–52.

142. Nakanishi H, Groskopf J, Fritsche HA, et al. PCA3 molecular urine assay correlates with prostate cancer tumor volume: implication in selecting candidates for active surveillance. J Urol 2008; 179:1804–9 [discussion: 1809–10].

143. van Poppel H, Haese A, Graefen M, et al. The relationship between prostate cancer gene 3 (PCA3) and prostate cancer significance. BJU Int 2012; 109(3):360–6.

144. Aubin SM, Reid J, Sarno MJ, et al. Prostate cancer gene 3 score predicts prostate biopsy outcome in men receiving dutasteride for prevention of prostate cancer: results from the REDUCE trial. Urology 2011;78:380–5.

145. Lin DW, Newcomb LF, Brown EC, et al. Urinary TMPRSS2:ERG and PCA3 in an active surveillance cohort: results from a baseline analysis in the canary prostate active surveillance study. Clin Cancer Res 2013;19:2442–50.

146. Stewart GD, Van Neste L, Delvenne P, et al. Clinical utility of an epigenetic assay to detect occult prostate cancer in histopathologically negative biopsies: results of the MATLOC study. J Urol 2013;189:1110–6.

147. Wanjala J, Taylor BS, Chapinski C, et al. Identifying actionable targets through integrative analyses of GEM model and human prostate cancer genomic profiling. Mol Cancer Ther 2015;14:278–88.

148. Kulik G. Precision therapy to target apoptosis in prostate cancer. Exp Oncol 2014;36:226–30.

149. Wen X, Deng FM, Wang J. MicroRNAs as predictive biomarkers and therapeutic targets in prostate cancer. Am J Clin Exp Urol 2014;2:219–30.

150. Ojemuyiwa MA, Madan RA, Dahut WL. Tyrosine kinase inhibitors in the treatment of prostate cancer: taking the next step in clinical development. Expert Opin Emerg Drugs 2014;19:459–70.

151. Courtney KD, Manola JB, Elfiky AA, et al. A phase I study of everolimus and docetaxel in patients with castration-resistant prostate cancer. Clin Genitourin Cancer 2015;13(2):113–23.

# Active Surveillance
## Pathologic and Clinical Variables Associated with Outcome

Mark Pomerantz, MD*

## KEYWORDS

• Prostate adenocarcinoma • Active surveillance • Gleason grade • PSA

## ABSTRACT

Over the past 10 years, active surveillance has emerged as a primary management option for men diagnosed with low-risk prostate cancer. Given the morbidity associated with curative treatment, active surveillance maintains quality of life for men whose disease may never become symptomatic. In order to confidently and safely offer this approach to as many patients as possible, improved metrics are needed to fully assess risk. While pathologic and clinical variables currently help determine whether active surveillance is a reasonable approach, emerging biomarkers and imaging technologies demonstrate promise for more precise identification of ideal candidates.

## OVERVIEW

Prostate cancer is exceedingly common among men in the United States. Autopsy series suggest that more than 50% of elderly men and as many as 30% to 40% of men in their 30s and 40s are harboring the disease.[1] Nonetheless, the vast majority of American men will experience no symptoms and will not succumb to the disease. With widespread adoption of prostate-specific antigen (PSA) screening in the early 1990s, many of these clinically occult cancers were revealed, and prostate cancer incidence dramatically increased.[2] This in turn has been associated with a marked increase in the procedures used to treat prostate cancer, such as radical prostatectomy and radiation therapy, and along with them, significant morbidity. It is now widely acknowledged that these aggressive treatments are often unwarranted, as each year thousands of men are needlessly exposed to life-altering side effects to cure prostate cancers that may never be destined to cause harm.

PSA testing has been held largely responsible for overdiagnosis and overtreatment of prostate cancer over the past 20 years. As a result, in the absence of clear evidence of a mortality benefit from PSA testing, the US Preventive Services Task Force released a level D recommendation against PSA screening (http://www.uspreventive servicestaskforce.org/uspstf12/prostate/prostateart. htm). Accordingly, screening rates in the United States have declined.[3] However, the PSA screening controversy has not yet been settled. Despite waning enthusiasm for PSA testing, several lines of evidence, while not yet definitive, suggest that PSA screening saves lives.[4] There is a clear need for early detection of aggressive prostate cancer, as the disease remains the second-leading cause of cancer-related death among men in the United States.[5] An overarching goal in the detection and subsequent management of localized prostate cancer, therefore, is to identify aggressive disease early while avoiding overtreatment of indolent cancer.

Active surveillance addresses the issue of overtreatment of newly detected disease. The approach has proven successful in safely managing nonaggressive prostate cancers, allowing physicians to withhold definitive local treatment until it is clearly necessary. A decision-analysis study, carefully taking quality of life into consideration, favored this approach for the average 65-year-old diagnosed with low-grade disease, when compared with radical prostatectomy or radiation

Disclosures: None.
Department of Medical Oncology, Dana-Farber Cancer Institute, 450 Brookline Avenue, D1230, Boston, MA 02115, USA
* Corresponding author.
E-mail address: Mark_Pomerantz@dfci.harvard.edu

Surgical Pathology 8 (2015) 581–585
http://dx.doi.org/10.1016/j.path.2015.09.002

surgpath.theclinics.com

therapy.[6] Identifying ideal candidates for active surveillance is critical, and the pathologist plays a central role in this determination (see also Adeniran and Humphrey, Morphologic Updates in Prostate Pathology, Surgical Pathology Clinics, 2015, vol 8, issue 4).

Active surveillance entails close monitoring of a biopsy-proven prostate cancer, proceeding with definitive local treatment if and when the disease appears more aggressive than initially anticipated. Several series of active surveillance cohorts have been reported.[7] Although data suggest that active surveillance can successfully avoid or meaningfully forestall aggressive therapies, data are limited regarding its safety after 10 to 15 years of follow-up. This is an important limitation in our current understanding of the approach, given the long natural history of the disease and the long life expectancy of many newly diagnosed patients.

## ACTIVE SURVEILLANCE OUTCOMES

Among the most extensively annotated cohorts is from the University of Toronto. In that cohort, 993 patients with Gleason score of 6 or lower and PSA of 10 ng/mL or lower (as well as patients with PSA 10–20 ng/mL and/or Gleason score 3 + 4 with a life expectancy of <10 years) have been followed with serial PSAs (every 3 months for 2 years, then every 6 months if stable), digital rectal examinations, and prostate biopsies (performed according to Vienna nomogram[8] within 1 year then every 3–4 years thereafter).[9] Patients have been referred for treatment due to any of the following factors: significant change in PSA kinetics (through 2008, PSA doubling time <3 years was an automatic trigger for treatment, although this is no longer an automatic trigger), histologic upgrade on repeat prostate biopsy, or development of a palpable prostate proven to represent progression.[9]

After median follow-up of 6.4 years from time of initial biopsy, including greater than 10 years of follow-up for 206 individuals, prostate cancer–specific deaths were rare. Among 993 patients, a total of 28 (2.8%) developed metastatic prostate cancer, and there were 15 (1.5%) prostate cancer–specific deaths. Of note, among the 28 who developed metastases, 12 were in the subset of 132 patients with Gleason 7 disease at diagnosis.[9] At 10 years' follow-up, approximately 38% of patients underwent definitive local treatment, most commonly due to a shortening PSA doubling time.[9]

Other series have reported active surveillance or watchful waiting outcomes, but information from these studies are generally limited because of relatively short follow-up time, inclusion of patients with higher-risk disease, or low proportion of patients undergoing definitive local treatment despite evidence of progression. A study from Sweden, for example, in which 223 men with localized disease underwent watchful waiting, showed a marked increase in mortality in the subset of patients reaching 15 years' follow-up.[10] However, only 70 of the 223 patients were considered low risk at the time of diagnosis and patients were not followed closely with intention of timely referral for curative treatment as in the Canadian cohort. In this series, patients were started on androgen deprivation therapy at the time of symptomatic progression.

## PATHOLOGIC AND CLINICAL VARIABLES ASSOCIATED WITH OUTCOME

As active surveillance is increasingly adopted by urologists and medical oncologists as an attractive approach for localized disease, appropriate patient selection is critically important. This entails thorough and accurate characterization of a patient's disease at the time of diagnosis (see also Adeniran and Humphrey, Morphologic Updates in Prostate Pathology, Surgical Pathology Clinics, 2015, vol 8, issue 4). It is clear that Gleason 3 + 3 prostate cancer has extraordinarily little metastatic potential.[11] In retrospective series of 14,123 Gleason 3 + 3 radical prostatectomy cases in which lymph nodes were sampled, only 22 cases (0.1%) had lymph node involvement. Histopathologic analysis of the 19 cases available for review demonstrated higher grade than originally reported.[12] However, these series were able to clearly establish low-grade disease based on examination of the entire prostate gland. Biopsy is only a sampling and a diagnosis of Gleason 3 + 3 disease at biopsy does not guarantee indolent disease.

One approach to help ensure the safety of active surveillance is to use conservative criteria for initiating this approach. In a series at Johns Hopkins, 769 men with very low risk cancers, defined by clinical stage T1c, PSA density less than 0.15 ng/mL, biopsy Gleason score 6 or lower, 2 or fewer positive biopsy cores, and 50% or less cancer involvement of any core, were followed for a median 2.7 years (range, 0.01–15.0). No prostate cancer–specific deaths have been reported.[13] However, the data from the University of Toronto, in which 13% had Gleason 7 disease on screening biopsy and many more had greater than 2 cores positive, strongly suggest that many men not meeting these stringent criteria may safely pursue and benefit from active surveillance (Box 1).[9]

**Box 1**
**Commonly used active surveillance criteria**

- Clinical stage T1c

- Prostate-specific antigen (PSA) density <0.15 ng/mL

- Gleason score ≤6

- ≤2 positive core biopsies

- ≤50% cancer involvement of any core

*Adapted from* Tosoian JJ, Trock BJ, Landis P, et al. Active surveillance program for prostate cancer: an update of the Johns Hopkins experience. J Clin Oncol 2011;29:2185–90.

Several variables available at the time of biopsy and initial diagnosis have been assessed for their ability to predict disease aggressiveness. In the University of Toronto series, 862 active surveillance patients were analyzed to determine which clinical variables could predict upgrading from low-grade or low-intermediate–grade disease at diagnosis to higher grade disease on repeat prostate biopsy.[14] Upgrading appears to be a clinically meaningful event, as high-grade disease triggers definitive treatment, and is associated with higher risk of advanced disease. In this series, 10-year treatment-free survival rate was 78.6% in those not upgraded versus 29.5% for those that were upgraded (hazard ratio 0.16, *P* <.01). Overall, 185 cases (31.3%) were upgraded at repeat biopsy. These results are consistent with rates of upgrading in several series comparing initial biopsy scores with subsequent radical prostatectomy scores among patients seeking local treatment.[15–17] In the active surveillance population, 15% of upgraded cases (n = 27) were upgraded to Gleason 8 or higher.[14]

Certain clinical factors were associated with risk of upgrading. These included T2 disease at diagnosis compared with T1 (odds ratio [OR] 2.4) and PSA velocity greater than 2 ng/mL per year (OR 3.3). Other variables that trended with increased risk were age, PSA level, number of biopsy cores positive, and percentage of involved core.[14] These risk variables are also consistent with larger series in which biopsy specimens were compared with subsequent radical prostatectomy specimens.[18] It is estimated that the likelihood of upgrading increases approximately 1% each year from the time of diagnosis, arguing for regular surveillance but providing reassurance that Gleason grade remains stable over several years of follow-up in most cases.

Other baseline characteristics, such as age and race, also have been examined. Active surveillance series suggest that patients younger than 60 years old are good candidates for active surveillance.[9] This reflects the fact that autopsy series demonstrate occult disease in a sizable percentage of men in their 40s and 50s. Low-risk disease discovered by biopsy in this population does not necessarily behave aggressively. West African ancestry, on the other hand, may be a factor that influences decisions regarding active surveillance. In a series of 256 African American and 1473 European American men with low-risk subjects at diagnosis, African Americans were significantly more likely to be upgraded on radical prostatectomy and exhibit positive surgical margins.[19]

Although it is not yet established how best to incorporate these clinical variables into practice, they can be used collectively to help guide decisions with patients. Nomograms have been developed,[14] and these should prove more valuable as data from active surveillance series mature.

## NOVEL BIOMARKERS AND IMAGING TECHNIQUES PREDICTING AGGRESSIVENESS OF LOW-RISK PROSTATE CANCER

New biomarkers have been developed to try to more accurately predict which newly diagnosed prostate cancers are likely to behave aggressively. The Oncotype DX Prostate Cancer Assay (Genomic Health, Redwood City, CA, USA) uses reverse-transcriptase polymerase chain reaction to measure expression in a set of 12 genes shown to correlate with prostate cancer aggressiveness.[20] Expression is measured using RNA derived from biopsy specimens, allowing, at the time of diagnosis, calculation of a Genomic Prostate Score used to predict outcome. The Polaris assay (Myriad Genetics, Salt Lake City, UT, USA) also uses RNA from paraffin-embedded biopsy tissue cores to measure expression of 31 cell cycle–related genes to calculate a cycle progression score that was showed to improve the prognostic information regarding aggressiveness provided by Gleason score and PSA.[21] High scores with either of these assays may dissuade researchers from recommending active surveillance. However, they have not yet been thoroughly tested prospectively to determine whether they predict long-term active surveillance outcomes. Additionally, it is not yet known how often false-positive or false-negative results are delivered to good active surveillance candidates.

Although the standard 12-core prostate biopsy allows in-depth pathologic assessment of the prostate tissue for tumor, it necessarily provides only a sampling of the gland. The possibility of not sampling the full extent of a patient's cancer is always a concern, given the multifocal nature of prostate cancer. In particular, the anterior and apical portions of the gland are often undersampled. Great strides have been made in prostate imaging, and the prostate MRI is increasingly used to measure the full extent and aggressiveness of newly diagnosed prostate cancer. The role for MRI in the initial workup of low-risk patients is not fully established, but recent data suggest a meaningful role.

Most major academic centers currently recommend using a multiparametric imaging and 3.0-T magnets, although clinically informative data have been generated using 1.5 T. Several centers also use an endorectal coil to optimize imaging, although it is not clear whether this procedure is necessary in the era of the 3.0-T magnet. A standardized scoring system, Prostate Imaging Reporting and Data System (PI-RADS), has been devised to characterize prostate lesions. Focal lesions are scored 1 to 5 based on predicted aggressiveness (http://www.acr.org/Quality-Safety/Resources/PIRADS/).

In one study of 388 low-risk patients undergoing MRI, 20% of patients were upgraded on repeat biopsy.[22] An independent radiologist assessed all patient MRIs and scored them on a scale of 1 to 5 based on the predicted presence of tumor. MRI scores correlated with disease aggressiveness, and a score of 5 was highly sensitive for predicting that a tumor would be upgraded. Low scores (1–2) had a negative predictive value of 0.96 to 1.0 for predicting an upgraded tumor. This suggests a potential usefulness for the test, as benign-appearing MRIs may provide reassurance that active surveillance is a preferred management option. Nevertheless, data are needed to validate and expand on these results. Also, experience reading prostate MRIs is currently limited to high-volume centers and it is not yet clear how generalizable data will be across operators of varying experience (**Box 2**).

## SUMMARY

Over the past 10 years, active surveillance has emerged as a primary management option for men diagnosed with low-risk prostate cancer. Given the morbidity associated with curative treatment, active surveillance maintains quality of life for men whose disease may never become symptomatic. Active surveillance also allays concern that prostate cancer screening inevitably leads to large-scale overtreatment.

The National Comprehensive Cancer Network recommends active surveillance as an option for all men with stage T1c, Gleason 3 + 3 disease with fewer than 3 positive biopsy cores and 50% or less cancer in each core and a PSA density less than 0.15 ng/mL/g. It is the preferred option for men with life expectancy of less than 20 years. For men with slightly more aggressive features, active surveillance remains a possibility, but improved metrics are needed to fully assess risk. Pathologic and clinical variables, such as T stage, number of positive cores, and PSA kinetics, as well as ethnicity, may help determine whether active surveillance is a reasonable approach. Emerging biomarkers and imaging technologies demonstrate promise in identifying ideal candidates for this approach.

**Box 2**
**Clinicopathologic factors that affect management of prostate cancer**

- PSA kinetics
- Gleason score
- Number of transrectal ultrasound (TRUS) prostate cores involved by carcinoma
- Volume of TRUS prostate cores involved by carcinoma
- Biomarkers
- Imaging
- Life expectancy (number of years)

## REFERENCES

1. Sakr WA, Grignon DJ, Crissman JD, et al. High grade prostatic intraepithelial neoplasia (HGPIN) and prostatic adenocarcinoma between the ages of 20-69: an autopsy study of 249 cases. In Vivo 1994;8:439–43.
2. Jemal A, Siegel R, Ward E, et al. Cancer statistics, 2009. CA Cancer J Clin 2009;59:225–49.
3. Drazer MW, Huo D, Eggener SE. National prostate cancer screening rates after the 2012 US Preventive Services Task Force recommendation discouraging prostate-specific antigen-based screening. J Clin Oncol 2015;33:2416–23.
4. Cooperberg MR. Implications of the new AUA guidelines on prostate cancer detection in the U.S. Curr Urol Rep 2014;15:420.
5. Siegel RL, Miller KD, Jemal A. Cancer statistics, 2015. CA Cancer J Clin 2015;65:5–29.
6. Hayes JH, Ollendorf DA, Pearson SD, et al. Active surveillance compared with initial treatment for men with low-risk prostate cancer: a decision analysis. JAMA 2010;304:2373–80.
7. Klotz L. Active surveillance for low-risk prostate cancer. Curr Urol Rep 2015;16:24.

8. Remzi M, Fong YK, Dobrovits M, et al. The Vienna nomogram: validation of a novel biopsy strategy defining the optimal number of cores based on patient age and total prostate volume. J Urol 2005; 174:1256–60 [discussion: 1260–1; author reply: 1261].

9. Klotz L, Vesprini D, Sethukavalan P, et al. Long-term follow-up of a large active surveillance cohort of patients with prostate cancer. J Clin Oncol 2015; 33:272–7.

10. Popiolek M, Rider JR, Andrén O, et al. Natural history of early, localized prostate cancer: a final report from three decades of follow-up. Eur Urol 2013;63:428–35.

11. Eggener SE, Badani K, Barocas DA, et al. Gleason 6 prostate cancer: translating biology into population health. J Urol 2015;194:626–34.

12. Ross HM, Kryvenko ON, Cowan JE, et al. Do adenocarcinomas of the prostate with Gleason score (GS) </=6 have the potential to metastasize to lymph nodes? Am J Surg Pathol 2012;36: 1346–52.

13. Tosoian JJ, Trock BJ, Landis P, et al. Active surveillance program for prostate cancer: an update of the Johns Hopkins experience. J Clin Oncol 2011; 29:2185–90.

14. Jain S, Loblaw A, Vesprini D, et al. Gleason upgrading with time in a large prostate cancer active surveillance cohort. J Urol 2015;194:79–84.

15. Pinthus JH, Witkos M, Fleshner NE, et al. Prostate cancers scored as Gleason 6 on prostate biopsy are frequently Gleason 7 tumors at radical prostatectomy: implication on outcome. J Urol 2006;176: 979–84 [discussion: 984].

16. Boorjian SA, Karnes RJ, Crispen PL, et al. The impact of discordance between biopsy and pathological Gleason scores on survival after radical prostatectomy. J Urol 2009;181:95–104 [discussion: 104].

17. Mehta V, Rycyna K, Baesens BM, et al. Predictors of Gleason Score (GS) upgrading on subsequent prostatectomy: a single institution study in a cohort of patients with GS 6. Int J Clin Exp Pathol 2012;5: 496–502.

18. Epstein JI, Feng Z, Trock BJ, et al. Upgrading and downgrading of prostate cancer from biopsy to radical prostatectomy: incidence and predictive factors using the modified Gleason grading system and factoring in tertiary grades. Eur Urol 2012;61: 1019–24.

19. Sundi D, Ross AE, Humphreys EB, et al. African American men with very low-risk prostate cancer exhibit adverse oncologic outcomes after radical prostatectomy: should active surveillance still be an option for them? J Clin Oncol 2013;31:2991–7.

20. Knezevic D, Goddard AD, Natraj N, et al. Analytical validation of the Oncotype DX prostate cancer assay—a clinical RT-PCR assay optimized for prostate needle biopsies. BMC Genomics 2013; 14:690.

21. Cuzick J, Berney DM, Fisher G, et al. Prognostic value of a cell cycle progression signature for prostate cancer death in a conservatively managed needle biopsy cohort. Br J Cancer 2012;106:1095–9.

22. Vargas HA, Akin O, Afaq A, et al. Magnetic resonance imaging for predicting prostate biopsy findings in patients considered for active surveillance of clinically low risk prostate cancer. J Urol 2012; 188:1732–8.

# Adult Renal Cell Carcinoma

## A Review of Established Entities from Morphology to Molecular Genetics

 CrossMark

Michelle S. Hirsch, MD, PhD*, Sabina Signoretti, MD,
Paola Dal Cin, PhD

**KEYWORDS**

- Renal cell carcinoma • Clear cell • Papillary • Chromophobe
- Mucinous tubular and spindle cell carcinoma • Translocation • Xp11.2 • Collecting duct

## ABSTRACT

According to the current World Health Organization (WHO), renal cell carcinomas (RCCs) that primarily affect adults are classified into 8 major subtypes. Additional emerging entities in renal neoplasia have also been recently recognized and these are discussed in further detail by Mehra et al (Emerging Entities in Renal Neoplasia, Surgical Pathology Clinics, 2015, Volume 8, Issue 4). In most cases, the diagnosis of a RCC subtype can be based on morphologic criteria, but in some circumstances the use of ancillary studies can aid in the diagnosis. This review discusses the morphologic, genetic, and molecular findings in RCCs previously recognized by the WHO, and provides clues to distinction from each other and some of the newer subtypes of RCC. As prognosis and therapeutic options vary for the different subtypes of RCC, accurate pathologic distinction is critical for patient care.

## OVERVIEW

Primary cancers of the kidney are a heterogeneous group of neoplasms that account for approximately 4% of newly diagnosed malignancies in men and women annually.[1] In the United States, this translates into approximately 65,000 new cases annually, approximately one-fifth (23%) of which will result in death from disease (~2.6% of all cancer deaths).[1] Renal epithelial neoplasms account for most renal tumors (80%–85%), and in 2004, the World Health Organization (WHO) recognized the following 8 adult renal epithelial malignancies: clear cell (conventional) renal cell carcinoma (CCRCC), multilocular CCRCC, papillary RCC (PRCC), chromophobe RCC (ChRCC), Xp11.2 translocation RCC, mucinous tubular and spindle cell carcinoma (MTSCC), collecting duct carcinoma, and unclassified RCC.[2] Overall, renal epithelial tumors occur more frequently in men than women, but some of the newer subtypes affect women more frequently than men. Renal epithelial neoplasms can be associated with a lack of early warning signs (based on their protected location in the retroperitoneum) and diverse clinical signs, and are frequently found incidentally with imaging studies for other clinical reasons. Accordingly, the average age of a patient with a renal epithelial neoplasm is now likely younger than originally thought (classically RCCs are thought to occur most frequently in the seventh to eighth decades). Although the overall 5-year survival for all renal malignancies has shown a trend toward improvement over the past 3 decades,[1] the actual prognosis based on RCC subtype can vary significantly with CCRCC, collecting duct carcinoma, unclassified RCC, and those with sarcomatoid differentiation having the worst survival rates.[3–7] For this reason, accurate subtyping of renal epithelial neoplasms is paramount to defining the most appropriate treatment options and predicting prognosis[8] (see also

Disclosures: The authors have no conflicts of interest or funding to disclose.
Department of Pathology, Brigham and Women's Hospital, Harvard Medical School, 75 Francis Street, Boston, MA 02115, USA
* Corresponding author. Department of Pathology, Brigham and Women's Hospital, 75 Francis Street, Amory-3, Boston, MA 02115.
E-mail address: mhirsch1@partners.org

Surgical Pathology 8 (2015) 587–621
http://dx.doi.org/10.1016/j.path.2015.09.003

Albiges et al., Diagnosis of Renal Cell Carcinoma: A Clinician's Perspective, Surgical Pathology Clinics, 2015, Volume 8, Issue 4).

## CLEAR CELL (CONVENTIONAL) RENAL CELL CARCINOMA

### CLINICAL PRESENTATION, GROSS FEATURES, AND PROGNOSIS

CCRCC is the most common variant of RCC, accounting for more than 70% of kidney malignancies. It can present as a small solitary lesion confined to the kidney or can grow quite large beyond the confines of the renal capsule (**Fig. 1**). Tumors can also be multifocal or bilateral; however, this is a less common occurrence. CCRCC has the highest propensity for renal vein involvement and can present with metastatic disease. Grossly, the tumors are often well circumscribed and may be surrounded by a thin fibrous pseudocapsule. The cut surface of CCRCC is typically golden yellow to tan (see **Fig. 1**); the former of which is due to lipid and glycogen within the cells. It is important to sample fleshy white appearing areas of a CCRCC as this may represent

sarcomatoid differentiation, which is associated with a worse prognosis.[3,5,9] As CCRCC is derived from cortically based tubules (thought to be the proximal convoluted tubules), the renal cortex is often the epicenter of the tumor, and growth typically occurs with a "pushing" front, displacing non-neoplastic renal parenchymal elements (nephrons) to the periphery (**Fig. 2**). However, high-grade tumors may demonstrate small satellite nodules or infiltrate between renal tubular structures beyond the confines of the main mass.[10] Areas of cystic change and hemorrhage within CCRCCs are frequently present. Necrosis has been shown to be associated with a worse prognosis,[11,12] and the presence should be mentioned in the final pathology report. Approximately half of CCRCCs are confined to the kidney at the time of surgery (pT1-pT2); nevertheless, approximately 30% of CCRCCs will recur or metastasize and this is not restricted to high-grade, high-stage disease. Although patients with von Hippel Lindau (VHL) disease may develop CCRCC, most CCRCCs are associated with a sporadic mutation on the short arm of chromosome 3 (3p), including the site of the *VHL* gene[13] (see below for more details).

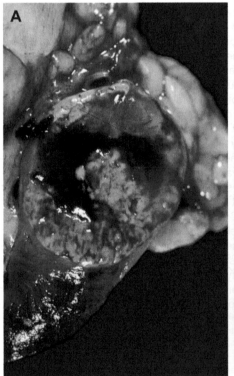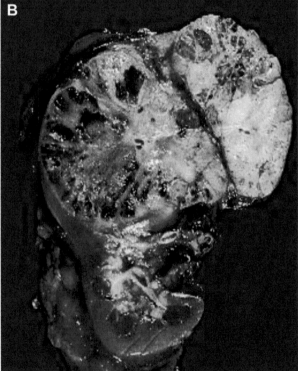

*Fig. 1.* Clear cell renal cell carcinoma. The gross appearance of a CCRCC is characteristically golden yellow, and it may be associated with variable amounts of hemorrhage and necrosis. Tumors arise from cortical tubules and can be (*A*) confined to the renal parenchyma or (*B*) extend beyond the capsule into perinephric soft tissue.

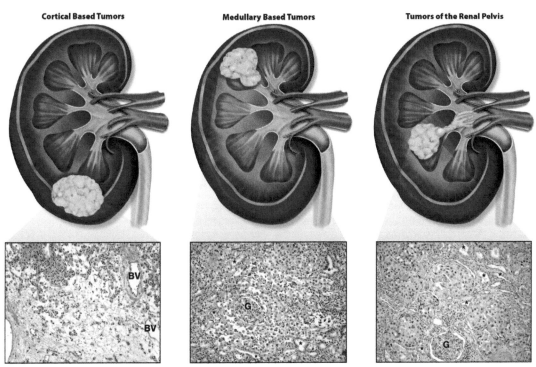

*Fig. 2.* This schematic diagram illustrates the growth pattern of cortical based tumors, medullary based tumors, and tumors of the renal pelvis. Cortical based tumors (*left*) are derived from proximal and distal convoluted tubules, and typically have an expansile growth pattern that pushes non-neoplastic nephrons to the periphery of the tumor. Note in the H&E example the absence of non-neoplastic tubular structures; however, stromal edema and blood vessels (BV) are present. In medullary based tumors (*middle*), the neoplasm arises from the distal nephron, predominantly the collecting tubules/ducts. A 'primary' tumor mass may be seen in the medulla or at the corticomedullary junction (also see **Fig. 20**); this may be obscured if the tumor grows very large. Neoplastic cells of medullary based tumors typically invade the renal cortex, and infiltrate between normal structures as seen in the H&E image (G, glomerulus; *, benign tubules); this invasive pattern can be a clue that a tumor originated in the renal medulla when the primary lesion is not evident. Renal pelvis tumors (*right*) originate from the overlying urothelium, and invasive tumors will demonstrate 2 common growth patterns: invasion through soft tissues and renal parenchyma, and retrograde growth up the collecting tubules. In the H&E image you can see both patterns, expanded round tubules filled with tumor (*middle of the image*) and invasion of renal parenchyma (*upper left*). Like medullary based tumors, invasive urothelial carcinomas will infiltrate between normal renal structures (G, glomerulus; *, benign tubules).

## MICROSCOPIC EXAMINATION

CCRCC can display a variety of growth patterns, including solid, alveolar, tubular, cystic, pseudo-papillary, and papillary architectures. Characteristically the cells have varying amounts of "clear" cytoplasm, as the glycogen and lipid in the cytoplasm is not visible with routine hematoxylin-eosin (H&E) stain (**Fig. 3**). However, some cells can have a more granular to eosinophilic appearance, and this may be seen focally as a component of a more conventional clear cell tumor, diffusely in tumors that were previously designated as "granular RCC" (a term that is no longer used), or in areas of higher nuclear grade (see **Fig. 3**). A delicate branching vascular network that surrounds clusters of tumor cells (the so-called "alveolar" vascular pattern) is quite characteristic and can be an important clue to making the correct diagnosis (see **Fig. 3**). Occasionally true fibrovascular cores are present within a CCRCC, but more frequently viable oxygenated cells are found clinging to the vessels when necrosis and/or poor preservation is present, resulting in a pseudopapillary architecture (see **Fig.** 3D).

Although some have proposed using a nucleolar grading system[14] plus or minus the presence of necrosis,[8] the International Society of Urologic Pathologists (ISUP) recommends using the Fuhrman nuclear grade (FNG) system for CCRCC, which is based on nuclear and nucleolar size.[15] FNG 1 through 4 nuclei are approximately 10, 15, 20 and larger than 20 μm in diameter, respectively,

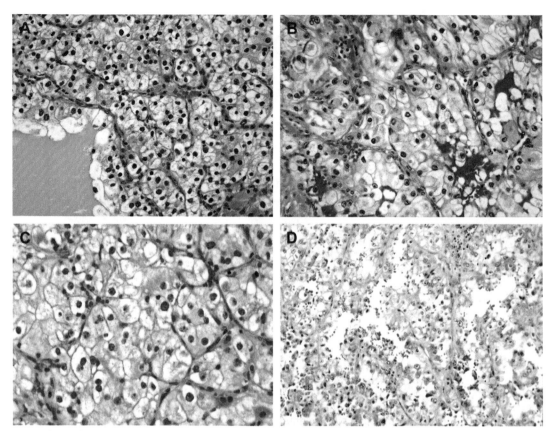

**Fig. 3.** Clear cell renal cell carcinoma. (*A*) Tumors frequently demonstrate a solid to nested growth pattern; however, intratumoral cystic change may also be present. Note the clear cytoplasm and small nuclei without obvious nucleoli, consistent with a Fuhrman nuclear grade 2 tumor. (*B*) A fine delicate, wrapping vascular pattern ('alveolar') is characteristically seen in clear cell renal cell carcinoma. (*C*) Some clear cell renal cell carcinomas have a more granular/eosinophilic appearance, and this is common in higher grade tumors (Fuhrman nuclear grade 3 shown). (*D*) Pseudopapillary architecture can be seen in high grade tumors.

and prominent nucleoli can be visualized at low power (×100) starting with FNG 3. Reproducible grading is possible when using a red blood cell, which is 7 μm in diameter, as a reference (ie, FNG 1–4 nuclei are ~1, 2, 3, and ≥4 times the diameter of a red blood cell, respectively). Tumors should be graded based on the highest grade present, and tumors with sarcomatoid and/or rhabdoid differentiation, both of which are associated with a poor prognosis, are always considered FNG 4.[15–18]

## GENETIC ALTERNATIONS

Loss of the short arm (p) of chromosome of 3 is the characteristic abnormality in CCRCC, and is rarely seen in other subtypes of RCC (**Fig. 4**). A variety of mechanisms have been described from simple, interstitial, or terminal deletions: unbalanced translocations with a der(3)t(3;5)(p11-p22;q13-q31) being the most frequent; and loss of 3pter-3q12 or 3pter-3q21 with a concurrent

translocation of the remaining 3q segment to other chromosomes.[19] There is no specific association between 3p loss and tumor size, nodal involvement, tumor grade, or metastasis; however, tumors with gains of 5q31-qter, most often through the der(3)t(3;5), have been reported to have a more favorable prognosis.[20]

The identification of a single critical region on 3p has proven difficult, as several 3p regions may be frequently lost or inactive. For example, 3p12 to 14, 3p21, and 3p25 are affiliated with several tumor suppressor genes or oncogenes, which are implicated in the etiology of sporadic CCRCC. Cytogenetically, several other nonrandom chromosomal abnormalities can also occur, including loss of chromosomes 8, 9, 13, and 14, gains of chromosomes 12 and 20, and structural aberrations affecting 5q, 6q, 8p, 9p, 10q, and 14q. Some studies have shown that specific chromosomal change (in chromosomes other than chromosome 3) may be related to tumor progression. For example, monosomy 9/9p has been associated with the presence of lymph

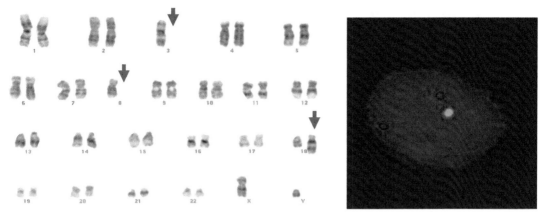

*Fig. 4.* Giemsa (G) banding of a renal cell carcinoma (*left*) yields a 44,XY,-3,-8,der(18)t(3;18)(q11;q11) karyotype, which includes the characteristic loss of the short arm of chromosome 3 (3p) seen in clear cell renal cell carcinoma. Fluorescence in situ hybridization (FISH) can be performed on formalin fixed paraffin embedded (FFPE) tissue to evaluate for a loss of 3p (*right*); in this example two copies of the long arm of chromosome 3 (3q) are present (two red fluorescent dots), whereas one copy of 3p is lost (only one green fluorescent dot is present).

node and distant metastasis, and therefore is considered a "biomarker" for aggressive CCRCC, especially in a patient who presents initially with localized disease.[21–23]

## MOLECULAR PATHWAYS

Important insights into the biology of CCRCC have been gained from studies of VHL disease. VHL disease is a rare, autosomal dominant, hereditary syndrome characterized by multiple tumors in several organs, including the kidney.[24] It is caused by a germline mutation in the *VHL* gene, located at 3p25.[25] Consistent with the Knudson 2-hit model, VHL disease-associated tumors, including CCRCC, arise from inactivation of the remaining normal (wild-type) *VHL* allele.[26,27] Importantly, it has also been demonstrated that *VHL* is bialleli-cally inactivated in most sporadic CCRCCs. Indeed, chromosome 3p loss encompassing the *VHL* locus is observed in more than 90% of sporadic CCRCC cases, and 60% to 80% of these cases also have mutation or promoter methylation of the second *VHL* allele.[28,29]

The VHL protein (pVHL) is part of an ubiquitin ligase complex that, in the presence of oxygen, targets the alpha subunit of the hypoxia-induced factor (HIF) for degradation via the proteasome. Loss of pVHL function leads to stabilization of HIF in normoxic conditions and promotes tumoro-genesis.[26,29] Although 3 HIF alpha subunits have been identified in humans (HIF-1a, HIF-2a, and HIF-3a), there is increasing evidence that HIF-2a is the major player in the pathogenesis of CCRCC.[30] HIF overexpression leads to the transcription of many genes involved in several pro-oncogenic pathways whose functions include cell survival, cell proliferation, and angiogenesis.[31,32]

Vascular endothelial growth factor (VEGF) is a HIF target that plays a critical role in vasculogenesis and angiogenesis. In recent years, antiangio-genic targeted therapies that inhibit VEGF function by either binding to the VEGF molecule (bevacizumab) or it receptors (sunitinib, sorafenib, and pazopanib) have shown to produce tumor shrinkage in most patients with kidney cancer and significantly prolong median progression-free survival[33–35] (see also Albiges et al., Diagnosis of Renal Cell Carcinoma: A Clinician's Perspective, Surgical Pathology Clinics, 2015, Volume 8, Issue 4). For these reasons, VEGF-targeted therapies were approved by the US Food and Drug Administration for the treatment of advanced RCC. It can be hypothesized that VEGF-targeted therapies are effective as single agents in advanced RCC because many tumors are highly dependent on VEGF-mediated angiogenesis due to constitutively high HIF levels secondary to *VHL* inactivation.[33] If this is true, patients whose tumors are characterized by dys-regulation of the VHL-HIF pathway should be most likely to respond to these therapies. A study from Choueiri and colleagues[36] found a positive association between the presence of *VHL* mutation in patients' tumors and responses to sorafenib. Similarly, it has been suggested that the hypoxia-inducible protein Carbonic Anhydrase IX (CAIX) might be a predictive biomarker for response to sorafenib treatment.[37] Larger studies in prospective clinical trial cohorts are needed to establish whether markers of activation of the VHL-HIF pathway can be successfully used to select patients for VEGF-directed therapy.

A recent effort directed at sequencing the protein coding exome in a series of primary CCRCCs has led to the identification of polybromo 1 (*PBRM1*) as a second major cancer gene in CCRCC.[38] *PBRM1* is located at 3p21 and encodes the BAF180 protein, which is the chromatin-targeting subunit of the PBAF SWI/SNF chromatin remodeling complex.[39] Varela and colleagues documented the presence of truncating *PBRM1* mutations in 92 of 227 (41%) CCRCC cases.[38] In all cases with available DNA copy-number data, *PBRM1* mutations were observed in association with 3p loss. Additionally, silencing of *PBRM1* expression in CCRCC cell lines produced a significant increase in cell proliferation as well as in an increase in colony formation in soft agar and in cell migration. These results seem to support the concept that *PBRM1* functions as a tumor suppressor gene in the kidney, and that genetic inactivation plays an important role in the pathogenesis and/or progression of CCRCC.

More recently, additional genomic studies of CCRCC have identified recurrent inactivating mutations in other genes involving chromatin-remodeling or histone modification, including BRCA1-associated protein-1 (*BAP1*),[40,41] SET domain-containing protein-2 (*SETD2*),[40,42] and *JARID1C/KDM5C/SMCX*.[40,42] Sequencing analyses have also demonstrated that a subset of CCRCCs harbor somatic mutations in *TSC1*, *MTOR*, and other genes in the mammalian target of rapamycin (mTOR) pathway (e.g. *PTEN*, *PIK3CA*, *RHEB*, *AKT1*) that lead to activation of mTOR signaling.[38,40,43,44] Accordingly, mTOR inhibitors such as everolimus and temsirolimus, are approved by the US Food and Drug Administration for the treatment of metastatic RCC (see also Albiges, et al. Diagnosis of Renal Cell Carcinoma: A Clinician's Perspective, Surgical Pathology Clinics, 2015, Volume 8, Issue 4). A recent analysis including a limited number of RCCs suggests that *TSC1* and *MTOR* mutations leading to mTOR signaling hyperactivation might identify patients that could experience long-term response to mTOR inhibition.[45] However, further investigations in larger patient cohorts are needed to establish if mutations in mTOR pathway genes can represent clinically useful/predictive biomarkers for mTOR-targeted therapy in RCC.

## ANCILLARY STUDIES

Classic morphologic features make CCRCC a histologic diagnosis in most cases; however, in a subset of cases, ancillary studies may be helpful to confirm the diagnosis or exclude other tumors in

---

**Box 1**
**Differential diagnosis of "clear cell lesions" in the kidney**

- Benign/Low malignant potential:
  - Cystic nephroma
  - Multilocular cystic renal cell neoplasm of low malignant potential (previously multilocular cystic clear cell RCC)
- Malignant:
  - Clear cell renal cell carcinoma
  - Clear cell (tubulo) papillary renal cell carcinoma
  - TCEB1-mutated ('monosomy 8') renal cell carcinoma
  - Papillary renal cell carcinoma with clear cell features
  - Xp11.2 translocation renal cell carcinoma
  - Chromophobe renal cell carcinoma
- Metastatic:
  - Adrenal cortical carcinoma
  - Ovarian clear cell carcinoma
- Non-neoplastic:
  - Xanthogranulomatous pyelonephritis

---

the differential diagnosis (**Box 1**). Biomarker analyses have shown that CCRCCs are typically negative for CK7, variable for alpha-methylacyl-CoA racemase (AMACR), and positive for CD10 and RCC antigen.[46,47] CK7 can be focally positive in a subset of cases, especially when the tumor demonstrates cystic change.[16] Carbonic anhydrase (CAIX) is diffusely positive in most CCRCCs, reflecting the downstream effect of a mutation in the VHL gene.[48] However, it should be noted that CAIX expression is not restricted to CCRCC and can be expressed in other RCC subtypes (ie, CAIX is sensitive but not entirely specific).[48–51] When available, conventional cytogenetics will demonstrate a loss of 3p with or without other chromosomal aberrations (as described previously). Loss of 3p also can be demonstrated by other modalities such as florescence in situ hybridization (FISH), comparative genomic hybridization (array CGH), and next-generation sequencing; the presence of such a loss is supportive of a CCRCC in most cases.

## DIFFERENTIAL DIAGNOSIS

The differential diagnosis for a CCRCC includes benign, malignant, and non-neoplastic renal lesions (see Box 1). Multilocular cystic renal cell neoplasm of low malignant potential (previously called "multilocular cystic renal cell carcinoma") is a predominantly cystic lesion, devoid of large solid mural tumor nodules, with atypical cytologic features that are indistinguishable from a FNG 1 CCRCC (Fig. 5).[11,52–56] Microscopic invasive tumor nests within cyst septae confirm the diagnosis, and also distinguish it from other benign cystic lesions such as cystic nephroma and simple cortical cysts. The latter diagnoses lack cytologic atypia and the cysts are typically lined by hobnail to cuboidal to flattened epithelial cells. In contrast to many CCRCCs, multilocular cystic renal cell neoplasm of low malignant potential is associated with a favorable prognosis.[55,57,58]

Clear cell (tubulo) papillary RCC is another low-grade, indolent tumor that has morphologic overlap with CCRCC, and in the past has likely been misdiagnosed as CCRCC or PRCC[11,49,50,56,59–61] (for further discussion see also Mehra et al., Emerging Entities in Renal Neoplasia, Surgical Pathology Clinics, 2015, Volume 8, Issue 4). Clear cell (tubulo) papillary RCC can be confused with CCRCC as both have characteristic clear cell cytology; the distinction, however, is in the arrangement of the nuclei: CCRCC has clustered, nested, and disorganized nuclei (see Fig. 3), whereas clear cell (tubulo) papillary RCCs have a more distinct tubular to tubulopapillary architecture with nuclei arranged in a "picket-fence"–like orientation in the mid to apical portion of the cells (Fig. 6). In difficult cases, immunohistochemistry can be used to distinguish these 2 cell types, as unlike CCRCC, clear cell (tubulo) papillary RCC is diffusely positive for CK7 (Fig. 6, inset), positive

for high molecular weight keratin 34BE12, negative to very focally positive for CD10, and negative for AMACR (Table 1). CAIX is not useful for distinguishing these 2 tumor types, as both are diffusely positive; however, CAIX in clear cell (tubulo) papillary RCC has been described as having a "cuplike" staining pattern.[49,60] No specific chromosomal abnormalities have been identified in clear cell (tubulo) papillary RCCs, and most are associated with 2 intact copies of 3p regions.

A third tumor type, the TCEB1-mutated RCC, has recently been described, and has overlapping features with both CCRCC and clear cell (tubulo) papillary RCC (Fig. 7). These features include a predominant tubular architecture containing well-organized cells with clear cytoplasm and a linear array of nuclei, intraluminal eosinophilic material, and diffuse expression of CAIX.[62,63] However, distinguishing features include a thick fibrous capsule, dissecting thick fibrous bands, and diffuse CK7 expression as well as immunoreactivity with AMACR and CD10 (see Table 1). Molecular and genetics studies have shown that these tumors contain a mutated TCEB1 gene (which encodes for the elongin protein) on chromosome 8 plus loss of heterozygosity of the second chromosome 8 allele (two-hit theory); no loss of 3p should be found in this tumor type (see also Mehra et al., Emerging Entities in Renal Neoplasia, Surgical Pathology Clinics, 2015, Volume 8, Issue 4).

Occasionally renal tumors with extensive papillary architecture also have clear cytology.[64,65] The differential diagnosis in this setting includes a CCRCC with papillary architecture, a PRCC with clear cell cytology, and an Xp11.2 translocation RCC (Fig. 14). A more thorough discussion of the

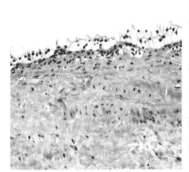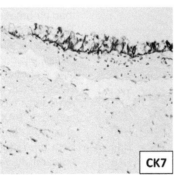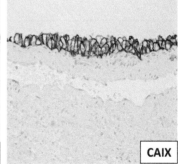

*Fig. 5.* Multilocular cystic renal cell neoplasm of low malignant potential (previously called "multilocular cystic renal cell carcinoma") is a low grade renal tumor that contains multiple cystic structures lined by atypical clear cells which are cytologically similar to that seen in low grade clear cell renal cell carcinoma. Small nests of atypical clear cells in the underlying stroma, as is seen focally in the upper right of this H&E, help distinguish these cystic tumors from cystic nephroma, simple cortical cysts, and other cystic lesions of the kidney. In contrast to non-cystic clear cell renal cell carcinomas, most multilocular cystic renal cell neoplasm of low malignant potential (as well as cystic components of bone fide clear cell renal cell carcinoma) express CK7. Like clear cell renal cell carcinoma, multilocular cystic renal cell neoplasm of low malignant potential also expresses CAIX.

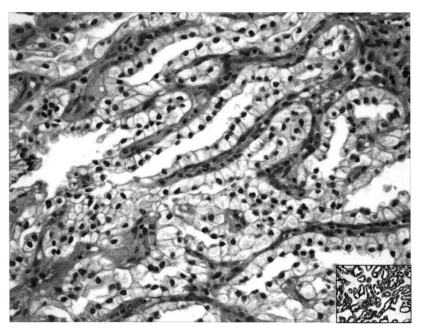

*Fig. 6.* Clear cell (tubulo) papillary renal cell carcinoma has overlapping cytologic and architectural features with clear cell and papillary renal cell carcinomas, respectively. However, the distinct picket fence-like nuclear arrangement and the presence of diffuse CK7 (inset) help distinguish it from clear cell renal cell carcinoma; the absence of AMACR and CD10 (not shown) help distinguish it from a papillary renal cell carcinoma.

latter 2 entities can be found later in this article, but in brief, unlike CCRCC, PRCC is typically positive for CK7, AMACR, and CD10 and negative for CAIX, whereas Xp11.2 translocation RCCs are negative for CK7 and CAIX, and should be positive for TFE3 (see **Table 1**).[46,51,52,66,67] If morphologic features and immunostains are not definitive, the presence of chromosomal changes, as determined with karyotype, FISH, or other mechanisms, can help confirm the diagnosis, as all 3 of these entities have distinct genetic findings: 3p loss in CCRCC (see **Fig. 4**), extra copies of chromosomes 7 and 17 in PRCC (**Fig. 10**), and TFE3 gene rearrangement in Xp11.2 RCCs.[68,69]

Other neoplasms that should be distinguished from CCRCC include chromophobe RCC and metastases from other sites. Morphologic features of chromophobe RCC that distinguish it from CCRCC include a more diffuse growth pattern in which sheets of cells are separated by long, linear, parallel vessels in a fibrotic stroma, prominent cell membranes, eosinophilic cytoplasm, and irregular-shaped and multinucleated "raisinoid" nuclei with perinuclear halos (**Fig. 12**). In cases of chromophobe RCC, in which the cells are more "clear" in appearance, the presence of patchy CK7, the absence of CD10 and CAIX, and the loss of multiple chromosomes other than chromosome 3 all support the diagnosis.[70,71] The distinction of primary and secondary tumors with clear cell features in the kidney requires suspicion, clinicopathologic correlation, and/or ancillary studies. Metastatic adrenal cortical carcinoma is positive for inhibin, MelanA, and steroidogenic factor 1 (SF1) and negative for PAX8. In contrast, PAX8 is not helpful for distinguishing clear cell carcinomas of the kidney and ovary, as both are diffusely positive; however, CK7 immunoreactivity would be expected more frequently in clear cell carcinoma of ovary and less frequently in CCRCC.

Lastly, non-neoplastic lesions in the kidney can be confused with CCRCC, and the most common is xanthogranulomatous pyelonephritis (XGP) (**Fig. 8**). XGP can present as a well-circumscribed mass, but instead of containing neoplastic cells, it is composed of numerous foamy histiocytes

**Table 1**
**Typical immunoprofile for renal tumors with "clear cell" features**

|          | CK7 | AMACR | CD10 | CAIX | TFE3 |
|----------|-----|-------|------|------|------|
| CCRCC    | Neg | Var   | Pos  | Pos  | Neg  |
| CCTPRCC  | Pos | Neg   | Neg  | Pos  | Neg  |
| TCEB1-RCC| Pos | Var   | Var  | Pos  | Neg  |
| PRCC     | Pos | Pos   | Pos  | Neg  | Neg  |
| Xp11.2 RCC | Neg | Pos | Var  | Neg  | Pos  |
| ChRCC    | Var | Var   | Neg  | Neg  | Neg  |

*Abbreviations:* AMACR, alpha-methylacyl-CoA racemase; CAIX, Carbonic Anhydrase IX; CCRCC, clear cell renal cell carcinoma; CCTPRCC, clear cell tubulopapillary renal cell carcinoma; ChRCC, chromophobe RCC; Neg, negative; Pos, positive; PRCC, papillary renal cell carcinoma; RCC, renal cell carcinoma; Var, variable.

*Fig. 7.* Recently described TCEB1-mutated renal cell carcinoma has morphologic features that overlap with clear cell renal cell carcinoma and clear cell (tubulo) papillary renal cell carcinoma, including a prominent tubular architecture and clear cell cytology. Nuclei are often arranged in a linear orientation, but slightly less organized when compared to clear cell (tubulo) papillary renal cell carcinoma (see Fig. 6 for comparison). Intraluminal eosinophillic material is frequently present. TCEB1-mutated renal cell carcinoma is

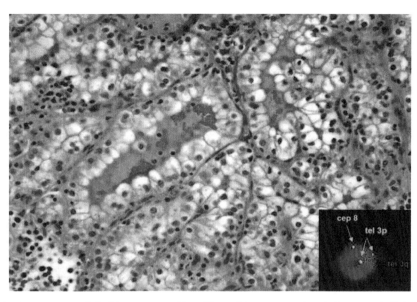

characterized by a mutated *TCEB1* on one allele (chromosome 8) and loss of heterozygosity of the second allele; the latter can be demonstrated with FISH analysis (inset, note monosomy 8 and diploid 3).

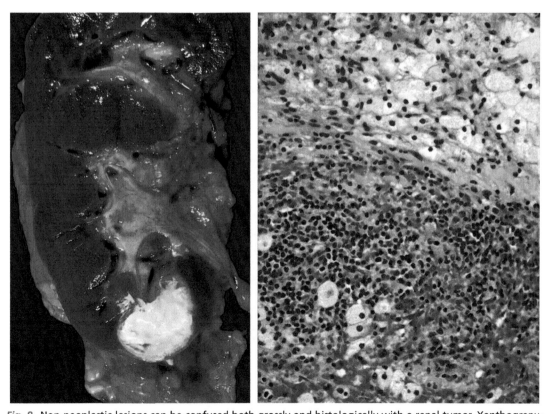

*Fig. 8.* Non-neoplastic lesions can be confused both grossly and histologically with a renal tumor. Xanthogranulomatous pyelonephritis (XGP) can form a mass-like lesion that is worrisome for neoplasia by imaging. The presence of numerous xanthoma cells (i.e., foamy histiocytes) can also be a mimic for the clear neoplastic cells in a clear cell renal cell carcinoma. Typically the distinction can be made by H&E analysis, but if necessary, keratin and histiocyte biomarkers can be used for a more definitive diagnosis.

(xanthomas cells, which may mimic the clear cells of a CCRCC), neutrophils, lymphocytes, and varying degrees of necrosis, fibrosis, and edema. The cells of XGP would be negative for epithelial markers and PAX8, and would be positive for histiocytic markers such as CD68, CD163, and PU1; the converse would be true for CCRCC.

## PAPILLARY RENAL CELL CARCINOMA

### CLINICAL PRESENTATION, GROSS FEATURES, AND PROGNOSIS

Papillary RCC (PRCC) is the second most common subtype of RCC, and accounts for approximately 15% of renal epithelial neoplasms in adults. Like CCRCC, PRCC occurs more frequently in men and may be found incidentally or secondary to nonspecific clinical symptoms. PRCC may occur spontaneously or in association with a germ line mutation (see later in this article); bilateral and multifocal unilateral tumors may occur with the latter. There is also an association of PRCC with end-stage kidney disease, and multiple papillary adenomas may be present.

Grossly, most PRCCs are cortical based and well circumscribed. The cut surface is typically a pale tan to brown color, and friable papillary structures may be evident. Some PRCCs may demonstrate hemorrhage, necrosis, and/or cystic degeneration. Many PRCCs are confined to the kidney (low stage) and are associated with a favorable prognosis. However, higher-stage tumors when present are more likely to recur and/or metastasize. In contrast to CCRCC, which often metastasizes distantly, PRCC often metastasizes locally to regional lymph nodes before metastasizing distantly. Similar to other RCCs, higher grade nuclear features and sarcomatoid differentiation are associated with a worse prognosis.

### MICROSCOPIC EXAMINATION

For most PRCCs, a papillary architecture predominates with tumors cells that rim fibrovascular cores; however, other architectures can also be present, including solid and tubular growth patterns (Fig. 9B–G). Other frequent, but nonspecific features include aggregates of foamy histiocytes within edematous fibrovascular cores (Fig. 9D), psammous calcifications, and intraepithelial

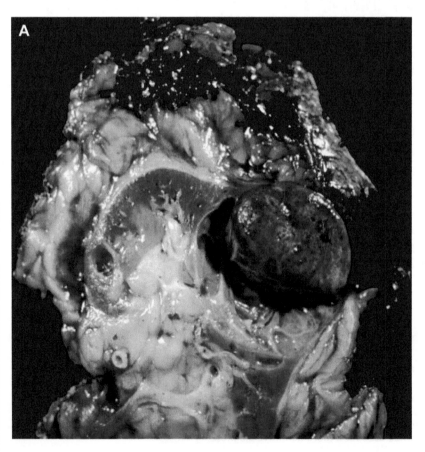

Fig. 9. Papillary renal cell carcinoma (PRCC) frequently forms a well-defined mass in the renal cortex. Like other renal neoplasms, it may be (A) low stage (i.e., confined to the renal parenchyma), or extend beyond the confines of the renal capsule (not shown). The cut surface of a PRCC is typically tan to brown in color, and may grossly demonstrate a rough papillary surface.

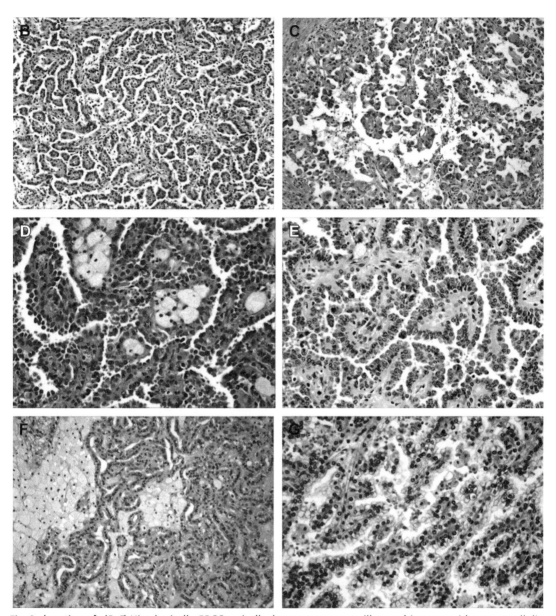

*Fig. 9.* (*continued*). (*B–E*) Histologically, PRCC typically demonstrates a papillary architecture with tumors cells lining the fibrovascular cores. (*B*) In so-called type I PRCC, a single cell layer of cuboidal to columnar basophilic-appearing cells line the fibrovascular cores. (*C*) In the so-called type II PRCC, tumor cells appear more eosinophilic, may be pseudostratified, and are typically of higher cytologic grade. (*D*) The presence of foamy histiocytes within the fibrovascular cores is a common, but not pathognomonic, feature in PRCC. (*E*) Intraepithelial pigment is another morphologic feature that is seen more often in PRCC when compared to other renal subtypes. (*F*) A tubular growth pattern can also been observed in PRCC, and this may be confused with a clear cell (tubulo) papillary renal cell carcinoma or a mucinous tubular and spindle cell carcinoma. In this example foamy histiocytes are present between tubules instead of within fibrovascular cores. (*G*) Some PRCCs have clear cell cytology, raising the possibility of a clear cell renal cell carcinoma, a translocation renal cell carcinoma, or a clear cell (tubulo) papillary renal cell carcinoma.

pigment (**Fig.** 9E) (in contrast to hemosiderin laden-macrophages). The cytology of the tumor cells has led some to separate PRCC into type 1 and type 2 tumors: type 1 tumors are described as having a more basophilic appearance with a single layer of cuboidal to columnar cells containing low-grade nuclei; in contrast, type 2 tumors are more eosinophilic, and have pseudostratified cells and higher-grade cytology with prominent nucleoli.[72] The difficulties lie in that some tumors are heterogeneous, containing areas consistent with type 1 features and other areas that are consistent with type 2 features within the same mass. Additionally, there is a controversial entity that is not currently included in the WHO classification of tumors, termed "oncocytic PRCC" that has overlapping features between type 1 and type 2 tumors; notably, a single cell layer of tumors cells lining fibrovascular cores with low-grade cytology, but prominent oncocytic/eosinophilic cytoplasm.[53] Regardless, grade has been shown to correlate with outcome, and will suffice in place of designating "the type" of PRCC as long as the highest grade is recorded (see **Fig. 9**B compared to 9C). Many pathologists continue to use FNG (see earlier in this article) for PRCC; however, some may choose to use the ISUP grading system, which is similar to FNG but places more emphasis on nucleoli and less on nuclear size.[15]

## GENETIC ALTERATIONS

A combination of trisomy/tetrasomy 7, trisomy 17, and loss of the Y chromosome are the most frequent cytogenetic aberrations found in PRCC, regardless of tumor size and grade (see **Fig. 10**). In fact, these findings are also associated with benign papillary cortical adenomas. However, in PRCC, additional trisomies, such as those involving chromosomes 12, 16, or 20, as well as +3/+3q, may also be present. Although some studies suggest that type 1 and type 2 PRCC are distinct variants of PRCC,[72] other cytogenetic analyses have also suggested that type 2 tumors evolve from type 1 tumors, as both show common chromosomal aberrations, including trisomy for chromosomes 3/3q, 7, 12, 16, 17, and 20.[73] However, unlike type 1 PRCCs, type 2 tumors show additional cytogenetic abnormalities (ie, loss of 1p, 8p, 9p, 11q, and 18, and gain of 1q) that are believed to reflect tumor progression. In terms of prognostic value, losses of 8p, 9p, and 11q have been reported to coincide with advanced clinical stage.[73]

## MOLECULAR PATHWAYS

Germline mutations in the tyrosine kinase domain of the *MET* gene located on chromosome 7 have been identified in the hereditary papillary renal carcinoma (HPRC) syndrome.[74] Patients with HPRC have a high risk of developing bilateral and/or multifocal PRCC.[75] HPRC tumors are characterized by trisomy 7 and harbor a nonrandom duplication of the mutant *MET* allele.[76] Of note, somatic *MET* mutations were also detected in a relatively small subset (~13%) of sporadic PRCCs.[74,77] *MET* encodes for a receptor tyrosine kinase that binds the hepatocyte growth factor (HGF). HGF-MET signaling is involved in various biological functions, including cell proliferation, survival, motility, and morphogenesis.[78] Importantly, functional studies demonstrated that activating *MET* mutations detected in hereditary and sporadic PRCCs are oncogenic and are thus likely to play a role in the pathogenesis of these tumors.[79] Clinical trials are currently being conducted to evaluate the efficacy of *MET* inhibitors in PRCC.[80]

Hereditary leiomyomatosis and renal cell carcinoma (HLRCC) is an autosomal dominant familial syndrome caused by germline mutations in the gene encoding the tricarboxylic acid cycle enzyme fumarate hydratase *(FH)*[81] (see also Mehra, et al., Emerging Entities in Renal Neoplasia, Surgical Pathology Clinics, 2015, Volume 8, Issue 4). Patients with HLRCC develop renal carcinomas that often display papillary

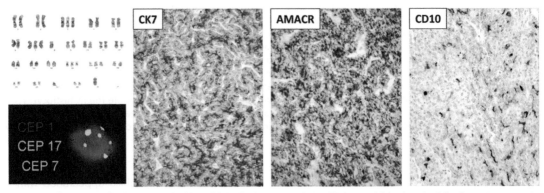

**Fig. 10.** Papillary renal cell carcinoma (PRCC) has distinct genetic and immunohistochemical findings. Extra copies of chromosomes 7 and 17 can be seen by G-band karyotype (47, X, -Y, +3, +7, -8, +16, +17, -21) and FISH analysis. Classically, PRCC is positive for CK7, AMACR, and CD10 by immunohistochemistry.

features and may resemble the so-called type 2 papillary RCC or collecting duct carcinoma.[82] Loss of heterozygosity is frequently detected in kidney cancers arising in HLRCC, suggesting that *FH* follows the 2-hit model for a tumor suppressor. Although somatic *FH* mutations are not detected in sporadic kidney tumors, a recent study indicates that germline *FH* mutations can be detected in patients presenting with isolated high-grade PRCC.[83] There is evidence that inactivation of FH leads to HIF stabilization through a mechanism that is mediated by reactive oxygen species and independent of pVHL.[84] These data suggest that targeting the HIF pathway might represent a viable therapeutic option for kidney tumors driven by inactivating *FH* mutations.

## ANCILLARY STUDIES

PRCC has a relatively distinct immunohistochemical profile; therefore, in a subset of RCC cases the use of biomarkers may be helpful. CK7, AMACR, and CD10 are the 3 most common biomarkers expected to positive in most PRCCs. The presence of CK7 helps distinguish it from most clear cell and translocation RCCs, the presence of AMACR and CD10 helps distinguish it from clear cell (tubulo) papillary RCC, and the presence of diffuse CD10 helps distinguish it from MTSCC.[46,47,71] A potential pitfall is that higher grade, more eosinophilic PRCCs may not express CK7 and are positive for CK20 at least focally in a subset of cases. The presence of BRAF by immunohistochemistry or mutational analysis argues against a PRCC and is consistent with a metanephric adenoma.[85,86]

Conventional cytogenetics and FISH can be useful in cases that are difficult to subtype (see **Fig. 10**). Most frequently this is required for the distinction of PRCC and MTSCC, which can have significant morphologic overlap (see also later in this article). PRCCs frequently demonstrate extra chromosomes (multiple "trisomies"), whereas MTSCC is associated with loss of genetic material (multiple "monosomies"), most frequently involving chromosomes 1, 6, 8, 14, 15, and 22 (**Fig. 18**); extra copies of chromosomes 7 and 17 are not found in MTSCC.[13,87–89] Distinction from CCRCC with papillary/pseudopapillary features and Xp11.2 RCC is also possible with FISH,[68,69] as a loss of 3p and the presence of a translocation involving the TFE3 gene supports the latter 2 diagnoses, respectively (see **Figs. 4** and **15**). FISH and karyotype are not helpful in distinguishing other subtypes of RCC, including collecting duct carcinoma, from PRCC.

## DIFFERENTIAL DIAGNOSIS

The differential diagnosis for PRCC includes other renal epithelial neoplasms with a papillary and/or tubular architecture (**Box 2**). Papillary adenomas are benign lesions that are morphologically and immunophenotypically identical to low-grade PRCCs, but are 1.5 cm or smaller (per the 2016 WHO classification of renal tumors) (see **Fig. 11**A). Tumors that are small but have higher nuclear grade (ie, ≥FNG3) should be described in a note or classified as PRCC. Papillary adenomas have been shown to harbor simple karyotypic changes, including extra copies of chromosomes 7 and 17, but lack the additional genetic changes seen in many PRCCs (see earlier in this article). Solitary or multiple papillary adenomas may be present in association with hereditary PRCC syndromes, end-stage kidney disease, or as an incidental finding accompanying any subtype of RCC.

Metanephric adenoma is a rare lesion of the kidney that can resemble PRCC (see **Fig. 11**B). In contrast to PRCC, it occurs more frequently in women (2:1 female preponderance) (**Box 3**) and may be associated with polycythemia. Metanephric adenoma grossly has a tan-white fleshy cut appearance (**Fig. 11**B, inset) secondary to being a highly cellular tumor composed of small tubular structures lined by monomorphic bland cuboidal cells. Psammous calcifications may be

> **Box 2**
> **Differential diagnosis of "papillary" lesions in the kidney**
>
> - Benign:
>   - Papillary adenoma
>   - Metanephric adenoma
> - Malignant:
>   - Papillary renal cell carcinoma
>   - Clear cell renal cell carcinoma with papillary/pseudopapillary architecture
>   - Xp11.2 translocation renal cell carcinoma
>   - Clear cell (tubulo) papillary renal cell carcinoma
>   - Mucinous tubular and spindle cell carcinoma
>   - Acquired cystic disease-related renal cell carcinoma
>   - Collecting duct carcinoma
>   - Fumarate hydratase-deficient renal cell carcinoma
>   - Metastatic carcinoma

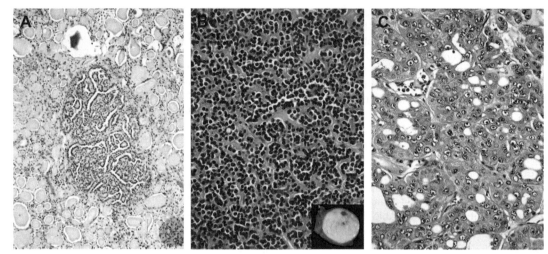

**Fig. 11.** The differential diagnosis for papillary renal cell carcinoma (PRCC) can include: (*A*) papillary adenoma, (*B*) metanephric adenoma, and (*C*) a fumarate hydratase-deficient renal cell carcinoma. (*A*) Papillary adenoma and PRCC have similar morphologic and immunophenotypic features; however, the former is 1.5 cm and smaller in size. (*B*) The low grade cuboidal cytology of a metanephric adenoma may be similar to the cytology of a PRCC, but typically metanephric adenomas have a nested to tubular growth pattern and lack the fibrovascular cores seen with a papillary architecture. The fleshy tan gross appearance of a metanephric adenoma (inset) is also distinct from that seen in PRCC. Although both tumor types are positive for PAX8 and CK7, the presence of BRAF and WT1 can distinguish metanephric adenoma from PRCC (not shown). (*C*) The high grade cytologic features and the presence of a papillary architecture in fumarate hydratase–deficient renal cell carcinoma can be similar to that seen in high grade PRCC. Note the characteristic perinucleolar halos in the tumor cells of this fumarate hydratase–deficient renal cell carcinoma. Confirmatory immunohistochemical and/or genetic studies (not shown) are required for the diagnosis of a fumarate hydratase–deficient renal cell carcinoma.

present, but there is an absence of cytologic atypia, necrosis, and mitoses. Distinction between metanephric adenoma and PRCC is clinically relevant, as metanephric adenoma is a benign tumor. Metanephric adenomas have recently been shown to harbor a *BRAF* mutation, and BRAF immunohistochemistry can be performed to distinguish these tumor types.[85,86] WT1 is also positive in metanephric adenoma and negative in PRCC.[71]

There are many other RCC subtypes that can be confused with PRCC secondary to overlapping architectural (papillary and tubulopapillary) features. High-grade clear cell RCC with clear to eosinophilic cytology, necrosis, and pseudopapillary architecture can be confused with a PRCC. Lower-grade "conventional" areas of clear cell RCC are the best clue to the correct diagnosis; however, when necessary, an absence

of CK7, the presence of CAIX, and a loss of 3p will confirm the diagnosis.[46,90] Xp11.2 translocation RCCs classically, although not exclusively, also have "clear cell cytology and papillary architecture," but differ from PRCC in that they occur more frequently in young female adults (**Box 3**), frequently present with metastatic disease in adults, and have distinct immunophenotypic and genetic features (see later in this article for a more detailed discussion) including an absence of CK7 expression (**Table 1**) and the presence of a translocation involving the *TFE3* gene (see **Figs. 14** and **15**).

Clear cell (tubulo) papillary RCC[49,59–61,91] is described previously and by Mehra and colleagues (Emerging Entities in Renal Neoplasia, Surgical Pathology Clinics, 2015, Volume 8, Issue 4), but in brief, can be distinguished from PRCC because of the clear cell cytology, picket-fence nuclei, and distinct immunoprofile, including an absence of AMACR and CD10 (see **Fig. 6** and **Table 1**). MTSCC is another RCC that occurs more frequently in women (see **Box 3**), and is not infrequently confused with PRCC, as both can have extensive tubulopapillary architecture and varying degrees of an edematous stroma.[53,56,89,92,93] However, MTSCC in classic

---

Box 3

Renal epithelial tumors that occur more frequently in women

- Mesonephric adenoma

- Xp11.2 translocation renal cell carcinoma

- Mucinous tubular and spindle cell carcinoma

cases has an associated myxoid matrix and a component of "spindle cells" (which likely represent collapsed tubules) (Figs. 16 and 17). As these 2 tumor types have a very similar immunoprofile, chromosomal changes as determined by karyotype or FISH (loss of multiple chromosome for MTSCC and gains of multiple chromosomes for PRCC) may be necessary to support the correct diagnosis (see Figs. 10 and 18). The presence of end-stage kidney disease and tumor-related oxalate crystals are supportive of an acquired cystic-disease–related RCC, which otherwise resembles a PRCC.[53,93]

Collecting duct carcinoma (Figs. 20 and 21) and fumarate hydratase (FH)-deficient RCC (see Fig. 11C) are 2 aggressive variants of RCC that can have papillary architecture and eosinophilic cytology, similar to that seen in the so-called type 2 PRCC.[53,56,93–95] Unfortunately, very few ancillary studies can be used to differentiate PRCC from collecting duct carcinoma and FH-deficient RCC; however, rare cases of collecting duct carcinoma have demonstrated loss of multiple chromosomes, so the presence of extra copies of chromosomes 7 and 17 could potentially help support the diagnosis of a PRCC.[96–98] Strong and diffuse nuclear and cytoplasmic staining for S-(2-succino)-cysteine (2SC, private antibody) and loss of staining with the FH antibody (commercially available) is highly sensitive and relatively specific for the diagnosis of FH-deficient RCC; however, studies have shown that approximately 20% of PRCCs can show focal or patchy cytoplasmic staining with 2SC, and FH is only lost in approximately 80% of FH-deficient RCCs.[94]

## CHROMOPHOBE RENAL CELL CARCINOMA

### CLINICAL PRESENTATION, GROSS FEATURES, AND PROGNOSIS

Chromophobe renal cell carcinoma (ChRCC) is a relatively uncommon subtype of RCC that accounts for approximately 5% of all renal epithelial tumors.[11,99,100] ChRCC has similar clinical characteristics when compared to most other RCC subtypes, including a lack of specific symptoms, incidental identification, and a large range in tumor sizes. Some renal oncocytic tumors that resemble ChRCC, at least partially, are associated with the Birt-Hogg-Dubé (BHD) syndrome.[101,102] Typically ChRCCs are well-circumscribed solid masses with a tan-brown cut surface (see Fig. 12). Most (~85%) ChRCCs are low grade and confined to the kidney (low stage), and have a favorable/indolent outcome; however, a small subset of cases behave aggressively and these cases are associated with significant cytologic atypia, including sarcomatoid differentiation, necrosis, and higher stage.[5,103–105]

## MICROSCOPIC EXAMINATION

Most ChRCCs are recognizable and can be easily diagnosed by H&E alone when classic features are present (see Fig. 12). In such cases, sheets of tumor cells (ie, solid growth) are present and are separated by long linear, parallel blood vessels in fibrotic septae. Between these linear vessels, small wrapping capillaries may cluster a subset of tumor cells, resembling the alveolar vascular pattern of CCRCC. Cytologically, the tumor cells are demarcated by well-formed cell membranes and have variable granular to eosinophilic to pale/clear cytoplasm. Nuclei can be variable in size but are typically small, round to oval, with a wrinkled nuclear membrane ("raisinoid" morphology) and may be multinucleated. Nucleoli are inconspicuous. Characteristic cytoplasmic clearing ("perinuclear halos") are present in well-preserved cases, with the halos representing the presence of perinuclear microvesicles that can be identified by electron microscopy but not by routine H&E stain.

The grading of ChRCC is a controversial topic, and to date a specific and accepted grading scheme has not been established. Traditionally, and until recently, FNG has been used for all/most subtypes of RCC including ChRCC[106,107]; however, multiple studies have shown that FNG of ChRCC may not be reproducible or clinically accurate secondary to irregular nuclear morphology.[108] Other schemes for grading ChRCC have been proposed (Box 4), including the nucleolar grading method,[15] grading based on geographic nuclear crowding and anaplasia ("chromophobe tumor grading"),[109] and a recently proposed 2-tier grading scheme,[110] but none of these methods is universally accepted at this time. Due to the lack of consensus, the International Society of Urological Pathologists (ISUP) has recently recommended that ChRCCs not be graded[15]; however, it is clear that a subset of ChRCCs are of higher grade and have metastatic potential, so there is still a need to distinguish in the pathology report such tumors from the more typical low-grade, indolent ChRCC. Regardless, the presence of sarcomatoid differentiation and high stage may be the most clinically relevant information needed with regard to prognosis.[103–105]

## GENETIC ALTERATIONS

Cytogenetic studies, array CGH, and microsatellite and DNA cytometric analyses have demonstrated

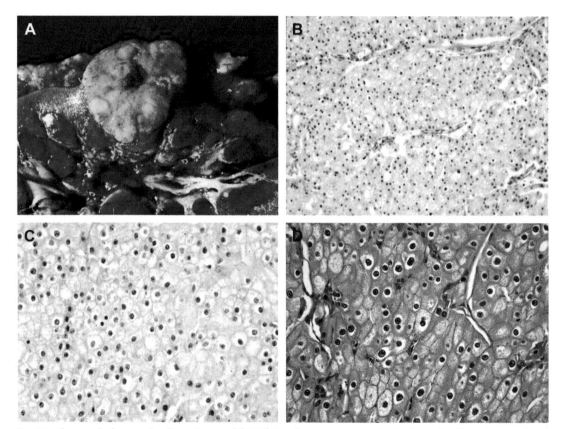

Fig. 12. Chromophobe renal cell carcinoma (ChRCC) is a less common variant of renal cell carcinoma that is known for its 'oncocytic features'. (A) Typically ChRCC are small, well circumscribed masses with a tan to brown cut surface; however, a smaller subset of ChRCC can grow large and extend beyond the confines of the renal capsule. (B) Architecturally, ChRCC often demonstrates a sheet like growth pattern that is separated by long linear vessels, which sometimes are surrounded by hyalinized stroma. (C) Cytologically, ChRCC tumor cells demonstrate well defined cell borders, round to irregular shaped nuclei, clear to granular to oncocytic cytoplasm, and perinuclear halos. (D) The eosinophilic variant of ChRCC demonstrates increased oncocytic features and cytoplasmic granularity; perinuclear halos are also more prominent.

that ChRCCs are typically hypodiploid, and contain a unique combination of monosomies, notably involving chromosomes 1, 2, 6, 10, 13, 17, and 21 (Fig. 13).[111] In contrast to CCRCC, the short arm of 3p is retained in ChRCC. Additionally, the loss of a sex chromosome, and monosomy of chromosome 1 and/or chromosome 11 are rearrangements more suggestive of oncocytoma than ChRCC.[111]

## MOLECULAR PATHWAYS

Recent molecular interrogation has broadened our understanding of ChRCC. These studies demonstrate that ChRCCs originate from the distal nephron, are affected by changes in mitochondrial function, and are associated with recurrent structural breakpoints within the telomerase reverse transcriptase (TERT) promoter region and TERT upregulation.[112] ChRCCs have also been shown to harbor P53 and PTEN mutations in approximately one-third and approximately one-fifth of

cases, respectively. As the latter is affiliated with the mammalian target of rapamycin (mTOR) pathway, there is implication for possible therapeutic options.

Burt-Hogg-Dube (BHD) syndrome is an inherited disease characterized by the development of renal neoplasias that morphologically resemble sporadic ChRCC and oncocytoma.[113] Germline mutations in the BHD gene (also known as folliculin, FLCN) have been identified in approximately 90% of affected families.[114,115] However, most sporadic renal tumors, including ChRCC, lack BHD mutations and show gene expression profiles and cytogenetic characteristics distinct from BHD-related tumors.[101]

## ANCILLARY STUDIES AND DIFFERENTIAL DIAGNOSIS

Most ChRCCs can be diagnosed based on classic morphologic features, as described previously (see Fig. 12). However, when necessary,

---

**Box 4**
**Proposed grading schemes for chromophobe renal cell carcinoma**

- Fuhrman nuclear grading
  - Grade 1: Small, ~10 μm, round uniform nuclei, inconspicuous nucleoli
  - Grade 2: Larger ~15 μm, mildly irregular nuclei, nucleoli visible at ×400
  - Grade3: Even larger, ~20 μm, nuclei with irregular outlines, nucleoli visible at ×100
  - Grade 4: Large, >20 μm, bizarre multilobated nuclei with or without spindle cells (sarcomatoid differentiation)
- Nucleolar grading
  - Grade 1: Small basophilic nucleolar condensations within the nucleus at ×400
  - Grade 2: Eosinophilic nucleolus at ×400, sometimes visible but inconspicuous at ×100
  - Grade 3: Eosinophilic, prominent nucleolus at ×100
- Chromophobe tumor grading
  - Grade 1: No significant nuclear crowding or anaplasia
  - Grade 2: Geographic nuclear crowding, including high N/C density detectable at ×100, nuclei in direct contact with other nuclei at ×400, nuclear pleomorphism (size variation ≥3-fold), and distinct nuclear chromatic irregularities
  - Grade 3: Presence of frank anaplasia (nuclear polylobation, tumor giant cells) or giant cell change
- 2-tier chromophobe tumor grading
  - Low grade: Monomorphic, hypochromatic nuclei, without necrosis or mitotic activity
  - High grade: Increased nuclear atypia, hyperchromasia, presence of necrosis, increased mitotic activity including atypical forms

---

immunostains can be used to support the diagnosis of a ChRCC or to exclude other tumors that have morphologic overlap (**Box 5**). A "textbook" ChRCC would be positive for CK7 (often patchy), but negative for AMACR, CD10, CAIX, S100a1, and HNF1b, and this immunoprofile is distinct from other tumor subtypes (see **Fig. 13**).[70,71,116–118] As S100a1 and HNF1b are positive for all other renal epithelial neoplasms (including oncocytoma), they are useful only when the differential diagnosis includes ChRCC. However, as focal S100a1 and HNF1b staining has been observed in a small subset of cases, one should rely on the combination of morphologic and immunophenotypc findings. Additionally, as S100a1 may have a multifocal staining pattern, use of this antibody can lead to false-negative results in core biopsies, and should be used with caution and in conjunction with HNF1b.[116] CD117 stains both ChRCC and oncocytoma; therefore, it is not useful for distinguishing these 2 tumor types.[70] When other oncocytic tumors, such as epithelioid PEComa or succinate dehydrogenase (SDH)-deficient RCC are being considered (see also Mehra et al., Emerging Entities in Renal Neoplasia, Surgical Pathology Updated, 2015, Volume 8, Issue 4), HMB45 or MelanA and SDH-

B antibodies, respectively, should be included in the panel of immunostains.[70,119,120]

Although relatively specific chromosomal abnormalities are present in ChRCC,[13,88] conventional cytogenetics and FISH are not typically necessary and may only help in a small subset of cases. When the differential diagnosis includes CCRCC and ChRCC, the presence of CAIX and the absence of CK7, and a loss of 3p by FISH if needed, would support the former diagnosis. The 3 tumors that can have overlapping karyotypic abnormalities (ie, multiple monosomies) with ChRCC are malignant PEComa, MTSCC, and collecting duct carcinoma. As malignant PEComa can also have overlapping morphologic features with high grade ChRCC (**Fig. 22**D), it requires a high sense of suspicion and the use of HMB45 and/or MelanA to make the correct diagnosis.[121] Although MTSCC is also associated with multiple monosomies (see later in this article for more detail),[88,89,122] the total number of chromosomes lost is typically fewer than that of ChRCC, and thankfully, there is very little morphologic overlap with ChRCC, so the distinction is quite straightforward; the same is true for collecting duct carcinoma. Unfortunately there are no biomarkers that distinguish a ChRCC from a sporadic or inherited (ie, BHD syndrome) "hybrid oncocytic tumor."

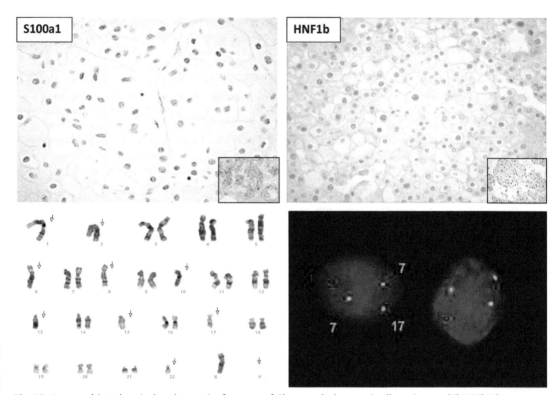

**Fig. 13.** Immunohistochemical and genetics features of Chromophobe renal cell carcinoma (ChRCC). There are no specific biomarkers which distinguish ChRCC from other renal cell carcinomas and importantly oncocytoma in all cases. However, the majority of ChRCC have been shown to lose expression of S100A1 and HNF1b, and this is in contrast to all the other renal epithelial neoplasms, including oncocytoma, which typically express these biomarkers (inset for both biomarkers is an example of oncocytoma). Genetically, ChRCCs are characterized by the loss of multiple chromosomes; an example is shown by G-band karyotype (36,X,-Y,-1,-2,-6,-8,-10,-13,-15,-17,-22). FISH can be used in FFPE tissue, to support a diagnosis of ChRCC, but the loss of chromosomes as determined by FISH alone is not entirely specific for ChRCC.

## Xp11.2 (TFE3) TRANSLOCATION RENAL CELL CARCINOMA

### OVERVIEW, GENETIC ALTERATIONS, AND PROGNOSIS

The Xp11.2 translocation RCC was included as a distinct entity in the 2004 WHO classification of renal tumors.[2] These carcinomas initially were described both in the pediatric and young adult populations, but are now recognized in older individuals as well.[123–125] The gene of interest at Xp11.2 is *TFE3*, a member of the microphthalmia transcription factor (MiTF) family, and several partner genes have been identified, including *ASPL* (17q25), *PRCC* (1q21.2), *CLTC* (17q23), *NONO* (Xq12), and *PSF* (1p34), with *ASPL* (t(X;1) (p11.2;q21)) and *PRCC* (t(X;17)(p11.2;q25)) accounting for the most frequent translocations.[124,126] PARP14 is a unique fusion partner for *TFE3* that has recently been reported.[127] Other

translocations have also been described, including t(X;10)(p11;q23) and t(X;19)(p11;q13), but the identity of the genes fused to *TFE3* in these examples are still unknown.

Although tumors with different translocation/fusion genes may have slightly different morphologic features, it has not been established whether different TFE3-fusion types display different biological behavior.[125] Nevertheless, multiple studies have shown that Xp11.2 RCCs in adults frequently present with metastatic disease and appear to have a more aggressive clinical course when compared with children in whom the tumors are more easily managed.[128–133] In children, previous exposure to cytotoxic chemotherapy has been shown to be associated with subsequent development of an Xp11.2 RCC.[126,134,135] Of interest, another member of the MiTF family, *TFEB*, is also involved in a specific translocation RCC, namely the t(6;11)(p21;q12) RCC. This tumor predominantly affects children and has only rarely been seen in adults.[53,70,124,134,136] The t(6;11)

- Benign:
  - Renal oncocytoma
- Malignant/low malignant potential:
  - Clear cell ("granular") renal cell carcinoma
  - Chromophobe renal cell carcinoma
  - Papillary renal cell carcinoma
  - Mucinous tubular and spindle cell carcinoma
  - Succinate dehydrogenase-deficient RCC
  - Epithelioid/malignant PEComa
  - Hybrid oncocytic tumors
    - Birt-Hogg-Dubé associated renal cell carcinoma
    - Renal oncocytic neoplasm, not otherwise specified
    - Oncocytosis

translocation RCC will be included in the updated WHO classification for renal tumors with Xp11.2 RCCs under the category of "MiTF/TFE-family translocation-associated RCC."

## CLINICAL PRESENTATION AND MORPHOLOGIC FEATURES

Xp11.2 RCC is a relatively rare subtype of RCC, accounting for approximately 4% of adult renal epithelial tumors. However, the incidence of Xp11.2 RCC is likely underestimated due to morphologic overlap with other RCCs and misdiagnosis. Xp11.2 RCC is one of the fewer subtypes of RCC that occur in females more frequently than males (2.5:1) (see Box 3), and the age at presentation is typically earlier than with other RCC subtypes (ie, in the third to fifth decades).[93] Tumors can be found incidentally or secondary to symptoms related to a renal mass; however, not infrequently, Xp11.2 RCCs in adults will present with metastatic disease, including lymph node and lung metastases.

Gross examination of Xp11.2 RCCs includes lesions that can range from small (1–2 cm) to quite large (up to 20 cm); smaller lesions tend to be well circumscribed, whereas larger lesions may be irregular in shape and extend beyond the confines of the kidney. Xp11.2 RCCs are typically tan-yellow, and they will have a solid to papillary cut surface. Hemorrhage and/or necrosis are frequent findings. Histologically, Xp11.2 RCCs are characterized by heterogeneous architectural and cytologic features. Architecturally, these tumors can contain papillary, nested, and solid growth patterns (see Fig. 14). Tumor cells are clear to eosinophilic with varying amounts of cytoplasm (moderate to voluminous). Nuclei are relatively large and often contain nucleoli (typically FNG 3 or 4). Psammous calcifications are a sensitive finding, but are not specific to Xp11.2 RCCs. As these histologic features can vary, and clinical distinction is relevant, it is simply important to add this tumor to the differential diagnosis of any young woman, and even man, who has a renal tumor with "mixed clear cell and papillary features."

## DIFFERENTIAL DIAGNOSIS AND ANCILLARY STUDIES

The differential diagnosis for an Xp11.2 includes any other renal neoplasm with clear cell and papillary features (see Boxes 1 and 2). This list includes CCRCC, PRCC, ChRCC, and clear cell (tubulo) papillary RCC. Xp11.2 RCCs are typically negative for keratins, so the absence of CK7 argues against PRCC and clear cell (tubulo) papillary RCC (see Table 1). The presence of S100a1 and HNF1b would be found in an Xp11.2 RCC and argues against a ChRCC. The most difficult distinction may be with CCRCC, as both are negative of CK7. CAIX has been shown to be present in a small subset of Xp11.2 RCCs and therefore may not be helpful with this differential diagnosis.[48] Some have suggested the use of cathepsinK for translocation RCC, as it effectively distinguishes translocation and nontranslocation RCCs (high specificity); however, cathepsinK stains only approximately 60% of Xp11.2 RCCs (moderate sensitively), and staining patterns vary with TFE3 translocation partners.[137] CathepsinK is also present in other MiTF tumors (angiomyolipomas and PEComas) and this could be a diagnostic pitfall. In contrast, the most confirmatory biomarker for an Xp11.2 RCC is the presence of diffuse and strong TFE3 (see Fig. 15). However, this antibody is not always reliable, so patchy, weak, or negative staining patterns may result in false-positive or false-negative diagnoses. Therefore, when suspicion is high, and staining patterns are equivocal, one should rely on either conventional karyotype or FISH to confirm the diagnosis; the latter can be performed in paraffin-embedded tissues, and has been shown to be both sensitive and specific for Xp11.2 renal tumors.[68,69]

## MOLECULAR PATHWAYS

The MiTF gene family comprises the *MITF*, *TFE3*, *TFEB*, and *TFEC* genes. In addition to kidney

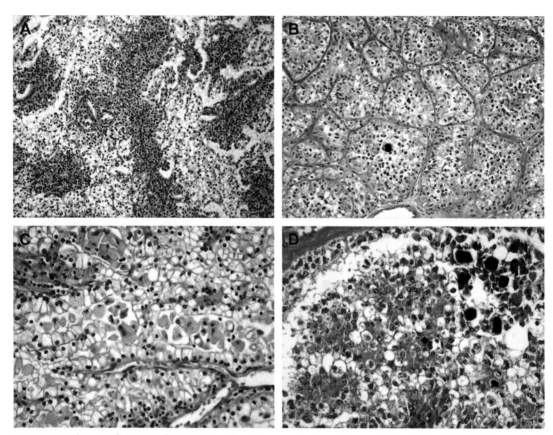

**Fig. 14.** Morphologic features of Xp11.2 translocation renal cell carcinoma. Typically Xp11.2 RCC demonstrates heterogeneous morphologic features that include both clear cell cytology and papillary architecture. (*A*) At low magnification, fibrovascular cores and biphasic cytology, including alternating regions with basophilic and clear cell cytology, can be appreciated. (*B*) Some Xp11.2 RCCs can have a more nested architecture with wrapping vessels that mimic a clear cell renal cell carcinoma. (*C*) Many Xp11.2 RCCs have wel defined cell borders and voluminous clear to eosinophilic cytology. (*D*) Psammomatous calcifications, although not pathognomonic, are a frequent and sensitive finding in Xp11.2 RCC.

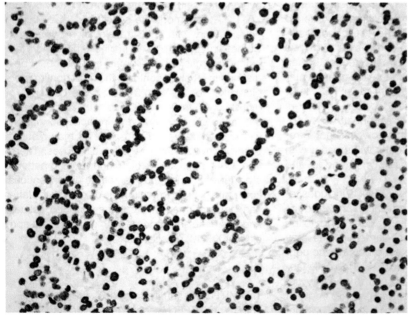

**Fig. 15.** Xp11.2 translocation renal cell carcinoma. Strong and diffuse expression with the TFE3 antibody is supportive of a translocation renal cell carcinoma. Patchy, focal and/or weak expression (not shown) requires additional evidence (i.e. a TFE3 rearrangement by FISH analysis) to confirm the diagnosis of a Xp11.2 translocation renal cell carcinoma.

cancer, mutations and/or dysregulated expression of MiTF genes have been observed in melanoma, clear cell sarcoma, alveolar soft part sarcoma, and angiomyolipoma (AML)/perivascular epithelioid cell tumor (PEComa).[124,138]

In Xp11.2 translocation RCC, at least 5 fusion partner genes of *TFE3* have been identified. These include PRCC (translocation-associated) (*PRCC*) at 1q21, alveolar soft part sarcoma chromosome region, candidate 1 (*ASPL*) at 17q25, splicing factor proline/glutamine-rich (*PSPQ*) at 1p34, non-POU domain–containing octamer-binding (*NONO*) at Xq13, and clathrin heavy-chain (*CLTC*) at 17q23.[135,139–141] It has been recently shown that TFE3 fusion proteins transactivate the *MET* promoter, and induce autophosphorylation of the MET protein and activation of downstream signaling. Importantly, inhibition of MET signaling (by RNA interference or by the inhibitor PHA665752) in cell lines containing endogenous TFE3 fusion proteins caused a decrease in cell growth.[142] These data suggest that MET might represent a therapeutic target for tumors with a TFE3 fusion.[142]

## MUCINOUS TUBULAR AND SPINDLE CELL CARCINOMA

### CLINICAL PRESENTATION, GROSS FEATURES, AND PROGNOSIS

MTSCC is a distinct low-grade, indolent neoplasm that was included in the previous 2004 WHO classification of renal tumors.[2] Unlike most renal epithelial tumors, MTSCC has a striking female to male predominance of approximately 4:1 (Box 3), and can occur across a wide range of ages (13–81, median 60). Its association to other renal epithelial tumors, especially PRCC and collecting duct carcinoma, has been debated due to overlapping morphologic and genetic features[143–145]; however, no definitive connection to any other RCC subtype has been proven to date, and fewer are convinced that there is a relationship with PRCC.[89]

Most MTSCCs are discovered incidentally, although signs and symptoms, such as hematuria, flank pain, and abdominal masses have been reported. The tumors are often grossly described as well-defined tan/yellow/brown masses with a solid consistency, located in the corticomedullary region of the kidney or in the cortex (Fig. 16). Necrosis and hemorrhage are absent in most cases. An accurate diagnosis is important for clinical care as these tumors typically have a favorable prognosis, especially when confined to the kidney and in the absence of bona fide sarcomatoid differentiation.

There are rare documented cases of regional lymph node and distant metastases, as well as sarcomatoid change; these findings are associated with more aggressive behavior.[92,146]

## MICROSCOPIC EXAMINATION

Classic morphologic features for MTSCC include low-grade epithelial cells organized in tubules and spindled cords, associated with abundant myxoid or mucinous extracellular matrix (see Fig. 16).[53,93] MTSCCs lack large hyperchromatic/pleomorphic nuclei, and significant mitotic activity, necrosis, and hemorrhage are uncommon. This is true for the spindle cells as well, and it is important to distinguish the low grade spindle cell component from areas of high-grade sarcomatoid differentiation. Expanded histologic features for MTSCC include "mucin-poor" variants, tumors with either tubular or spindle cell predominance, and oncocytic cytology (see Fig. 17).[147] The architectural and morphologic findings for MTSCC have overlapping features with other renal epithelial neoplasms, most frequently PRCC (especially the tubular variant), and possibly oncocytoma (when oncocytic cytology is present in the MTSCC). The percentage of spindle versus epithelioid cuboidal cells may vary, and tumors that have large areas of the spindle cell component may be misdiagnosed as mesenchymal lesions or sarcomatoid variants of other renal epithelial tumors (such as CCRCC or PRCC), especially in core biopsies. As tumors with sarcomatoid differentiation behave very differently from those without, it is important not to overdiagnose the bland spindle cell component as such. Suspicion for bona fide sarcomatoid differentiation would require increased cytologic atypia, necrosis, and mitoses.

### ANCILLARY STUDIES

A few reports have attempted to define a distinct immunophenotypic profile for MTSCC. Although not entirely sensitive or specific, CD10 appears to be the most affective biomarker for distinguishing MTSCC and PRCC, as it is absent in the former and present in the latter; in contrast, both tumors are positive for CK7 and AMACR (Fig. 18).[46,71,72,148–150] If an oncocytic variant of MTSCC and a tubular variant of oncocytoma are being considered, the absence of CK7, AMACR, and CD10 would be supportive of an oncocytoma diagnosis.

A few previously reported karyotypes for MTSCC have described multiple monosomies (see below); however, fewer than typically seen in ChRCC. Additionally, loss of 3p and chromosomal gains seen in CCRCC and PRCC,

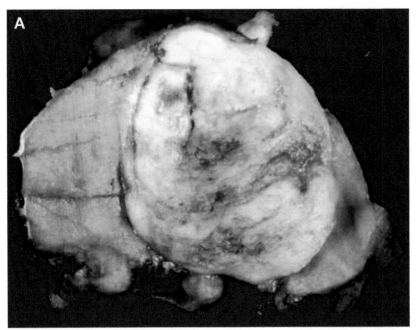

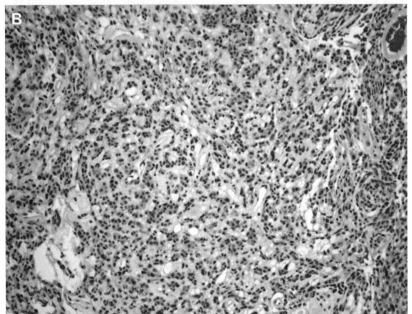

*Fig. 16.* Mucinous Tubular and Spindle Cell Carcinoma (MTSCC). (*A*) Most MTSCCs are well circumscribed, tan to white, soft masses that are located at the corticomedullary junction or within the renal cortex. Necrosis is an infrequent finding. (*B*) Histologically, most MTSCCs consist of a low grade epithelial proliferation that is associated with a prominent myxoid matrix.

respectively, are not frequently found in MTSCC. Therefore, and if necessary, due to overlapping morphologic features and an absence of definitive immunohistochemical findings, FISH can be performed to distinguish CCRCC and PRCC from MTSCC (see **Fig. 18**). As ChRCCs, collecting duct carcinomas, and malignant PEComas have also been reported to demonstrate a loss of multiple chromosomes, FISH cannot be used for these distinctions.

## GENETIC ALTERATIONS

Both array CGH and/or FISH investigations have found a loss of several chromosomes in MTSCC, mostly 1, 4q, 6, 8p, 9p, 11q, 13, 14, 15, and 22.[88,89,92,122,145,149,151,152] This is in contrast to PRCC which remonstrates extra copies of multiple chromosomes, including, but not limited to, chromosomes 7 and 17 (see above for more details). A combination of FISH probes including chromosomes 7, 15, 17, and 22 has been

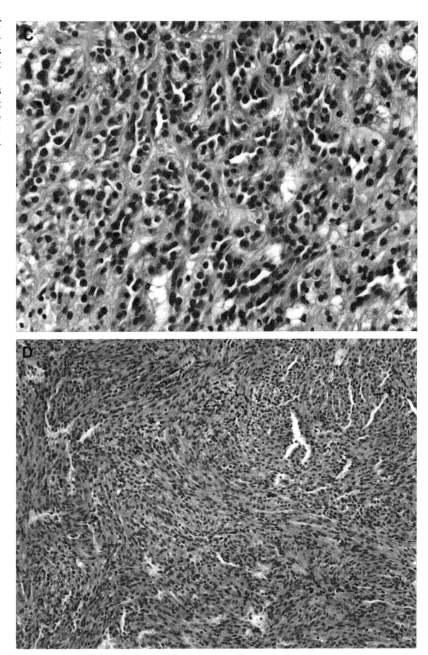

*Fig. 16. (continued).* (C and D) Tumor cells are typically arranged into tubules or present as a compact spindle cell component. The absence of necrosis and significant mitotic activity distinguishes the low grade spindle cell component from sarcomatoid differentiation.

suggested to help distinguish MTSCC from PRCC.[149] However, monosomies 15 and 22 with disomy 7 and 17, have been described to occur in a few renal tumors classified as collecting duct carcinoma.[96] Therefore, morphologic evaluation and interpretation should not be ignored. Additionally, chromosomal changes using cytogenetic and array CGH analyses have been reported when sarcomatoid differentiation is present within an MTSCC; these changes have been reported to include gains of 1q, 2, 3, 5, 7, 12, 16, 19q, 20, and Y, and loss of chromosome 1p, 6p, 8p, 11q, 13, and 15.[153]

## DIFFERENTIAL DIAGNOSIS

The differential diagnosis for MTSCC is relatively broad, and includes both epithelial and mesenchymal neoplasms (**Box 6**). As mentioned, overlapping morphologic features with PRCC can make the distinction from MTSCC difficult. This is especially true for those PRCCs with a tubular

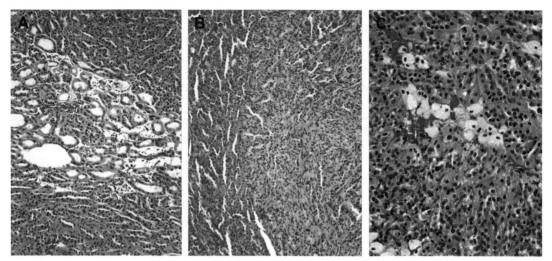

**Fig. 17.** Mucinous Tubular and Spindle Cell Carcinoma (MTSCC). (*A*, *B*) Less commonly, MTSCC can demonstrate oncocytic cytology, and this can causes confusion with oncocytoma when there is prominent tubular architecture. (*C*) Foamy histiocytes can be seen in MTSCC and should not be confused with a papillary renal cell carcinoma.

architecture, those with focal myxoid stroma, and especially with the so-called "PRCC with low-grade spindle cell foci."[154] This latter tumor, however, unlike MTSCC, is characterized by a strong male predominance and foci of bland-appearing spindle cells dispersed among more conventional-appearing PRCC. As these tumors, and other PRCCs with divergent morphology, demonstrate the typical gains in chromosomes 7 and 17 associated with PRCC, FISH analysis can

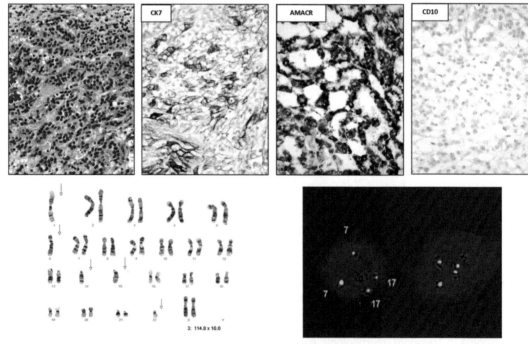

**Fig. 18.** The classic immunoprofile for mucinous tubular and spindle cell carcinoma (MTSCC) includes the presence of CK7 and AMACR, and an absence of CD10; however, focal CD10 can be seen in a subset of cases. G-band karyotype yields a loss of multiple chromosomes, similar (although typically fewer in number) to that seen in chromophobe renal cell carcinoma. Although chromosomal changes are similar in these two tumor types, the morphologic features are quite distinct (see also **Figures 12** and **16**) causing little confusion. FISH analysis may be used to evaluated for chromosomal changes especially when the differential diagnosis include a papillary renal cell carcinoma as extra copies of chromosomes 7 and 17 are not see in MTSCC.

be used in previously fixed tissue to support the diagnosis if needed.[89,149,155]

The more critical distinction for an atypical spindle cell proliferation in a kidney tumor is the presence of a sarcomatoid component accompanying an RCC, because all subtypes of RCC are able to de-differentiate.[5,9,52,103,105,146,156,157] It is important to understand that the WHO no longer recognizes a separate category for "sarcomatoid RCC"; instead, studies have shown that sarcomatoid differentiation both morphologically and genetically will be associated with an underlying classic subtype of RCC, most commonly CCRCC, as well as unclassified RCC and collecting duct carcinoma.[2] Sarcomatoid differentiation within an RCC is a morphologic diagnosis, and is made when an area of the epithelial tumor undergoes de-differentiation into spindle cells, and is associated with increased cytologic atypia, mitoses, and necrosis (Fig. 19). Such areas of the tumor will demonstrate a white/tan fleshy appearance that may be relatively distinct at gross examination from the adjacent nonsarcomatous components. As the presence of sarcomatoid differentiation in

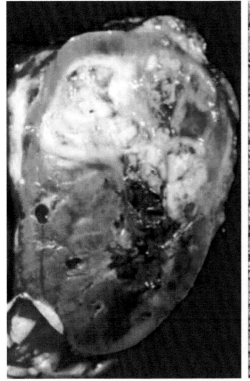
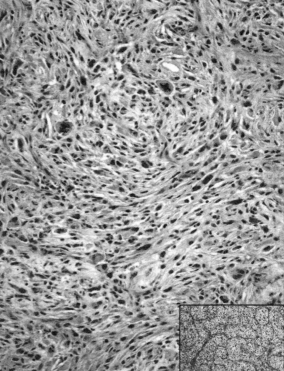

*Fig. 19.* Renal Cell Carcinoma with Sarcomatoid Differentiation. All subtypes of renal cell carcinoma are able to de-differentiate into a malignant spindle cell neoplasm, referred to as 'sarcomatoid differentiation'. Grossly such tumors are characterized by the presence of a white fleshy component (from focal to extensive) that accompanies the underlying renal cell carcinoma. In the gross photo shown, the focal yellow golden area suggests an underlying clear cell component, but the tumor is predominantly sarcomatoid. Histologically the areas of sarcomatoid differentiation contain a high grade spindle cell proliferation that includes significant cytologic atypia, increased mitotic activity, and necrosis (the latter is not shown). Focally, features consistent with clear cell renal cell carcinoma (inset) were present, confirming the underlying RCC subtype. Sarcomatoid differentiation is associated with a poor prognosis.

any RCC is associated with a dismal prognosis, sampling such "fleshy" areas in a renal mass is critical for diagnostic, prognostic, and therapeutic reasons. Of course, the presence of an atypical spindle cell neoplasm in the kidney also warrants consideration of a primary benign or malignant mesenchymal neoplasm; this discussion, however, is beyond the scope of this review.

## COLLECTING DUCT CARCINOMA

### CLINICAL PRESENTATION, MORPHOLOGIC FEATURES, AND PROGNOSIS

Collecting duct carcinoma (CDCA) is a rare tumor of the distal nephron that accounts for fewer than 1% of all renal epithelial tumors.[53,93] Its original name, "Bellini duct carcinoma," reflects the presumed cell of origin in the collecting duct of Bellini. Tumors are seen more frequently in men (2:1), and patients typically present in the sixth decade. CDCA is a clinically aggressive tumor with a very poor 5-year survival rate, and patients with stage 3 or 4 disease often succumb to their disease within 1 to 2 years. Therefore, it is critically

important for the pathologist to be aware of the gross and histologic features, so that an accurate diagnosis can be made. Nevertheless, CDCA remains a diagnosis of exclusion combined with supporting diagnostic features.

Features that support the diagnosis of a CDCA include a medullary based tumor, tubular/acinar architecture with high-grade cytology, and an infiltrative growth pattern with an associated desmoplastic stroma (see Fig. 21). The cut surface of a CDCA is typically firm, homogeneous, and tan/white in color (secondary to the desmoplastic stroma); a "fleshy" appearance suggests the presence of a sarcomatoid component. Origination in the medulla can be determined by gross evaluation in a subset of cases when a smaller "primary" lesion is centered in a pyramid or at the corticomedullary interface (Fig. 20); in other cases, this can be difficult to determine when the tumor has grown large, obliterating the "primary site" (Box 8). Histologically, in the absence of grossly identifiable "primary lesion," a good indication that a tumor originates in the medulla is an infiltrative pattern that extends between non-neoplastic tubules in the renal cortex (see Fig. 2). This type of growth pattern can be seen

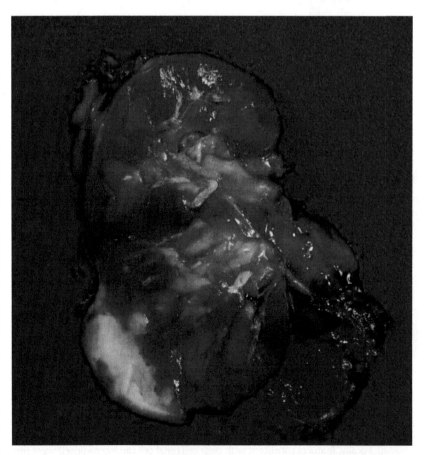

Fig. 20. Collecting Duct Carcinoma. Collecting duct carcinoma is a high grade aggressive tumor that originates from the collecting ducts of Bellini in the renal medulla. Grossly, tumors have a homogeneous white cut surface, and associated necrosis is common. In some cases the tumor can be seen originating in the renal medulla; in this example the small white nodule at the corticomedullary junction represents the 'primary' tumor. However, frequently a CDCA will extend into the renal cortex, and possibly overgrow the "primary" medullary lesion, grossly mimicking a renal cortical tumor (not shown).

with CDCA, medullary carcinoma, and invasive urothelial carcinoma; metastatic tumors and lymphoma may also show a similar growth pattern and can be a diagnostic pitfall for a primary kidney tumor.

Architecturally, an acinar/tubular/tubulopapillary growth pattern typically predominates (Fig. 21A), but solid growth, true papillary formation, and satellite nodules may also be present. Necrosis and mitoses are common, and sarcomatoid differentiation can be present in at least half of the cases (Fig. 21B). Tumor cells often have hobnail nuclei and eosinophilic cytoplasm. By definition, the cells have high-grade nuclear features, so there is no need to apply a specific tumor grade.

There is some evidence to suggest that MTSCC may represent a "low-grade" CDCA, and there are morphologic and genetic findings that support this

Fig. 21. Collecting Duct Carcinoma. Morphologically, collecting duct carcinoma is typically comprised of a high grade invasive adenocarcinoma that is associated with an inflamed/desmoplastic stroma. Tumors often infiltrate between nonneoplastic structure (see also Figs. 2 and 22) and this can be a clue to the diagnosis. (A) Although acinar structures typically predominate, papillary and solid growth patterns may also be present (not shown). (B) Reflective of the aggressive nature of this tumor, the presence of sarcomatoid differentiation is frequently present as a component of collecting duct carcinoma.

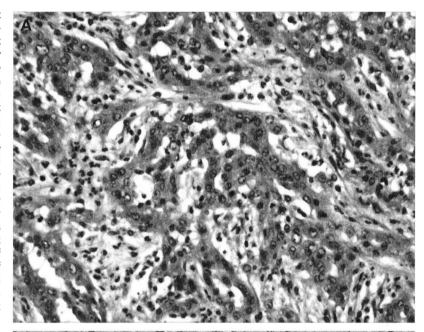

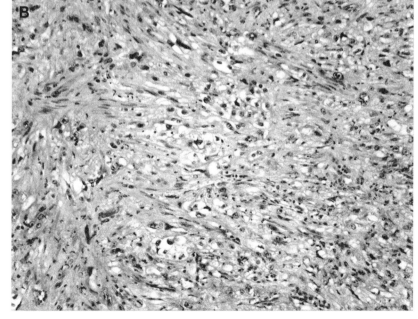

theory (**Box 7**). However, more definite studies are required to be certain.

## ANCILLARY STUDIES AND DIFFERENTIAL DIAGNOSIS

The differential diagnosis for a CDCA includes other medullary/renal pelvis–based tumors, such medullary carcinoma and urothelial carcinoma, PRCC, unclassified RCC, and a metastatic poorly differentiated neoplasm. Ancillary studies, such as immunohistochemistry and FISH, are not typically helpful for confirming a diagnosis of CDCA, but can be used to exclude these other entities in the differential diagnosis. If a final determination cannot be made, the designation of "unclassified RCC" should be considered.[46,47,156]

The only biomarkers that are consistently positive in CDCA are PAX8 and INI1/SMARCB.[46,158–160] PAX8 confirms that the tumor is of renal origin but does not help with tumor subtyping. Immunohistochemistry can be used when the differential diagnosis includes a renal pelvis urothelial carcinoma, but one must be aware that up to 20% of renal pelvis urothelial carcinomas can be at least focally positive for PAX8 (**Box 8**).[161] To avoid this pitfall, including GATA3 and p63 in the panel of immunostains should help with the distinction, as both should be negative in CDCAs and

---

**Box 7**
**Comparison of features: mucinous tubular and spindle cell carcinoma and collecting duct carcinoma**

- Mucinous tubular and spindle cell carcinoma
  - Tubular/acinar/spindle cell components
  - Low grade cytology
  - Distinctive stroma: myxoid
  - Expansile growth pattern
  - Infrequent sarcomatoid component
  - Typically CD10-
  - Hypodiploid
- Collecting duct carcinoma
  - Tubular/acinar/papillary/solid components
  - High-grade cytology
  - Distinctive stroma: desmoplastic
  - Expansile and infiltrative growth pattern
  - Frequent sarcomatoid component
  - Typically CD10-
  - Hypodiploid

---

**Box 8**
**Pitfalls for collecting duct carcinoma**

- Large growth obscures medullary primary, confused with a cortical-based tumor
- Infiltrative pattern of melanoma, lymphoma, or metastasis between non-neoplastic tubules and glomeruli is confused with a renal primary
- PAX8 can be expressed in a subset of renal pelvis urothelial primaries
- High-grade tumor with a loss of INI1 in the absence of sickled red blood cells is misclassified as a collecting duct carcinoma

---

positive in urothelial carcinomas (GATA3 has greater sensitivity than p63 for poorly differentiated urothelial tumors).[158,159,162] Additionally, the presence of retrograde tumor within collecting tubules is morphologically supportive of an urothelial primary (see **Fig. 2**; **Fig. 22**B).

Another medullary based tumor, medullary carcinoma, has significant morphologic overlap with CDCA, but is associated with a different clinical scenario (ie, typically a younger patient with sickle cell trait).[133,163–165] In difficult cases, the presence of INI1 is supportive of a CDCA as well as other subtypes of RCC, and excludes medullary carcinoma where loss of INI1 expression is expected.[46,166] OCT3/4 is also positive in medullary carcinoma and negative in CDCA and urothelial carcinomas.[167] Recently it has been suggested that tumors with overlapping features of CDCA and medullary carcinoma (ie, medullary based tumor with an absence of INI1 but in older patients without sickle cell trait) be designated as "unclassified RCC with medullary features" (**Box 8**).[168]

## GENETIC ALTERATIONS

Cytogenetic reports on CDCA are limited secondary to the rarity of the tumor and the absence of a prospective diagnosis leading to tissue sampling for cytogenetic analysis. Additionally, the data that are in the literature contain conflicting results. Most studies detect a combination of several monosomies,[96–98] whereas others find more trisomies and structural abnormalities.[169,170] However, the findings in the latter 2 studies may represent misclassification of the tumors, especially as some of the chromosomal aberrations present can also be seen in PRCC. It is likely that more information on genetic and molecular data will be collected for CDCA now that paraffin-embedded tissue can be used for other techniques, such as array CGH and next-generation sequencing.

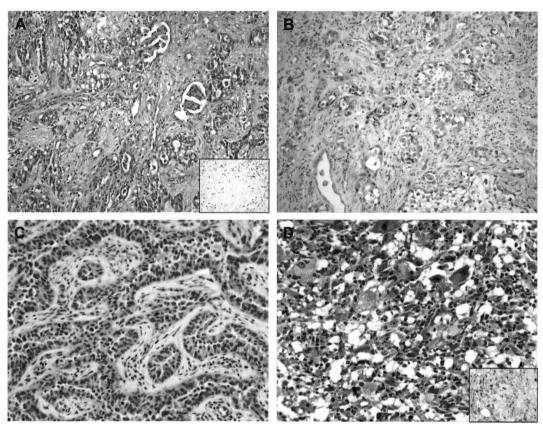

*Fig. 22.* The Differential Diagnosis of Medullary Based Tumors. Many high grade neoplasms can be included in the differential diagnosis with collecting duct carcinoma and other medullary based tumors. (*A*) Renal medullary carcinoma typically occurs in children and is associated with sickle cell trait. Morphologically, it has similar architectural, infiltrative, and cytologic features when compared to collecting duct carcinoma. The distinction from collecting duct carcinoma includes the clinical presentation, the presence of sickle cell trait, and the loss of INI1 (inset). (*B*) Urothelial carcinoma can have overlapping features with other medullary based tumors, especially including an invasive growth pattern between non-neoplastic tubules; however, the presence of retrograde intratubular growth and urothelial biomarkers (i.e., GATA3 and p63) are supportive of a urothelial carcinoma. (*C*) Unclassified renal cell carcinoma is a WHO recognized renal epithelial tumor subtype. The histologic features found in an unclassified RCC do not fit into any other category of RCC based on morphologic, immunophenotypic, and genetic findings. Mostly, it is a diagnosis of exclusion, and tumors of this subtype can be found in the renal cortex or medulla. (*D*) Malignant PEComas usually have distinct morphological and immunophenotypic findings when compared to collecting duct carcinoma; however, multiple chromosomal losses have been seen in rare cases of malignant PEComa and this result could cause confusion with collecting duct carcinoma, mucinous tubular and spindle cell carcinoma, and chromophobe renal cell carcinoma; the latter has the greatest morphologic overlap with malignant PEComa.

## ACKNOWLEDGMENTS

The authors wish to thank Mr. Michael Cooper of Cooper Graphics (www.cooper247.com) for his assistance with schematic illustration.

## REFERENCES

1. Siegel RL, Miller KD, Jemal A. Cancer statistics, 2015. CA Cancer J Clin 2015;65:5–29.

2. Eble JN, Sauter G, Epstein JI, et al. World Health Organization (WHO) classification of tumors. Lyon (France): IARC Press; 2004.

3. Motzer RJ, Bacik J, Mariani T, et al. Treatment outcome and survival associated with metastatic renal cell carcinoma of non-clear-cell histology. J Clin Oncol 2002;20:2376–81.

4. Leibovich BC, Lohse CM, Crispen PL, et al. Histological subtype is an independent predictor of outcome for patients with renal cell carcinoma. J Urol 2010;183:1309–15.

5. Amin MB, Amin MB, Tamboli P, et al. Prognostic impact of histologic subtyping of adult renal epithelial neoplasms: an experience of 405 cases. Am J Surg Pathol 2002;26:281–91.

6. Cheville JC, Lohse CM, Zincke H, et al. Comparisons of outcome and prognostic features among histologic subtypes of renal cell carcinoma. Am J Surg Pathol 2003;27:612–24.

7. Delahunt B, Bethwaite PB, Nacey JN. Outcome prediction for renal cell carcinoma: evaluation of prognostic factors for tumours divided according to histological subtype. Pathology 2007;39:459–65.

8. Delahunt B, McKenney JK, Lohse CM, et al. A novel grading system for clear cell renal cell carcinoma incorporating tumor necrosis. Am J Surg Pathol 2013;37:311–22.

9. Lohse CM, Gupta S, Cheville JC. Outcome prediction for patients with renal cell carcinoma. Semin Diagn Pathol 2015;32:172–83.

10. Kapur P, Christie A, Raman JD, et al. BAP1 immunohistochemistry predicts outcomes in a multi-institutional cohort with clear cell renal cell carcinoma. J Urol 2014;191:603–10.

11. Delahunt B, Srigley JR, Montironi R, et al. Advances in renal neoplasia: recommendations from the 2012 International Society of Urological Pathology Consensus Conference. Urology 2014;83:969–74.

12. Pichler M, Hutterer GC, Chromecki TF, et al. Histologic tumor necrosis is an independent prognostic indicator for clear cell and papillary renal cell carcinoma. Am J Clin Pathol 2012;137:283–9.

13. Presti JC Jr, Rao PH, Chen Q, et al. Histopathological, cytogenetic, and molecular characterization of renal cortical tumors. Cancer Res 1991;51:1544–52.

14. Lloreta-Trull J, Bielsa-Gali O, Dominguez-Sola D, et al. Ultrastructural morphometry of nucleoli: potential usefulness for objective grading of clear cell renal cell carcinoma. Ultrastruct Pathol 2001;25:105–10.

15. Delahunt B, Cheville JC, Martignoni G, et al. The International Society of Urological Pathology (ISUP) grading system for renal cell carcinoma and other prognostic parameters. Am J Surg Pathol 2013;37:1490–504.

16. Kuroda N, Karashima T, Inoue K, et al. Review of renal cell carcinoma with rhabdoid features with focus on clinical and pathobiological aspects. Pol J Pathol 2015;66:3–8.

17. Przybycin CG, McKenney JK, Reynolds JP, et al. Rhabdoid differentiation is associated with aggressive behavior in renal cell carcinoma: a clinicopathologic analysis of 76 cases with clinical follow-up. Am J Surg Pathol 2014;38:1260–5.

18. Ito K, Yoshii H, Asakuma J, et al. Clinical impact of the presence of the worst nucleolar grade in renal cell carcinoma specimens. Jpn J Clin Oncol 2009;39:588–94.

19. Balzarini P, Dal Cin P, Roskams T, et al. Histology may depend on the presence of partial monosomy or partial trisomy 3 in renal cell carcinoma. Cancer Genet Cytogenet 1998;105:6–10.

20. Gunawan B, Huber W, Holtrup M, et al. Prognostic impacts of cytogenetic findings in clear cell renal cell carcinoma: gain of 5q31-qter predicts a distinct clinical phenotype with favorable prognosis. Cancer Res 2001;61:7731–8.

21. Brunelli M, Eccher A, Gobbo S, et al. Loss of chromosome 9p is an independent prognostic factor in patients with clear cell renal cell carcinoma. Mod Pathol 2008;21:1–6.

22. La Rochelle J, Klatte T, Dastane A, et al. Chromosome 9p deletions identify an aggressive phenotype of clear cell renal cell carcinoma. Cancer 2010;116:4696–702.

23. de Oliveira D, Dall'Oglio MF, Reis ST, et al. Chromosome 9p deletions are an independent predictor of tumor progression following nephrectomy in patients with localized clear cell renal cell carcinoma. Urol Oncol 2014;32:601–6.

24. Maher ER, Kaelin WG Jr. von Hippel-Lindau disease. Medicine (Baltimore) 1997;76:381–91.

25. Latif F, Tory K, Gnarra J, et al. Identification of the von Hippel-Lindau disease tumor suppressor gene. Science 1993;260:1317–20.

26. Kaelin WG Jr. The von Hippel-Lindau tumor suppressor gene and kidney cancer. Clin Cancer Res 2004;10:6290S–5S.

27. Kim WY, Kaelin WG. Role of VHL gene mutation in human cancer. J Clin Oncol 2004;22:4991–5004.

28. Beroukhim R, Brunet JP, Di Napoli A, et al. Patterns of gene expression and copy-number alterations in von-Hippel Lindau disease-associated and sporadic clear cell carcinoma of the kidney. Cancer Res 2009;69:4674–81.

29. Nickerson ML, Jaeger E, Shi Y, et al. Improved identification of von Hippel-Lindau gene alterations in clear cell renal tumors. Clin Cancer Res 2008;14:4726–34.

30. Gordan JD, Lal P, Dondeti VR, et al. HIF-alpha effects on c-Myc distinguish two subtypes of sporadic VHL-deficient clear cell renal carcinoma. Cancer Cell 2008;14:435–46.

31. Kaelin WG Jr. Treatment of kidney cancer: insights provided by the VHL tumor-suppressor protein. Cancer 2009;115:2262–72.

32. Linehan WM, Srinivasan R, Schmidt LS. The genetic basis of kidney cancer: a metabolic disease. Nat Rev Urol 2010;7:277–85.

33. Atkins MB, Choueiri TK, Cho D, et al. Treatment selection for patients with metastatic renal cell carcinoma. Cancer 2009;115:2327–33.

34. Choueiri TK, Bellmunt J. Sunitinib in renal-cell carcinoma: expanded indications. Lancet Oncol 2009;10:740.

35. Ward JE, Stadler WM. Pazopanib in renal cell carcinoma. Clin Cancer Res 2010;16:5923–7.

36. Choueiri TK, Vaziri SA, Jaeger E, et al. von Hippel-Lindau gene status and response to vascular endothelial growth factor targeted therapy for metastatic clear cell renal cell carcinoma. J Urol 2008;180: 860–5 [discussion: 865–6].

37. Choueiri TK, Regan MM, Rosenberg JE, et al. Carbonic anhydrase IX and pathological features as predictors of outcome in patients with metastatic clear-cell renal cell carcinoma receiving vascular endothelial growth factor-targeted therapy. BJU Int 2013;106:772–8.

38. Varela I, Tarpey P, Raine K, et al. Exome sequencing identifies frequent mutation of the SWI/SNF complex gene PBRM1 in renal carcinoma. Nature 2011;469:539–42.

39. Reisman D, Glaros S, Thompson EA. The SWI/SNF complex and cancer. Oncogene 2009;28:1653–68.

40. Creighton CJ, Morgan M, Gunaratne PH, et al and the Cancer Genome Atlas Research Network. Comprehensive molecular characterization of clear cell renal cell carcinoma. Nature 2013;499(7456): 43–9.

41. Peña-Llopis S, Vega-Rubín-de-Celis S, Liao A, et al. BAP1 loss defines a new class of renal cell carcinoma. Nat Genet 2012;44(7):751–9.

42. Dalgliesh GL, Furge K, Greenman C, et al. Systematic sequencing of renal carcinoma reveals inactivation of histone modifying genes. Nature 2010; 463(7279):360–3.

43. Gerlinger M, Rowan AJ, Horswell S, et al. Intratumor heterogeneity and branched evolution revealed by multiregion sequencing. N Engl J Med 2012;366(10):883–92.

44. Kucejova B, Peña-Llopis S, Yamasaki T, et al. Interplay between pVHL and mTORC1 pathways in clear-cell renal cell carcinoma. Mol Cancer Res 2011;9(9):1255–65.

45. Voss MH, Hakimi AA, Pham CG, et al. Tumor genetic analyses of patients with metastatic renal cell carcinoma and extended benefit from mTOR inhibitor therapy. Clin Cancer Res 2014;20(7): 1955–64.

46. Reuter VE, Argani P, Zhou M, et al. Best practices recommendations in the application of immunohistochemistry in the kidney tumors: report from the International Society of Urologic Pathology consensus conference. Am J Surg Pathol 2014;38:e35–49.

47. Tan PH, Cheng L, Rioux-Leclercq N, et al. Renal tumors: diagnostic and prognostic biomarkers. Am J Surg Pathol 2013;37:1518–31.

48. Genega EM, Ghebremichael M, Najarian R, et al. Carbonic anhydrase IX expression in renal neoplasms: correlation with tumor type and grade. Am J Clin Pathol 2010;134:873–9.

49. Aron M, Chang E, Herrera L, et al. Clear cell-papillary renal cell carcinoma of the kidney not associated with end-stage renal disease: clinicopathologic correlation with expanded immunophenotypic and molecular characterization of a large cohort with emphasis on relationship with renal angiomyoadenomatous tumor. Am J Surg Pathol 2015;39:873–88.

50. Williamson SR, Eble JN, Cheng L, et al. Clear cell papillary renal cell carcinoma: differential diagnosis and extended immunohistochemical profile. Mod Pathol 2013;26:697–708.

51. Alshenawy HA. Immunohistochemical panel for differentiating renal cell carcinoma with clear and papillary features. Pathol Oncol Res 2015;21: 893–9.

52. Kristiansen G, Delahunt B, Srigley JR, et al. Vancouver classification of renal tumors: recommendations of the 2012 consensus conference of the International Society of Urological Pathology (ISUP). Pathologe 2015;36:310–6.

53. Srigley JR, Delahunt B, Eble JN, et al. The International Society of Urological Pathology (ISUP) Vancouver classification of renal neoplasia. Am J Surg Pathol 2013;37:1469–89.

54. Kuroda N, Ohe C, Mikami S, et al. Multilocular cystic renal cell carcinoma with focus on clinical and pathobiological aspects. Histol Histopathol 2012;27:969–74.

55. Williamson SR, Halat S, Eble JN, et al. Multilocular cystic renal cell carcinoma: similarities and differences in immunoprofile compared with clear cell renal cell carcinoma. Am J Surg Pathol 2012;36: 1425–33.

56. Kuroda N, Tanaka A. Recent classification of renal epithelial tumors. Med Mol Morphol 2014;47:68–75.

57. Delahunt B, Srigley JR. The evolving classification of renal cell neoplasia. Semin Diagn Pathol 2015; 32:90–102.

58. Winters BR, Gore JL, Holt SK, et al. Cystic renal cell carcinoma carries an excellent prognosis regardless of tumor size. Urol Oncol 2015. [Epub ahead of print].

59. Aydin H, Chen L, Cheng L, et al. Clear cell tubulopapillary renal cell carcinoma: a study of 36 distinctive low-grade epithelial tumors of the kidney. Am J Surg Pathol 2010;34:1608–21.

60. Deml KF, Schildhaus HU, Comperat E, et al. Clear cell papillary renal cell carcinoma and renal angiomyoadenomatous tumor: two variants of a morphologic, immunohistochemical, and genetic distinct entity of renal cell carcinoma. Am J Surg Pathol 2015;39:889–901.

61. Gobbo S, Eble JN, Grignon DJ, et al. Clear cell papillary renal cell carcinoma: a distinct

histopathologic and molecular genetic entity. Am J Surg Pathol 2008;32:1239–45.

62. Hakimi AA, Tickoo SK, Jacobsen A, et al. TCEB1-mutated renal cell carcinoma: a distinct genomic and morphological subtype. Mod Pathol 2015;28: 845–53.

63. Hirsch MS, Barletta J, Gorman M, et al. Renal cell carcinoma with monosomy 8 and CAIX expression: a distinct entity or another member or the clear cell tubulopapillary RCC/RAT family? Mod Pathol 2015; 28(s2):229A.

64. Gobbo S, Eble JN, Maclennan GT, et al. Renal cell carcinomas with papillary architecture and clear cell components: the utility of immunohistochemical and cytogenetical analyses in differential diagnosis. Am J Surg Pathol 2008;32:1780–6.

65. Ross H, Martignoni G, Argani P. Renal cell carcinoma with clear cell and papillary features. Arch Pathol Lab Med 2012;136:391–9.

66. Komai Y, Fujiwara M, Fujii Y, et al. Adult Xp11 translocation renal cell carcinoma diagnosed by cytogenetics and immunohistochemistry. Clin Cancer Res 2009;15:1170–6.

67. Argani P, Hicks J, De Marzo AM, et al. Xp11 translocation renal cell carcinoma (RCC): extended immunohistochemical profile emphasizing novel RCC markers. Am J Surg Pathol 2010;34: 1295–303.

68. Green WM, Yonescu R, Morsberger L, et al. Utilization of a TFE3 break-apart FISH assay in a renal tumor consultation service. Am J Surg Pathol 2013; 37:1150–63.

69. Mosquera JM, Dal Cin P, Mertz KD, et al. Validation of a TFE3 break-apart FISH assay for Xp11.2 translocation renal cell carcinomas. Diagn Mol Pathol 2011;20:129–37.

70. Kryvenko ON, Jorda M, Argani P, et al. Diagnostic approach to eosinophilic renal neoplasms. Arch Pathol Lab Med 2014;138:1531–41.

71. Kuroda N, Tanaka A, Ohe C, et al. Recent advances of immunohistochemistry for diagnosis of renal tumors. Pathol Int 2013;63:381–90.

72. Delahunt B, Eble JN. Papillary renal cell carcinoma: a clinicopathologic and immunohistochemical study of 105 tumors. Mod Pathol 1997;10: 537–44.

73. Gunawan B, von Heydebreck A, Fritsch T, et al. Cytogenetic and morphologic typing of 58 papillary renal cell carcinomas: evidence for a cytogenetic evolution of type 2 from type 1 tumors. Cancer Res 2003;63:6200–5.

74. Schmidt L, Duh FM, Chen F, et al. Germline and somatic mutations in the tyrosine kinase domain of the MET proto-oncogene in papillary renal carcinomas. Nat Genet 1997;16:68–73.

75. Zbar B, Tory K, Merino M, et al. Hereditary papillary renal cell carcinoma. J Urol 1994;151:561–6.

76. Zhuang Z, Park WS, Pack S, et al. Trisomy 7-harbouring non-random duplication of the mutant MET allele in hereditary papillary renal carcinomas. Nat Genet 1998;20:66–9.

77. Schmidt L, Junker K, Nakaigawa N, et al. Novel mutations of the MET proto-oncogene in papillary renal carcinomas. Oncogene 1999;18:2343–50.

78. Weidner KM, Sachs M, Birchmeier W. The Met receptor tyrosine kinase transduces motility, proliferation, and morphogenic signals of scatter factor/hepatocyte growth factor in epithelial cells. J Cell Biol 1993;121:145–54.

79. Jeffers M, Fiscella M, Webb CP, et al. The mutationally activated Met receptor mediates motility and metastasis. Proc Natl Acad Sci U S A 1998;95: 14417–22.

80. Giubellino A, Linehan WM, Bottaro DP. Targeting the Met signaling pathway in renal cancer. Expert Rev Anticancer Ther 2009;9:785–93.

81. Launonen V, Vierimaa O, Kiuru M, et al. Inherited susceptibility to uterine leiomyomas and renal cell cancer. Proc Natl Acad Sci U S A 2001;98: 3387–92.

82. Merino MJ, Torres-Cabala C, Pinto P, et al. The morphologic spectrum of kidney tumors in hereditary leiomyomatosis and renal cell carcinoma (HLRCC) syndrome. Am J Surg Pathol 2007;31:1578–85.

83. Gardie B, Remenieras A, Kattygnarath D, et al. Novel FH mutations in families with hereditary leiomyomatosis and renal cell cancer (HLRCC) and patients with isolated type 2 papillary renal cell carcinoma. J Med Genet 2011;48:226–34.

84. Sudarshan S, Sourbier C, Kong HS, et al. Fumarate hydratase deficiency in renal cancer induces glycolytic addiction and hypoxia-inducible transcription factor 1alpha stabilization by glucose-dependent generation of reactive oxygen species. Mol Cell Biol 2009;29:4080–90.

85. Choueiri TK, Cheville J, Palescandolo E, et al. BRAF mutations in metanephric adenoma of the kidney. Eur Urol 2012;62:917–22.

86. Pinto A, Signoretti S, Hirsch MS, et al. Immunohistochemical staining for BRAF V600E supports the diagnosis of metanephric adenoma. Histopathology 2015;66:901–4.

87. Klatte T, Pantuck AJ, Said JW, et al. Cytogenetic and molecular tumor profiling for type 1 and type 2 papillary renal cell carcinoma. Clin Cancer Res 2009;15:1162–9.

88. Dal Cin P. Genetics in renal cell carcinoma. Curr Opin Urol 2003;13:463–6.

89. Cossu-Rocca P, Eble JN, Delahunt B, et al. Renal mucinous tubular and spindle carcinoma lacks the gains of chromosomes 7 and 17 and losses of chromosome Y that are prevalent in papillary renal cell carcinoma. Mod Pathol 2006;19: 488–93.

90. Amin MB, Epstein JI, Ulbright TM, et al. Best practices recommendations in the application of immunohistochemistry in urologic pathology: report from the International Society of Urological Pathology consensus conference. Am J Surg Pathol 2014; 38:1017–22.

91. Rohan SM, Xiao Y, Liang Y, et al. Clear-cell papillary renal cell carcinoma: molecular and immunohistochemical analysis with emphasis on the von Hippel-Lindau gene and hypoxia-inducible factor pathway-related proteins. Mod Pathol 2011;24: 1207–20.

92. Ferlicot S, Allory Y, Comperat E, et al. Mucinous tubular and spindle cell carcinoma: a report of 15 cases and a review of the literature. Virchows Arch 2005;447:978–83.

93. Srigley JR, Delahunt B. Uncommon and recently described renal carcinomas. Mod Pathol 2009; 22(Suppl 2):S2–23.

94. Chen YB, Brannon AR, Toubaji A, et al. Hereditary leiomyomatosis and renal cell carcinoma syndrome-associated renal cancer: recognition of the syndrome by pathologic features and the utility of detecting aberrant succination by immunohistochemistry. Am J Surg Pathol 2014;38: 627–37.

95. Kiuru M, Launonen V. Hereditary leiomyomatosis and renal cell cancer (HLRCC). Curr Mol Med 2004;4:869–75.

96. Fuzesi L, Cober M, Mittermayer C. Collecting duct carcinoma: cytogenetic characterization. Histopathology 1992;21:155–60.

97. Becker F, Junker K, Parr M, et al. Collecting duct carcinomas represent a unique tumor entity based on genetic alterations. PLoS One 2013;8: e78137.

98. Antonelli A, Portesi E, Cozzoli A, et al. The collecting duct carcinoma of the kidney: a cytogenetical study. Eur Urol 2003;43:680–5.

99. Przybycin CG, Cronin AM, Darvishian F, et al. Chromophobe renal cell carcinoma: a clinicopathologic study of 203 tumors in 200 patients with primary resection at a single institution. Am J Surg Pathol 2011;35:962–70.

100. Amin MB, Paner GP, Alvarado-Cabrero I, et al. Chromophobe renal cell carcinoma: histomorphologic characteristics and evaluation of conventional pathologic prognostic parameters in 145 cases. Am J Surg Pathol 2008;32:1822–34.

101. Klomp JA, Petillo D, Niemi NM, et al. Birt-Hogg-Dube renal tumors are genetically distinct from other renal neoplasias and are associated with up-regulation of mitochondrial gene expression. BMC Med Genomics 2010;3:59.

102. Pavlovich CP, Walther MM, Eyler RA, et al. Renal tumors in the Birt-Hogg-Dube syndrome. Am J Surg Pathol 2002;26:1542–52.

103. Lauer SR, Zhou M, Master VA, et al. Chromophobe renal cell carcinoma with sarcomatoid differentiation: a clinicopathologic study of 14 cases. Anal Quant Cytopathol Histpathol 2013; 35:77–84.

104. Cheville JC, Lohse CM, Sukov WR, et al. Chromophobe renal cell carcinoma: the impact of tumor grade on outcome. Am J Surg Pathol 2012;36: 851–6.

105. Gong Y, Sun X, Haines GK 3rd, et al. Renal cell carcinoma, chromophobe type, with collecting duct carcinoma and sarcomatoid components. Arch Pathol Lab Med 2003;127:e38–40.

106. Delahunt B, Egevad L, Samaratunga H, et al. Gleason and Fuhrman no longer make the grade. Histopathology 2015. [Epub ahead of print].

107. Delahunt B. Advances and controversies in grading and staging of renal cell carcinoma. Mod Pathol 2009;22(Suppl 2):S24–36.

108. Delahunt B, Sika-Paotonu D, Bethwaite PB, et al. Fuhrman grading is not appropriate for chromophobe renal cell carcinoma. Am J Surg Pathol 2007;31:957–60.

109. Paner GP, Amin MB, Alvarado-Cabrero I, et al. A novel tumor grading scheme for chromophobe renal cell carcinoma: prognostic utility and comparison with Fuhrman nuclear grade. Am J Surg Pathol 2010;34:1233–40.

110. Coulson H, Dal Cin P, Choueiri TK, et al. Chromophobe renal Cell carcinoma – A simplified and reproducible two tier approach to tumor grading. Mod Pathol 2015;28(s2):213A.

111. Yusenko MV, Kuiper RP, Boethe T, et al. High-resolution DNA copy number and gene expression analyses distinguish chromophobe renal cell carcinomas and renal oncocytomas. BMC Cancer 2009;9:152.

112. Rathmell KW, Chen F, Creighton CJ. Genomics of chromophobe renal cell carcinoma: implications from a rare tumor for pan-cancer studies. Oncoscience 2015;2:81–90.

113. Pavlovich CP, Grubb RL 3rd, Hurley K, et al. Evaluation and management of renal tumors in the Birt-Hogg-Dube syndrome. J Urol 2005;173: 1482–6.

114. Schmidt LS, Linehan WM. Molecular genetics and clinical features of Birt-Hogg-Dube syndrome. Nat Rev Urol 2015;12(10):558–69.

115. Nickerson ML, Warren MB, Toro JR, et al. Mutations in a novel gene lead to kidney tumors, lung wall defects, and benign tumors of the hair follicle in patients with the Birt-Hogg-Dube syndrome. Cancer Cell 2002;2:157–64.

116. Conner JR, Hirsch MS, Jo VY. HNF1beta and S100A1 are useful biomarkers for distinguishing renal oncocytoma and chromophobe renal cell carcinoma in FNA and core needle biopsies. Cancer Cytopathol 2015;123:298–305.

117. Kuroda N, Kanomata N, Yamaguchi T, et al. Immunohistochemical application of S100A1 in renal oncocytoma, oncocytic papillary renal cell carcinoma, and two variants of chromophobe renal cell carcinoma. Med Mol Morphol 2011;44: 111–5.

118. Li G, Barthelemy A, Feng G, et al. S100A1: a powerful marker to differentiate chromophobe renal cell carcinoma from renal oncocytoma. Histopathology 2007;50:642–7.

119. Gill AJ, Hes O, Papathomas T, et al. Succinate dehydrogenase (SDH)-deficient renal carcinoma: a morphologically distinct entity: a clinicopathologic series of 36 tumors from 27 patients. Am J Surg Pathol 2015;38:1588–602.

120. Williamson SR, Eble JN, Amin MB, et al. Succinate dehydrogenase-deficient renal cell carcinoma: detailed characterization of 11 tumors defining a unique subtype of renal cell carcinoma. Mod Pathol 2015;28:80–94.

121. Pan CC, Jong YJ, Chai CY, et al. Comparative genomic hybridization study of perivascular epithelioid cell tumor: molecular genetic evidence of perivascular epithelioid cell tumor as a distinctive neoplasm. Hum Pathol 2006;37:606–12.

122. Brandal P, Lie AK, Bassarova A, et al. Genomic aberrations in mucinous tubular and spindle cell renal cell carcinomas. Mod Pathol 2006;19:186–94.

123. Argani P, Olgac S, Tickoo SK, et al. Xp11 translocation renal cell carcinoma in adults: expanded clinical, pathologic, and genetic spectrum. Am J Surg Pathol 2007;31:1149–60.

124. Argani P. MiT family translocation renal cell carcinoma. Semin Diagn Pathol 2015;32:103–13.

125. Ellis CL, Eble JN, Subhawong AP, et al. Clinical heterogeneity of Xp11 translocation renal cell carcinoma: impact of fusion subtype, age, and stage. Mod Pathol 2014;27:875–86.

126. Argani P, Ladanyi M. The evolving story of renal translocation carcinomas. Am J Clin Pathol 2006; 126:332–4.

127. Huang W, Goldfischer M, Babyeva S, et al. Identification of a novel PARP14-TFE3 gene fusion from 10-year-old FFPE tissue by RNA-seq. Genes Chromosomes Cancer 2015. [Epub ahead of print].

128. Kuroda N, Mikami S, Pan CC, et al. Review of renal carcinoma associated with Xp11.2 translocations/TFE3 gene fusions with focus on pathobiological aspect. Histol Histopathol 2012;27:133–40.

129. Ross H, Argani P. Xp11 translocation renal cell carcinoma. Pathology 2010;42:369–73.

130. Bruder E, Passera O, Harms D, et al. Morphologic and molecular characterization of renal cell carcinoma in children and young adults. Am J Surg Pathol 2004;28:1117–32.

131. Meyer PN, Clark JI, Flanigan RC, et al. Xp11.2 translocation renal cell carcinoma with very aggressive course in five adults. Am J Clin Pathol 2007;128:70–9.

132. Komai Y, Fujii Y, Iimura Y, et al. Young age as favorable prognostic factor for cancer-specific survival in localized renal cell carcinoma. Urology 2011; 77:842–7.

133. Perlman EJ. Pediatric renal cell carcinoma. Surg Pathol Clin 2010;3:641–51.

134. Ramphal R, Pappo A, Zielenska M, et al. Pediatric renal cell carcinoma: clinical, pathologic, and molecular abnormalities associated with the members of the MiT transcription factor family. Am J Clin Pathol 2006;126:349–64.

135. Argani P, Antonescu CR, Illei PB, et al. Primary renal neoplasms with the ASPL-TFE3 gene fusion of alveolar soft part sarcoma: a distinctive tumor entity previously included among renal cell carcinomas of children and adolescents. Am J Pathol 2001;159:179–92.

136. Argani P, Yonescu R, Morsberger L, et al. Molecular confirmation of t(6;11)(p21;q12) renal cell carcinoma in archival paraffin-embedded material using a break-apart TFEB FISH assay expands its clinicopathologic spectrum. Am J Surg Pathol 2012; 36:1516–26.

137. Martignoni G, Pea M, Gobbo S, et al. Cathepsin-K immunoreactivity distinguishes MiTF/TFE family renal translocation carcinomas from other renal carcinomas. Mod Pathol 2009;22:1016–22.

138. Davis IJ, Fisher DE. MiT transcription factor associated malignancies in man. Cell Cycle 2007;6: 1724–9.

139. Argani P, Lui MY, Couturier J, et al. A novel CLTC-TFE3 gene fusion in pediatric renal adenocarcinoma with t(X;17)(p11.2;q23). Oncogene 2003;22:5374–8.

140. Clark J, Lu YJ, Sidhar SK, et al. Fusion of splicing factor genes PSF and NonO (p54nrb) to the TFE3 gene in papillary renal cell carcinoma. Oncogene 1997;15:2233–9.

141. Weterman MA, Wilbrink M, Geurts van Kessel A. Fusion of the transcription factor TFE3 gene to a novel gene, PRCC, in t(X;1)(p11;q21)-positive papillary renal cell carcinomas. Proc Natl Acad Sci U S A 1996;93:15294–8.

142. Tsuda M, Davis IJ, Argani P, et al. TFE3 fusions activate MET signaling by transcriptional up-regulation, defining another class of tumors as candidates for therapeutic MET inhibition. Cancer Res 2007;67: 919–29.

143. Shen SS, Ro JY, Tamboli P, et al. Mucinous tubular and spindle cell carcinoma of kidney is probably a variant of papillary renal cell carcinoma with spindle cell features. Ann Diagn Pathol 2007;11:13–21.

144. MacLennan GT, Farrow GM, Bostwick DG. Low-grade collecting duct carcinoma of the kidney: report of 13 cases of low-grade mucinous

tubulocystic renal carcinoma of possible collecting duct origin. Urology 1997;50:679–84.

145. Rakozy C, Schmahl GE, Bogner S, et al. Low-grade tubular-mucinous renal neoplasms: morphologic, immunohistochemical, and genetic features. Mod Pathol 2002;15:1162–71.

146. Dhillon J, Amin MB, Selbs E, et al. Mucinous tubular and spindle cell carcinoma of the kidney with sarcomatoid change. Am J Surg Pathol 2009;33:44–9.

147. Fine SW, Argani P, DeMarzo AM, et al. Expanding the histologic spectrum of mucinous tubular and spindle cell carcinoma of the kidney. Am J Surg Pathol 2006;30:1554–60.

148. Crumley SM, Divatia M, Truong L, et al. Renal cell carcinoma: evolving and emerging subtypes. World J Clin Cases 2013;1:262–75.

149. Kuroda N, Hes O, Michal M, et al. Mucinous tubular and spindle cell carcinoma with Fuhrman nuclear grade 3: a histological, immunohistochemical, ultrastructural and FISH study. Histol Histopathol 2008;23:1517–23.

150. Kuroda N, Toi M, Hiroi M, et al. Review of papillary renal cell carcinoma with focus on clinical and pathobiological aspects. Histol Histopathol 2003; 18:487–94.

151. Dal Cin P, Espinet B, Galeote M, et al. Expanding genetic and molecular findings in mucinous tubular and spindle cell carcinoma. Mod Pathol 2015; 28(s2):214A.

152. Weber A, Srigley J, Moch H. Mucinous spindle cell carcinoma of the kidney. A molecular analysis. Pathologe 2003;24:453–9.

153. Kuroda N, Naroda T, Tamura M, et al. High-grade mucinous tubular and spindle cell carcinoma: comparative genomic hybridization study. Ann Diagn Pathol 2011;15:472–5.

154. Argani P, Netto GJ, Parwani AV. Papillary renal cell carcinoma with low-grade spindle cell foci: a mimic of mucinous tubular and spindle cell carcinoma. Am J Surg Pathol 2008;32:1353–9.

155. Brunelli M, Gobbo S, Cossu-Rocca P, et al. Fluorescent cytogenetics of renal cell neoplasms. Pathologica 2008;100:454–60.

156. Lopez-Beltran A, Kirkali Z, Montironi R, et al. Unclassified renal cell carcinoma: a report of 56 cases. BJU Int 2012;110:786–93.

157. Shuch B, Bratslavsky G, Shih J, et al. Impact of pathological tumour characteristics in patients with sarcomatoid renal cell carcinoma. BJU Int 2012;109:1600–6.

158. Albadine R, Schultz L, Illei P, et al. PAX8 (+)/p63 (-) immunostaining pattern in renal collecting duct carcinoma (CDC): a useful immunoprofile in the differential diagnosis of CDC versus urothelial carcinoma of upper urinary tract. Am J Surg Pathol 2010;34:965–9.

159. Carvalho JC, Thomas DG, McHugh JB, et al. p63, CK7, PAX8 and INI-1: an optimal immunohistochemical panel to distinguish poorly differentiated urothelial cell carcinoma from high-grade tumours of the renal collecting system. Histopathology 2012;60:597–608.

160. Laury AR, Perets R, Piao H, et al. A comprehensive analysis of PAX8 expression in human epithelial tumors. Am J Surg Pathol 2011;35:816–26.

161. Tong GX, Yu WM, Beaubier NT, et al. Expression of PAX8 in normal and neoplastic renal tissues: an immunohistochemical study. Mod Pathol 2009;22:1218–27.

162. Gonzalez-Roibon N, Albadine R, Sharma R, et al. The role of GATA binding protein 3 in the differential diagnosis of collecting duct and upper tract urothelial carcinomas. Hum Pathol 2013;44:2651–7.

163. Swartz MA, Karth J, Schneider DT, et al. Renal medullary carcinoma: clinical, pathologic, immunohistochemical, and genetic analysis with pathogenetic implications. Urology 2002;60:1083–9.

164. Agaimy A. The expanding family of SMARCB1(INI1)-deficient neoplasia: implications of phenotypic, biological, and molecular heterogeneity. Adv Anat Pathol 2014;21:394–410.

165. Wesche WA, Wilimas J, Khare V, et al. Renal medullary carcinoma: a potential sickle cell nephropathy of children and adolescents. Pediatr Pathol Lab Med 1998;18:97–113.

166. Elwood H, Chaux A, Schultz L, et al. Immunohistochemical analysis of SMARCB1/INI-1 expression in collecting duct carcinoma. Urology 2011;78:474.e1–5.

167. Rao P, Tannir NM, Tamboli P. Expression of OCT3/4 in renal medullary carcinoma represents a potential diagnostic pitfall. Am J Surg Pathol 2012;36:583–8.

168. Amin MB, Smith SC, Agaimy A, et al. Collecting duct carcinoma versus renal medullary carcinoma: an appeal for nosologic and biological clarity. Am J Surg Pathol 2015;38:871–4.

169. Cavazzana AO, Prayer-Galetti T, Tirabosco R, et al. Bellini duct carcinoma. A clinical and in vitro study. Eur Urol 1996;30:340–4.

170. Gregori-Romero MA, Morell-Quadreny L, Llombart-Bosch A. Cytogenetic analysis of three primary Bellini duct carcinomas. Genes Chromosomes Cancer 1996;15:170–2.

# Emerging Entities in Renal Neoplasia

Rohit Mehra, MD[a], Steven C. Smith, MD[b], Mukul Divatia, MD[b], Mahul B. Amin, MD[b,*]

## KEYWORDS

- Renal cell carcinoma • Tubulocystic • Translocation • Acquired cystic disease
- Thyroid-like follicular • Hereditary • Leiomyomatosis

## ABSTRACT

This article reviews emerging entities in renal epithelial neoplasia, including tubulocystic carcinoma, clear-cell–papillary renal cell carcinoma (RCC), thyroid-like follicular RCC, ALK-related RCC, translocation RCC, acquired cystic disease–related RCC, succinate dehydrogenase–deficient RCC, and hereditary leiomyomatosis-RCC syndrome–associated RCC. Many of these rarer subtypes of RCC were recently studied in more depth and are included in the upcoming version of the World Health Organization classification of tumors. Emphasis is placed on common gross and morphologic features, differential diagnoses, use of ancillary studies for making accurate diagnoses, molecular alterations, and predicted biologic behavior based on previous studies.

clinicopathologic features of these unique tumors in 2009.[2,3] Tubulocystic carcinomas are an invariably well-circumscribed subtype of RCC and, as the name suggests, demonstrate a pure tubular and cystic architectural growth pattern. These tumors occur in adults across a wide age range (mean age = 54 years) and show a strong male preponderance (male:female ratio = 7:1). Most tubulocystic carcinomas present in an asymptomatic fashion; however, a subset may present with hematuria or abdominal discomfort. The overall literature describing the clinicopathologic and biological features of these tumors is sparse, and studies addressing its underlying molecular pathogenesis are even more limited.

## TUBULOCYSTIC CARCINOMA

### INTRODUCTION

In 1956, Pierre Masson described a cystic neoplasm of the kidney with hobnail cells in the central region of the kidney that he designated as Bellinien epithelioma or carcinoma of Bellini (collecting) duct. Examples of this distinctive tubulocystic neoplasm were more recently recognized by Dr George Farrow in the third series of the Armed Forces Institute of Pathology fascicle and were designated as "renal cell carcinoma, collecting duct type." The term tubulocystic carcinoma was first coined in 2004 by Amin and colleagues[1] to separate this tumor from collecting duct carcinoma; subsequently they described the detailed

### GROSS FEATURES

Tubulocystic carcinoma is invariably well circumscribed and demonstrates multiple cystic spaces of variable size, containing clear serous fluid, which imparts a spongy or "bubble wrap" appearance (**Fig. 1**).[1] More than half of these tumors arise in a subcapsular location, with the rest being cortico-medullary or medullary. Although most tubulocystic carcinomas measure 2 cm or less (mean size = 4.2 cm), tumors up to 17 cm in greatest dimension have been reported in the literature.

### MICROSCOPIC FEATURES

Tubulocystic carcinoma demonstrates a distinctive histology composed of variably sized tubules and cysts, lined by a single layer of cuboidal to flat eosinophilic epithelial cells and embedded in a fibrotic stroma (**Fig. 2**). In some areas, the lining

[a] Department of Pathology, University of Michigan Hospital and Health Systems, 1500, East Medical Center Drive, Ann Arbor, MI 48109, USA; [b] Department of Pathology & Laboratory Medicine, Cedars-Sinai Medical Center, 8700 Beverly Boulevard, Los Angeles, CA 90048, USA
* Corresponding author. Department of Pathology & Laboratory Medicine, Cedars-Sinai Medical Center, 8700 Beverly Boulevard, S. Tower Suite 8707, Los Angeles, CA 90048.
*E-mail address:* mahul.amin@cshs.org

Surgical Pathology 8 (2015) 623–656
http://dx.doi.org/10.1016/j.path.2015.08.004
1875-9181/15/$ – see front matter © 2015 Elsevier Inc. All rights reserved.

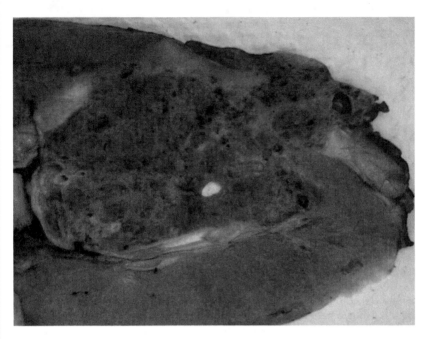

*Fig. 1.* Macroscopic image of tubulocystic carcinoma demonstrating a spongy cut surface with cysts of varying sizes.

epithelial cells might exhibit a hobnail appearance; however, cellular stratification and papillations are uncommon or very focal (**Fig. 3**). The cell nuclei are often large and have irregular nuclear membranes and prominent nucleoli, which are reminiscent of Fuhrman nuclear grade 3 tumors (**Fig. 4**). However, mitotic activity is generally low, and necrosis is only rarely present.[1]

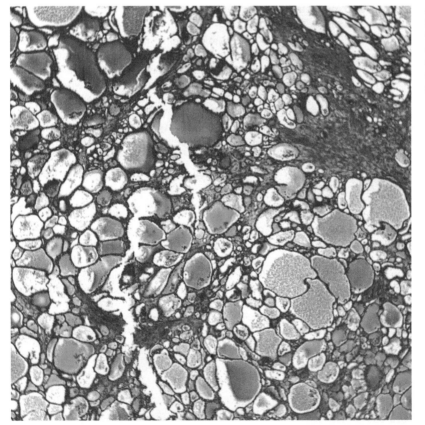

*Fig. 2.* Tubulocystic carcinoma with its characteristic histologic appearance of variably sized tubules and cysts (hematoxylin-eosin [H&E], original magnification ×10).

*Fig. 3.* Tubulocystic carcinoma showing tubules and cysts lined by a single layer of cuboidal to flat eosinophilic tumor cells exhibiting a hobnail appearance focally with surrounding fibrotic stroma (H&E, original magnification ×20).

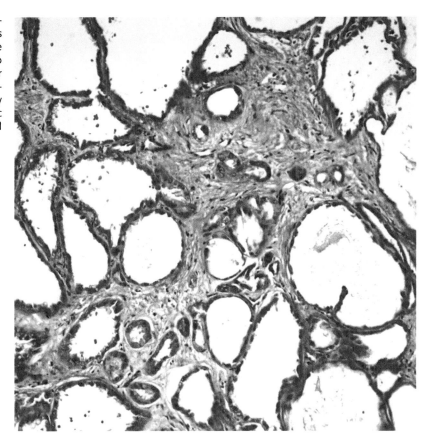

## DIFFERENTIAL DIAGNOSIS

The differential diagnosis for tubulocystic carcinoma includes other renal tumors that might exhibit a prominent tubular and cystic growth pattern, including mixed epithelial and stromal tumor (MEST, or cystic nephroma; see also Arias-Stella and Williamson, Updates in Benign Lesions of the Genitourinary Tract, Surgical Pathology Clinics, 2015, Volume 8, Issue 4), multilocular cystic renal tumor of low malignant potential (formerly multilocular RCC), and oncocytoma. MEST shows greater variability in size and shape of cysts and contains a variable, often solid, component histologically represented by ovarian or fibrotic stroma. In contrast to tubulocystic carcinoma, MEST shows a striking female preponderance. Multilocular cystic renal tumor of low malignant potential demonstrates a multicystic architecture with variably sized cystic spaces lined by flattened to cuboidal clear cells akin to those found in conventional (clear-cell) RCC. The presence of groups of clear cells within the fibrous septae is a defining characteristic for this entity, and the nuclei generally exhibit Fuhrman nuclear grade

1 or 2 features. An exclusive tubulocystic architecture is uncommon in renal oncocytoma, and, when present, the tubules are typically uniformly small. Additionally, nuclei of renal oncocytoma, in contrast to tubulocystic carcinoma, demonstrate round nuclei with evenly dispersed chromatin spread and occasionally prominent small nucleoli. In addition, the stroma of renal oncocytomas is often hypocellular and edematous, as opposed to the more fibrotic stroma seen in tubulocystic carcinoma. Rarely, translocation-associated RCC might present with tubular features and eosinophilic cells; however, these tumors more commonly occur in young adults and are associated with underexpression of cytokeratins. In these cases, rearrangements involving the *TFE3* or *TFEB* genes can be detected by fluorescence in situ hybridization.[4–7] Finally, a tubulocystic pattern may be seen in hereditary leiomyomatosis and RCC-associated RCC (HLRCC-associated RCC), although this pattern is focal and not always present in these rare and recently described tumors.[8] Cases described as dedifferentiated tubulocystic carcinoma likely represent HLRCC-associated RCC.[9]

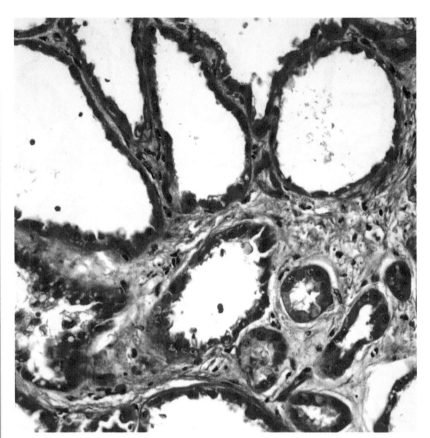

*Fig. 4.* High-power view of tubulocystic carcinoma with tumor cells demonstrating irregular nuclear membranes and prominent nucleoli (H&E, original magnification ×40).

## MOLECULAR PATHOGENESIS, IMMUNOHISTOCHEMISTRY, AND DIAGNOSIS

Radiologically, tubulocystic carcinoma may present as a Bosniak type II, type III, or type IV cystic mass and, therefore, may pose a clinical diagnostic dilemma because of significant radiologic overlap with other benign or malignant renal entities. The salient pathologic features that might contribute to reaching a diagnosis of tubulocystic RCC include a "bubble wrap" gross appearance and histologic features including variably sized cysts and tubules lined by hobnail cells with eosinophilic cytoplasm and enlarged nuclei with irregular nuclear membranes and prominent nucleoli. The intervening stroma is often fibrotic. Exclusion of other entities in the differential diagnosis can generally be performed on the basis of clinicopathologic features, as described in the previous paragraph.

Although the histogenetic relationship between tubulocystic carcinoma and collecting duct carcinoma is still largely unresolved, recent gene expression profiling data support the idea that tubulocystic carcinoma is a distinct entity from collecting duct carcinoma.[10] Finally, in a subset of cases in the literature, tubulocystic carcinoma has been reported in association with papillary RCC, and these tumors might share similar recurrent cytogenetic alterations involving chromosomes 7, 17, and Y.[11] In addition, based on recent gene expression profiling data, tubulocystic carcinoma is closely related to papillary RCC (and different from collecting duct carcinoma),[12] although the significance of these findings remains a subject of future studies.

No ancillary immunohistochemical or molecular tools are currently available for absolute confirmation of a diagnosis of tubulocystic carcinoma; however, in the correct clinicopathologic and histologic contexts, positive expression of CK7, alpha-methylacyl-CoA racemase (AMACR), and CD10 is supportive of this diagnosis.

## PROGNOSIS

Tubulocystic carcinoma demonstrates indolent behavior with a low but definite risk of metastatic dissemination. Metastatic sites include bone and liver (Fig. 5). A single case of tubulocystic carcinoma with sarcomatoid features has been reported.[13] The overall recurrence and metastatic rate is, however, considered to be less than 10% for these tumors.[2] Of note, most tubulocystic

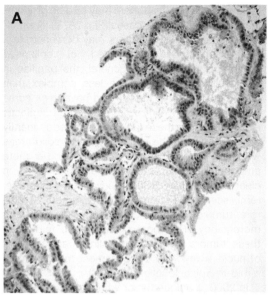
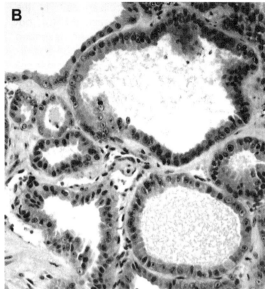

*Fig. 5.* (*A, B*) Metastatic tubulocystic carcinoma of the kidney in a core biopsy from the liver (H&E, original magnification ×10 [*A*] and ×20 [*B*]).

carcinomas demonstrate Fuhrman nuclear grade 3 features; however, this nuclear grading system does not seem to be prognostic for these tumors.

The histogenesis of tubulocystic carcinoma remains uncertain. Electron microscopy has demonstrated features of both proximal convoluted tubules and collecting ducts of the kidney.[1] Because of the rarity of this tumor and lack of associated intensive molecular studies, no established therapeutic guidelines beyond surgery are currently formulated for the management of tubulocystic RCC.

**Pathologic Key Feature**

1. Tubulocystic carcinomas are mostly detected incidentally, and most are low stage at the time of resection.

2. Grossly, tubulocystic carcinomas are well circumscribed and have a spongy or "bubble wrap" appearance.

3. Microscopically, tubulocystic carcinomas demonstrate exclusively tubular and cystic growth patterns and are composed of cells with eosinophilic cytoplasm and large nuclei with irregular membranes and prominent nucleoli; a fibrotic stroma is characteristic.

4. Most tubulocystic carcinomas have a good prognosis; however, a small subset might demonstrate an aggressive clinical course.

**Differential Diagnosis**

1. Cystic nephroma/MEST: These tumors are multicystic with ovarian-type stroma and demonstrate low-grade nuclei.

2. Multilocular cystic neoplasm of low malignant potential: These tumors are multicystic but are lined by clear cells with low-grade nuclei and, characteristically, have nests of clear cells within the fibrous septae.

3. Renal oncocytoma: These tumors might rarely demonstrate a predominantly tubular and cystic morphologic appearance; however, in contrast to tubulocystic carcinoma, the stroma is usually hypocellular and edematous.

4. Translocation-associated RCC: These tumors, in contrast to tubulocystic carcinoma, often occur in children and young adults and are associated with gene rearrangements involving *TFE3* or *TFEB*.

## CLEAR-CELL–PAPILLARY RENAL CELL CARCINOMA/RENAL ANGIOMYODENOMATOUS TUMOR CATEGORY OF TUMORS

### INTRODUCTION

Clear-cell–papillary RCC (also referred to by some as "clear-cell tubulopapillary RCC") was initially described by Tickoo and colleagues[14] in the setting of end-stage renal disease (ESRD), but subsequently these tumors have been described in patients without ESRD as well.[15–17] Clear-cell–papillary RCC demonstrates exquisite clear-cell cytology with low-grade nuclei that are aligned away from the basement membrane in a linear arrangement, which imparts a distinct morphologic appearance. These tumors have a male predominance (male-to-female ratio of 2:1), and most patients with clear-cell–papillary RCC occur in a sporadic setting and have adequate renal function. Current data indicate that clear-cell–papillary RCC is a distinct molecular entity from other renal neoplasia, including clear-cell (conventional) RCC and papillary RCC, although its exact molecular underpinnings have yet to be elucidated.

## GROSS FEATURES

Clear-cell–papillary RCCs are generally well circumscribed and may be encapsulated. They often demonstrate a partial to predominantly cystic appearance, although a subset of these tumors may form purely solid masses[16] (Fig. 6).

## MICROSCOPIC FEATURES

Similar to the gross appearance, clear-cell–papillary RCCs usually show a combination of cystic and solid growth patterns. As the name suggests, areas with papillary architecture are present in most of these tumors, although this finding may be very focal in some cases and conspicuous in others. The growth pattern may also be predominantly tubular in some cases (Fig. 7A, B). A significant subset of these tumors may demonstrate a solid appearance composed of collapsed papillae/tubules/acini. In general, the papillae in clear-cell–papillary RCC are less complex than other papillary renal tumors and have thick cores with cellular to hyalinized stroma. The neoplastic epithelial cells in these tumors have predominantly clear cytoplasm, the exception being solid areas where cytoplasm is scant and may be more amphophilic in character. The nuclei seen in clear-cell–papillary RCC are invariably low-grade, reminiscent of Fuhrman nuclear grade 2. Only rare tumors exhibit Fuhrman nuclear grade 3 morphology. The most characteristic feature of these tumors, however, is a linear arrangement of nuclei away from the basement membrane, in a mid-to-apical location (Fig. 7C).

In 2000, a unique tumor with intermixture of an epithelial component and smooth muscle–rich angioleiomyomatous stroma was designated as a benign neoplasm called renal angiomyoadenomatous tumor (RAT) (Figs. 8 and 9).[18,19] Recent studies show that RAT and clear-cell–papillary RCC belong to the same category of tumors due to the overlapping epithelial morphology and immunohistochemical profile. Clear-cell–papillary RCC may have variable smooth muscle stroma.

## DIFFERENTIAL DIAGNOSIS

The most common differential diagnosis for clear-cell–papillary RCC includes clear-cell

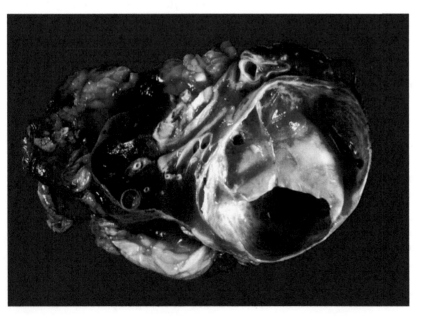

*Fig. 6.* Macroscopic appearance of clear-cell–papillary RCC with prominent cystic change. This well circumscribed multilocular cystic lesion contains thin septations and is encapsulated.

*Fig. 7.* (*A*) Low-power image of clear-cell–papillary RCC with an admixture of papillary and tubular patterns, composed of cells with clear and eosinophilic cytoplasm (H&E, original magnification ×10). (*B*) Clear-cell–papillary RCC with cystic change and hierarchical branching of tumoral papillae containing fibrovascular cores (H&E, original magnification ×10). (*C*) Clear-cell–papillary RCC exhibiting a tubular growth pattern of tumor cells with clear cytoplasm showing orientation of nuclei away from the basement membrane (H&E, original magnification ×40).

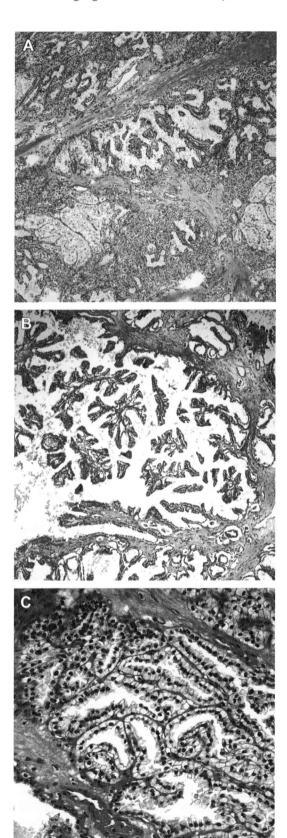

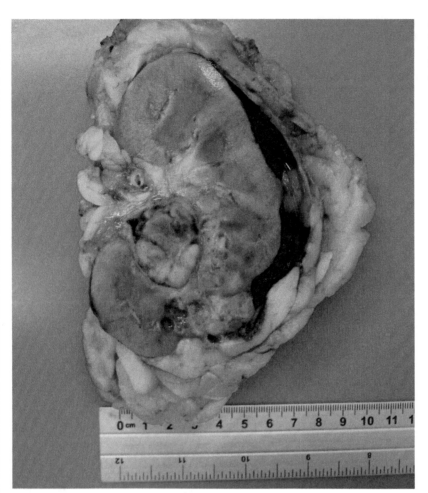

*Fig. 8.* Gross image of a case of RAT, highlighting the well-circumscribed encapsulated and fleshy appearance of the tumor.

(conventional) RCC, papillary RCC, and translocation-associated RCC. There is an entire spectrum of emerging tumors that may have similar or identical histology but different immunohistochemical profile, mutational status, or familial predisposition; these are described in the subsequent paragraph. Clear-cell RCC often demonstrates a prominent acinar/nested architecture with an intricate capillary vascular network and cells with clear cytoplasm (especially in areas with low Fuhrman-grade nuclei). Although papillary architecture is rarely identified in clear-cell RCC, the exception is in higher nuclear-grade areas, where a pseudopapillary growth pattern and cells with granular or eosinophilic cytoplasm may predominate; these papillary areas are distinct from the low-grade tubulopapillary areas of clear-cell–papillary RCC. Indeed, some clear-cell carcinomas may have very prominent clear-cell–papillary RCC-like areas. The designation of clear-cell carcinoma in such tumors is based on the recognition of more typical areas with clear-cell RCC histology and appropriate immunohistochemical support (CK7 negative, CD10 positive). Although areas of cytoplasmic clearing can be seen in papillary RCC, such areas are generally focal in extent, and an associated conventional papillary component be easily identified. Nuclear grade may be low or high in papillary RCC.[20] Translocation-associated RCC can be often distinguished from clear-cell–papillary RCC by the presence of cells with voluminous clear to eosinophilic cytoplasm and high-grade nuclei. These tumors also more often occur in younger patients.

The subject of tumors with clear cells and papillary architecture with prominent smooth muscle stroma is a matter of debate, as not all tumors

*Fig. 9.* Smooth muscle rich stroma in a case of RAT with a tubular growth pattern (H&E, original magnification ×10).

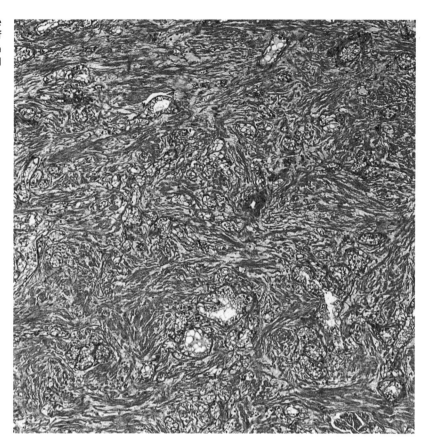

with these features represent clear-cell–papillary RCC. Recently, a subset of RCCs with a unique genomic profile including transcription elongation factor B, polypeptide 1 (TCEB1) mutation (TCEB-mutated RCC) has been described.[21,22] Also, a subset of tumors with clear-cell morphology and papillary architecture with CD10 positivity has been described as RCC with angioleiomyomalike stroma, and these may be a distinct tumor type.[18] Interestingly, patients with tuberous sclerosis might demonstrate a subset of renal tumors to have overlapping morphology with such tumors.[23] Finally, tumors with clear-cell–papillary RCC histology occurring in patients with Von Hippel-Lindau (VHL) disease may not represent clear-cell–papillary RCC.[24–26]

## MOLECULAR PATHOGENESIS, IMMUNOHISTOCHEMISTRY, AND DIAGNOSIS

Clear-cell–papillary RCC is a distinct entity with unique clinicopathologic features. Little is currently known about the molecular pathogenesis

of clear-cell–papillary RCC; however, they have been shown to lack the chromosomal 7 and 17 gains frequently seen in papillary RCC. A small subset of these tumors has been shown to harbor VHL gene mutations or chromosome 3p alterations, which are characteristic of clear-cell RCC.[16,17] Clear-cell–papillary RCC and RAT tumors do not show recurrent chromosomal imbalances by virtual karyotyping.[16] Seven cases of clear-cell–papillary RCC were interrogated by comparative genomic hybridization array and demonstrated a "silent" genomic profile with no characteristic chromosomal imbalances.[27] Munari and colleagues[28] demonstrated that clear-cell–papillary RCC lacks dysregulation of important microRNAs, which have been characteristically associated with a poor clinical outcome.

Immunophenotypic patterns further highlight the differences among clear-cell RCC, papillary RCC, and clear-cell–papillary RCC.[29] In contrast to clear-cell RCC, clear-cell–papillary RCC usually shows strong and diffuse expression of CK7, and unlike papillary RCC, clear-cell–papillary RCC is generally negative for AMACR expression. In addition, clear-cell–papillary RCC demonstrates a characteristic pattern of carbonic anhydrase IX (CAIX) expression, which includes the presence of basolateral membranous staining but absence of apical membranous staining, yielding a "cuplike" CAIX pattern in clear-cell–papillary RCC. This contrasts with the complete membranous CAIX staining pattern in clear-cell RCC and lack of CAIX expression in papillary RCC. Focal CD10 expression might be seen especially in the apical cell membrane of cyst epithelium in a subset of clear-cell–papillary RCC. This immunohistochemical profile, especially a uniform CAIX and CK7 expression, helps confirm the diagnosis of clear-cell–papillary RCC in the correct histologic context. Another marker, useful in the differential diagnosis, is high molecular weight cytokeratin, positive in more than 90% of clear-cell–papillary RCCs but typically negative in clear-cell RCC and most papillary RCC.[16]

## PROGNOSIS

Clear-cell–papillary RCCs typically have an indolent clinical course, as the vast majority are low clinical grade/stage tumors. Coupled with the lack of documented high-risk molecular alterations, these low-risk clinicopathologic features likely account for the fact that no clear-cell–papillary RCC recurrences or metastases have been reported to date.

### Pathologic Key Features

1. Clear-cell–papillary RCCs are clinically low-grade/stage tumors with unique morphologic and immunophenotypic features.

2. Grossly, these tumors are usually well circumscribed, may be encapsulated, and may have a predominantly cystic component.

3. Microscopically, clear-cell–papillary RCCs demonstrate a papillary and focally "solid" architecture of cells with clear cytoplasm and low-grade nuclei linearly arranged away from the basement membrane. These tumors characteristically express CK 7 and high molecular weight cytokeratin (strong and diffuse) and CAIX (in a "cuplike" pattern).

### △△ Differential Diagnosis

1. Clear-cell RCC: Cells with predominantly clear cytoplasm arranged in nests surrounded by an intricately branching vasculature. A small subset of tumors may rarely have a clear-cell–papillary RCC-like histology, and in such cases, the diagnosis is made on the recognition of more typical clear-cell RCC areas. Associated with VHL mutations and chromosome 3p alterations. Usually lack CK7 and high molecular weight cytokeratin expression.

2. Papillary RCC: Predominantly eosinophilic cells with papillary, tubular, and "solid" growth patterns and fibrovascular cores with foamy macrophages. Associated with chromosome 7 and 17 alterations. Usually express AMACR with variable CAIX expression.

3. RCC with angioleiomyomalike stroma: The tumors proposed under this entity have prominent smooth muscle stroma, low to high nuclear grade with positive CD10 immunoexpression.

4. Translocation-associated RCC: Cells with voluminous clear to eosinophilic cytoplasm and high-grade nuclei. Associated with TFE3 and TFEB gene rearrangements. Often occurs in younger patients.

5. TCEB1-mutated RCC: The cells have more voluminous cytoplasm and focal papillary architecture. Polarization of tumor nuclei or cuplike distribution of CAIX (features of clear-cell–papillary RCC) are absent. CK7 and CAIX are positive in TCEB1-muted RCC, and AMACR and CD10 are typically focally positive.

## THYROID-LIKE FOLLICULAR CARCINOMA OF THE KIDNEY

### INTRODUCTION

Thyroid-like follicular carcinoma of the kidney (TLFCK) is a recently described subtype of RCC that microscopically resembles follicular neoplasms or follicular carcinoma of the thyroid. A case report in 1996 first suggested the existence of TLFCK, and this initial observation was subsequently expanded in a case series by Amin and colleagues in 2009.[30] TLFCK is a rare tumor that is usually discovered incidentally during radiography performed for other reasons. Limited data are available regarding the molecular biology or clinical behavior of these tumors, but most appear to be indolent in nature. This tumor is regarded as an "emerging entity" in the contemporary classification of RCC.

## GROSS FEATURES

TLFCK is generally well circumscribed, with a tan-yellow cut surface and a wide size range (2–12 cm).

## MICROSCOPIC FEATURES

TLFCK can be microscopically indistinguishable from follicular neoplasms or follicular carcinomas of the thyroid. They usually have a distinct fibrous capsule and demonstrate small and large follicles filled with colloidlike material (**Fig. 10**). These follicles are lined by cuboidal to columnar cells with eosinophilic to amphophilic cytoplasm and nuclei with variable pseudoinclusions and grooves. A marked lymphocytic infiltrate, sometimes with reactive germinal center formation, may be present (**Fig. 11**). Tumors demonstrate a thyroid-like morphology throughout the neoplasm.

## DIFFERENTIAL DIAGNOSIS

The primary differential diagnosis for TLFCK is metastatic thyroid cancer. Both papillary and follicular thyroid carcinomas can metastasize to the kidney and present as a diagnostic challenge when trying to differentiate from TLFCK. Metastatic thyroid cancers are generally associated with a history of previous thyroid neoplasia, presence of concurrent tumor at other metastatic sites, and demonstrate positive expression for TTF1 and thyroglobulin by IHC. Also in the differential diagnosis are renal tumors with conspicuous colloid-like secretions and tubular architecture, such as renal oncocytoma and some papillary and clear-cell RCCs, and the recently described TCEB1-mutated RCC (see earlier in this article).

## MOLECULAR PATHOGENESIS, IMMUNOHISTOCHEMISTRY, AND DIAGNOSIS

Genetic studies in TLFCK are limited but have demonstrated multiple chromosomal gains and losses.[31] These tumors are usually negative for PAX2 expression. PAX8 expression has not been extensively studied; however, at least one case reportedly showed PAX8 expression.[32] These tumors are also usually negative for CK7, AMACR, RCC, and CD10 expression. This immunohistochemical profile, along with absence of TTF-1

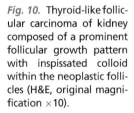

*Fig. 10.* Thyroid-like follicular carcinoma of kidney composed of a prominent follicular growth pattern with inspissated colloid within the neoplastic follicles (H&E, original magnification ×10).

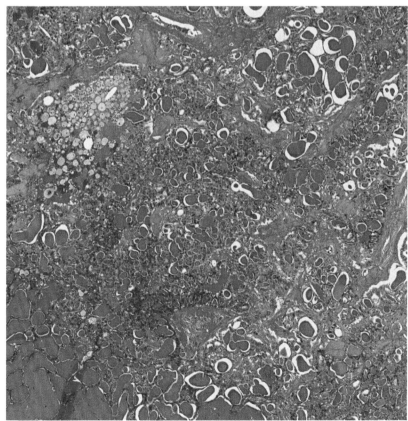

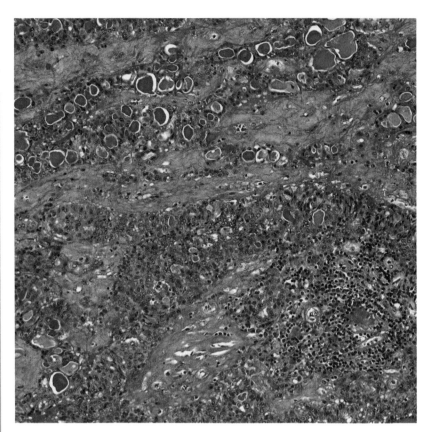

Fig.        11. Morphologic features of tumor cells in thyroid-like follicular carcinoma of kidney exhibiting cells with eosinophilic cytoplasm, round nuclei with uniform chromatin distribution, and occasional nucleoli. Note the accompanying lymphoid inflammatory infiltrate at the bottom right (H&E, original magnification ×20).

and thyroglobulin expression, helps confirm the diagnosis of TLFCK in suspected cases.

## PROGNOSIS

TLFCK is predominantly low clinical grade/stage tumors. Rare cases with metastatic spread have been described, and in these cases, the primary and metastatic tumors demonstrated similar morphologic features.[32]

 **Pathologic Key Features**

1. TLFCKs are well-circumscribed tumors with a fibrous capsule and morphologically resemble thyroid follicular neoplasms.

2. TLFCKs are usually negative for CK7 and PAX2 expression and may show PAX8 expression. TTF-1 and thyroglobulin are not expressed in TLFCK.

3. Most tumors have been confined to the kidney, with only rare reported metastases.

 **Differential Diagnosis**

1. Metastatic thyroid carcinoma: May be indistinguishable morphologically from TLFCK, but are often associated with a history of primary thyroid neoplasia and demonstrate positive TTF1 and thyroglobulin expression by IHC.

2. Renal oncocytoma, papillary RCC, and clear-cell RCC with prominent colloid secretions: Although areas may mimic TLFCK, a proportion of the tumor will typically demonstrate classic features of oncocytoma, papillary RCC, or clear-cell RCC.

## ANAPLASTIC LYMPHOMA KINASE– ASSOCIATED RENAL CELL CARCINOMA

### INTRODUCTION

Gene fusions involving the anaplastic lymphoma kinase (ALK) gene have been implicated in a variety of neoplasms, including inflammatory myofibroblastic tumor, lung adenocarcinoma, and a subset of high-grade lymphomas. The ALK protein inhibitor, crizotinib, has been recently approved by the US Food and Drug Administration for treatment of patients with lung adenocarcinoma harboring an *ALK* rearrangement. These developments are important for the field of renal oncology due to the recent discovery of a small subset of patients with RCCs with *ALK* rearrangements (ie, *ALK*-associated RCC)[33,34] who may be eligible for targeted therapy with ALK inhibitors. *ALK* rearrangements have been reported in renal tumors from younger patients with sickle cell trait (where they form a *VCL-ALK* gene fusion), as well as in patients without sickle cell trait.[35] In a recent survey of more than 500 renal tumors, the overall frequency of *ALK* rearrangement was less than 1%.[36] This tumor is regarded as an "emerging entity" in the contemporary classification of RCC.

## GROSS FEATURES

Little is known about the gross appearance of *ALK*-associated RCC; however, patients with sickle cell trait often have tumors based in the renal collecting system, where the differential diagnosis may include renal medullary carcinoma (RMC).

## MICROSCOPIC FEATURES

In tumors harboring the *VCL-ALK* gene fusion, the cells are polygonal to spindled with eosinophilic cytoplasm and intracytoplasmic vacuolation and have vesicular nuclei; prominent intratumoral lymphocytic infiltration also is present, and sickled red blood cells may be identified (**Figs. 12** and **13**).[35] Based on a limited number of reported cases, tumors without *VCL* as fusion partner for *ALK* may be associated with papillary, tubular, and/or cribriform morphology, which may or may not exhibit some cytoplasmic clearing; however, these tumors are not associated with sickled red blood cells. Interestingly, at least one *ALK*-associated RCC without *VCL* as the fusion partner demonstrated cribriform morphology with mucin production, which was somewhat similar to some *ALK*-rearrangement–positive lung adenocarcinomas.[37]

## DIFFERENTIAL DIAGNOSIS

RMC shares some clinicopathologic features with *ALK*-associated RCC, including its association with sickle cell trait, medullary location, and some overlapping morphologic features. RMCs, however, are associated with loss of nuclear INI-1 expression and demonstrate a very high Ki-67 index.[35] In addition, RMC have a very poor clinical prognosis, which contrasts with the indolent clinical pattern seen in renal tumors with the *VCL-ALK* fusion.

## MOLECULAR PATHOGENESIS, IMMUNOHISTOCHEMISTRY, AND DIAGNOSIS

*ALK* rearrangements in renal tumors have been described in 2 settings: young patients with sickle cell trait, where *ALK* is fused to *VCL*, and patients

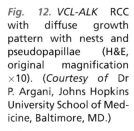

*Fig. 12. VCL-ALK* RCC with diffuse growth pattern with nests and pseudopapillae (H&E, original magnification ×10). (*Courtesy of* Dr P. Argani, Johns Hopkins University School of Medicine, Baltimore, MD.)

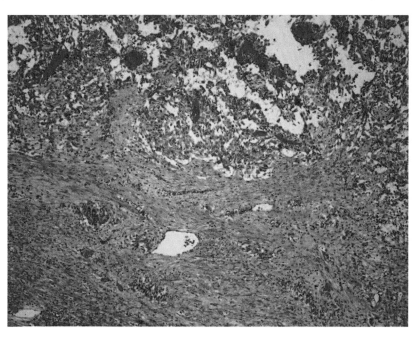

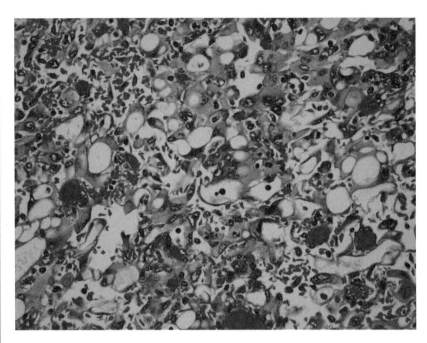

*Fig. 13.* Polygonal and focally spindled tumor cells in *VCL-ALK* RCC with intracytoplasmic vacuoles. Note the sickled erythrocytes in the background (H&E, original magnification ×20). (*Courtesy of* Dr P. Argani, Johns Hopkins University School of Medicine, Baltimore, MD.)

without sickle cell trait, where *EML4* and *TPM3* have been implicated as the partner fusion gene. In these tumors, cytoplasmic and subplasmalemmal ALK expression can be detected by IHC (**Fig. 14**); *ALK*-associated RCC usually also expresses cytokeratin and, in contrast to RMC, demonstrates retained nuclear INI-1 expression.

Apart from genomic rearrangement, *ALK* copy number gain also is implicated in the molecular pathogenesis of *ALK*-associated RCC.[36,38] Additional studies are needed to validate the relationship of these different genomic alterations with clinical response to targeted ALK inhibitor therapy.

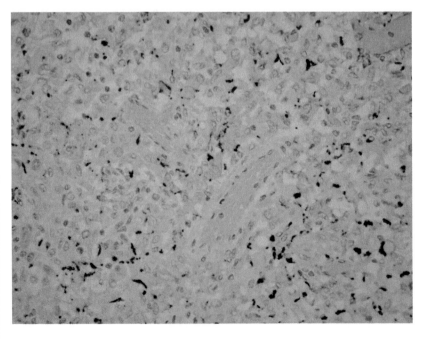

*Fig. 14.* ALK immunostaining demonstrating positivity with localization underneath the cell membrane (original magnification ×40). (*Courtesy of* Dr P. Argani, Johns Hopkins University School of Medicine, Baltimore, MD.)

## PROGNOSIS

Although a limited number of patients have been described in the literature with *ALK*-associated RCC, no recurrences were seen in limited follow-up of patients with sickle cell trait and *VCL-ALK* rearranged tumors. Recently, a study of more than 500 renal tumors identified *ALK* rearrangements in fewer than 1% of patients and *ALK* copy number gain in another 10% of patients with clear-cell RCC. In that study, both groups of patients with *ALK* aberrations had poorer outcome.[36] Thus, based on the currently available literature, patients with *ALK*-associated RCC may have a variable clinical course, with a more favorable outcome for patients with sickle cell trait and a *VCL-ALK* gene fusion.

### *Pathologic Key Features*

1. *ALK*-associated RCC may or may not be associated with sickle cell trait.

2. Patients with sickle cell trait and *ALK*-associated RCC often harbor a *VCL-ALK* fusion, have a medullary location, and demonstrate spindled and polygonal cells containing eosinophilic cytoplasm. These tumors express cytokeratins and showed retained INI-1 expression.

3. *ALK*-associated RCC may have a variable clinical course, with the *VCL-ALK* cases in patients with sickle cell trait having a more favorable outcome.

### *Differential Diagnosis*

1. Renal medullary carcinoma: A medulla-based tumor with high-grade morphologic features that may overlap with *VCR-ALK*–rearranged tumors in patients with sickle cell trait. Show loss of INI-1 expression by IHC, positivity for OCT 3/4 with a very high proliferation index.

## RENAL CELL CARCINOMA WITH t(6;11) TRANSLOCATION

### INTRODUCTION

RCCs demonstrating the characteristic t(6;11)-(p21;q12) translocation were first described by Argani and colleagues[39] in 2001. The t(6;11) RCCs have been recently accepted by the 2013 International Society of Urologic Pathology Vancouver Classification of Renal Neoplasia as a member of the Microphthalmia transcription (MiT)/transcription factor E3 (TFE3) family of translocation RCC, which also includes the more common Xp11.2 translocation RCC.[40] These tumors occur in any age group, including patients in the sixth decade, but most cases reported to date have occurred in young adults (mean age = 28.5 years). There is no specific gender predilection. Fewer than 50 cases of this rare entity have previously been described in the literature.[40]

### GROSS FINDINGS

RCCs with t(6;11) translocation exhibit a wide size range, with some tumors measuring up to 20 cm in diameter. The cut surface is similar to clear-cell RCC, with a solid yellow-tan appearance.[41,42] Variable amounts of cystic degeneration may be present in addition to foci of hemorrhage and necrosis. Melanotic translocation RCCs may exhibit varying degrees of pigmentation over the cut surface on gross examination.[41–43]

### MICROSCOPIC APPEARANCE

t(6;11) RCCs usually demonstrate a solid or alveolar architecture and are composed of larger epithelioid cells with clear to voluminous cytoplasm surrounding distinctive groups of smaller cells with dense chromatin, which are clustered around hyaline basement membrane material (rosette-forming) (**Figs. 15** and **16**). TFEB RCCs may demonstrate unusual morphologic features resembling papillary RCC, chromophobe RCC, clear-cell RCC, and epithelioid angiomyolipoma-like structures (**Fig. 17**). A multilocular cystic phenotype has also been reported in these tumors.[39–43] Although the tumors initially had features as characteristically described here, recent experience suggests that these tumors may have overlapping histology with Xp11 translocation-associated carcinoma (see later in this article).[44]

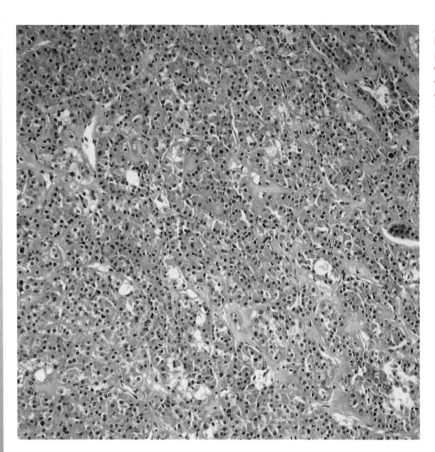

**Fig. 15.** t(6;11) RCC with a broad nested growth pattern of epithelioid cells with abundant eosinophilic cytoplasm (H&E, original magnification ×20).

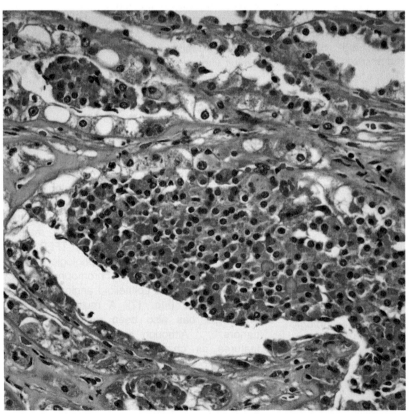

**Fig. 16.** Distinctive group of smaller cells in t(6;11) RCC with dense chromatin showing clustering around hyaline basement membrane material (rosette-forming) seen at the center of nests. Larger cells may vary from having eosinophilic to clear cytoplasm (H&E, original magnification ×40).

## MOLECULAR PATHOGENESIS, IMMUNOHISTOCHEMISTRY, AND DIAGNOSIS

t(6;11) RCCs have a relatively distinctive immuno-profile that is compatible with renal tubular origin or differentiation.[39–43,45,46] Smith and colleagues[46] demonstrated consistent expression of melanocytic markers Melan A and HMB45 in t(6;11) RCC, with diffuse Melan A, whereas HMB45 is usually only focally positive. These tumors are either negative or only focally positive for cytokeratins and may label for CD117. In addition, the t(6;11) RCC tumor cells also exhibit positivity for cathepsin K, a protease that is expressed in osteoclasts but that is not present in non–MiT/TFE3 family translocation RCCs.[45] A variable degree of positivity for PAX8, RCC marker antigen, CD10, Ksp-cadherin, and Cam5.2 cytokeratin has been documented.

*TFE3*, *TFEB*, *TFEC*, and *MiTF* are members of the MiTF-TFE family of basic helix-loop-helix zipper (bHLH-Zip) factors that bind DNA as homodimers and heterodimers. The t(6;11) translocation results in fusion of the first intron of transcription factor EB (*TFEB*) with *alpha*, an untranslated gene of unknown function, which ultimately leads to overexpression of native TFEB protein.[41–43] Overexpression of TFEB in the t(6;11) RCC is thought to result in expression of proteins normally driven by MiTF in other cell types. Regardless, detection of TFEB protein overexpression by IHC is currently a commonly used diagnostic technique for t(6;11) RCC in clinical practice. However, IHC detection is significantly dependent on adequate fixation and subject to variations with varying or suboptimal fixation time. Nontranslocated TFEB RCCs also may be associated with false-positive cytoplasmic staining and therefore always should be interpreted in context with morphologic and clinicopathologic features.[41–43,46]

TFEB RCCs are often diagnosed based on their distinctive morphology and immunophenotype; however, molecular methods, such as reverse-transcriptase polymerase chain reaction (PCR) and FISH, are extremely helpful and often mandated for an accurate diagnosis. *TFEB* break-apart FISH assays have been developed to detect *TFEB* gene rearrangements and can be performed on archival formalin-fixed, paraffin-embedded tissues. Detection by PCR is not as reliable as detection by other molecular methods owing to the variable breakpoints and amplification of large size range. The potential risk for false negatives and inefficient PCR amplifications are factors complicating the analysis.[4,42,43,46]

## DIFFERENTIAL DIAGNOSIS

The differential diagnosis of t(6; 11) RCCs, in both adults and children, includes other renal tumors with clear-cell or papillary morphology, such as clear-cell, papillary, and Xp11.2 RCC[40–43]; however, the biphasic pattern of large epithelioid cells and clusters of smaller cells seen in t(6;11) is less frequently seen in these other RCC subtypes. IHC may be helpful, as unlike t(6;11), clear-cell and papillary RCC are typically positive for pancytokeratin (AE1/AE3), Cam5.2, and EMA, whereas TFEB is negative in both these tumor types.[40,41,43,45,46] The presence on TFE3 staining or rearrangement using IHC or FISH, respectively, distinguishes Xp11.2 (TFE3) from t(6;11) (TFEB) RCCs.

Epithelioid angiomyolipoma (EAML) (also known as epithelioid PEComa; see also Arias-Stella and Williamson, Updates in Benign Lesions of the Genitourinary Tract, Surgical Pathology Clinics, 2015, Volume 8, Issue 4) represents another diagnosis mandating distinction from TFEB RCC.[46] Morphologically, EAML grows in solid sheets or in a large alveolar pattern. EAMLs may show clear cells with finely granular cytoplasm and small monomorphic nuclei, as well as eosinophilic cells with abundant cytoplasm (epithelioid morphology) and large nuclei with prominent nucleoli, thus raising a diagnostic consideration of t(6;11) RCCs. EAML may not always demonstrate a significant amount of intratumoral fat and malformed vessels, which may add to this diagnostic dilemma. PAX8 is extremely useful in making this distinction, as it is a very specific (95%) IHC marker for RCC and is typically absent in EAML. Additionally, *TFEB* FISH assay may be the most useful test in distinguishing EAML from t(6;11) RCC when necessary[46]; cathepsin K is not helpful, as it is positive in both EAML and t(6;11) RCC.

## PROGNOSIS

There still remains a degree of uncertainty regarding the final clinical outcome of patients in this group of rare tumors because of the relatively small number of documented cases. Of the approximately 30 genetically confirmed cases that have been reported, metastasis leading to death has been reported in 3 cases.[40] Metastatic involvement of lymph nodes and other sites, including lung and bone, also has been reported.[40–43] However, most studies have shown that TFEB RCCs are associated with a good prognosis, and therefore thought to be a relatively indolent tumor.[41–43,46] Further studies are warranted to determine long-term clinical outcomes.

## Pathologic Key Features

1. t(6;11) RCC typically demonstrates biphasic morphology, composed of larger epithelioid cells and smaller cells often clustered around basement membrane material; nevertheless, the full spectrum of morphologic appearances is not known and overlaps with Xp11.2 translocation RCC.

2. t(6;11) RCCs consistently express melanocytic markers such as HMB-45 and Melan-A, which are detectable by IHC but are either negative or only focally positive for epithelial markers such as cytokeratins; cathepsin K is frequently positive.

3. These tumors are characterized by the t(6;11) (p21;q12), which results in an *Alpha-TFEB* gene fusion.

4. A relatively sensitive and specific assay for t(6;11) RCCs is nuclear labeling for TFEB protein using IHC. However, IHC is largely fixation dependent, and break-apart FISH assays for *TFEB* gene fusion have thus been developed for archival material and currently remain the confirmatory assay of choice for these tumors.

## Differential Diagnosis

1. Clear-cell RCC with prominent eosinophilic cytoplasm: lacks the biphasic pattern of t(6;11) RCCs. Clear-cell RCCs are typically positive for pancytokeratin and EMA and they are negative for *TFEB* by IHC and FISH.

2. Papillary RCCs: are positive for AMACR and strongly express cytokeratins, including cytokeratin 7. Papillary RCCs are negative for TFEB rearrangement and frequently demonstrate trisomies of chromosome 7 and 17.

3. Xp11.2 translocation RCC: shares overlapping morphologic and immunophenotypic findings, except for TFE3 expression/translocation.

4. Epithelioid angiomyolipoma (EAML): shares an overlapping immunoprofile with t(6;11) RCC in that both tumors may express melanocytic markers (HMB45 and Melan A); however, EAML does not demonstrate a TFEB rearrangement by FISH and is negative for PAX8 expression by IHC.

## ACQUIRED CYSTIC DISEASE–ASSOCIATED RENAL CELL CARCINOMA

### INTRODUCTION

Acquired cystic kidney disease (ACKD) is the term used to refer to renal tubular cystic changes that develop in ESRD. An increased prevalence of RCC has been recorded in kidneys with ESRD with or, less frequently, without ACKD. Patients with ACKD are at a significantly greater risk for developing RCC (>100 times) than the general population, although the incidence is less than 10%.[47] A previous history of dialysis (especially a prolonged duration) is often associated with the development of ACKD and RCC.[14]

Traditionally, the different types of renal tumors encountered in cases with ESRD include the 3 common subtypes of RCC; that is, clear-cell (conventional) RCC, papillary RCC, and chromophobe RCC, as well as less common subtypes or renal neoplasia, including oncocytoma, angiomyolipoma, and mixed epithelial and stromal tumor (see also Arias-Stella and Williamson, Updates in Benign Lesions of the Genitourinary Tract, Surgical Pathology Clinics, 2015, Volume 8, Issue 4). More recently, at least 2 other subtypes of RCC have been described in association with ESRD: ACKD-associated RCC and clear-cell–papillary RCC (see earlier in this article for the latter). Acquired cystic disease (ACD)-associated RCC, first described by Tickoo and colleagues, has been reported only in patients with ESRD and ACKD; whereas clear-cell–papillary RCC can be seen in patients with both cystic and non-cystic ESRD, as well as in sporadic cases without ESRD.[14,16,48] These tumors occur in patients spanning a wide age range (30–78 years) but are most common in the fifth decade and affect more men than women (male:female ratio = 2:1).[14,48]

### GROSS FEATURES

ACD-associated RCC may be incidentally discovered on radiologic studies or in nephrectomy specimens in which surgery was performed for renal cysts with complications or renal parenchymal bleeding. In nephrectomy specimens from ACKD cases, hemorrhagic cysts or cysts containing blood clots should be sampled, as these areas may contain foci of tumor. Most tumors are well circumscribed, and often appear to arise within cysts (two-thirds of all cases). Large-sized tumors may be grossly solid with a thick, fibrous capsule and may be accompanied by foci of necrosis and hemorrhage (**Fig. 18**). Multifocal (>50%) and bilateral (>20%) tumors have been frequently reported in this subtype of RCC.[14,48]

*Fig. 17.* t(6;11) RCC composed of cells with clear cytoplasm and an arborizing vascular network resembling clear-cell RCC; this morphology also overlaps with Xp11.2 translocation RCC (H&E, original magnification ×10).

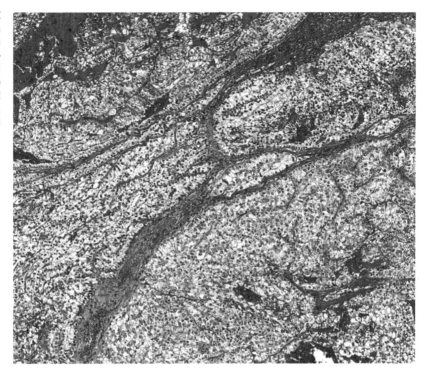

*Fig. 18.* Macroscopic appearance of a hemorrhagic ACD-associated RCC (*arrows*) located in the upper pole of the kidney and developing in a background of acquired cystic disease of the kidney.

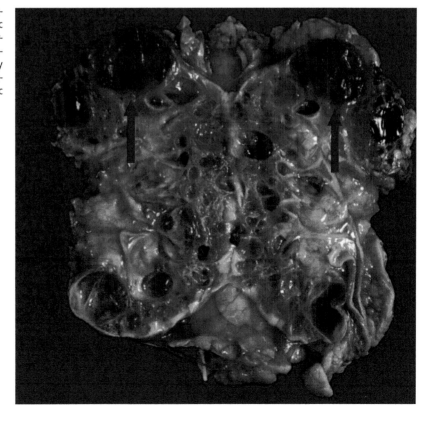

## MICROSCOPIC FEATURES

These tumors may demonstrate diverse architectural patterns with acinar, alveolar, solid, cystic, and papillary features (**Fig. 19**). In many cases, the presence of irregular lumens imparts a cribriform or sievelike appearance to the tumor (**Fig. 20**). Characteristic features include cells with abundant granular, eosinophilic cytoplasm and large nuclei with prominent nucleoli (**Fig. 21**). The cytoplasm may be vacuolated or focally clear cells are present. Most cases also show intratumoral oxalate crystals, a relatively specific feature observed in ACD-associated RCC distinct from other tumor types (see **Figs. 20** and **21**).[14,48] Rarely, psammoma bodies may be seen. It is also important to note that the background nonneoplastic renal parenchyma often contains cysts lined with large eosinophilic cells (clustered microcystic lesions) that show an immunophenotype similar to that of ACD-associated RCC.[14] Rare case reports of sarcomatoid transformation and aggressive behavior in this group of tumors have been documented.[49]

## MOLECULAR PATHOGENESIS, IMMUNOHISTOCHEMISTRY, AND DIAGNOSIS

The vast majority of ACD-associated RCC cases are diagnosed incidentally on radiologic follow-up in patients with chronic renal disease, or at the time of nephrectomy/transplantation. These tumors may be detected earlier owing to constant surveillance and regular radiological examination done as routine follow-up for these patients. ACD-associated tumors are positive for α-methylacyl-coenzyme A racemase (AMACR) and vinculin. They also demonstrate variable to focal staining for cytokeratin 7 and parvalbumin. Stains for cytokeratin AE1/AE3, CD10, RCC antigen, and glutathione S-transferase A are also reported to be positive, whereas variable positivity is noted for vimentin and CAM 5.2.[50] Staining for EMA and high molecular weight cytokeratins is reportedly negative. Ancillary immunohistochemical stains (diffuse positivity for AMACR and negative/focal positivity for CK7) are of assistance in distinguishing these tumors from papillary RCC.

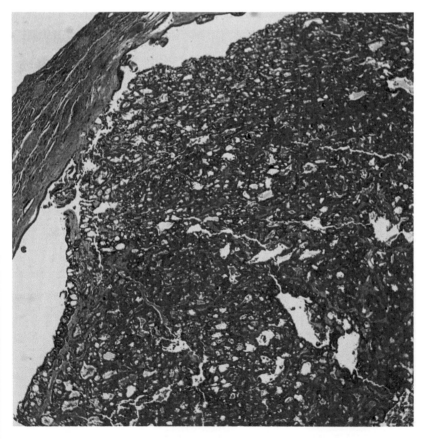

*Fig. 19.* ACD-associated RCC with characteristic sievelike appearance on low power (H&E, original magnification ×4). The lesions are frequently encapsulated.

*Fig. 20.* Anastomosing acinar and sievelike growth pattern in ACD-associated RCC comprising of tumor cells with abundant eosinophilic cytoplasm and intratumoral calcium oxalate crystals (H&E, original magnification ×20).

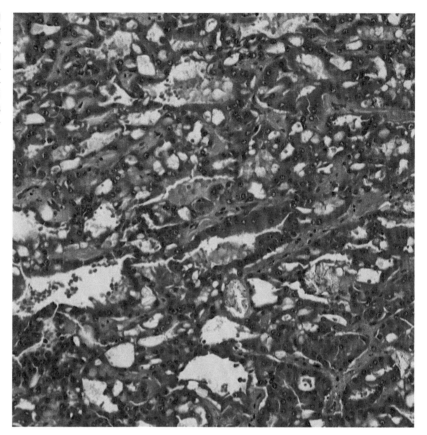

Although genetic studies in this category are limited, tumors diagnosed as ACD-associated RCC have been shown to be negative for extra copies (trisomy) of chromosomes 7 and 17 or loss of 3p, characteristic findings in papillary and clear-cell RCC, respectively. A recent study by Pan and colleagues[50] on 9 cases of ACD-associated RCC showed variable combined gains of chromosomes 3, 7, 16, 17, and Y using FISH and comparative genomic hybridization. The exact mechanisms underlying the increased incidence of RCC in ESRD, especially in those with superimposed ACKD are not completely understood. Possible precursor lesions in ESRD include papillary adenomas, dilated tubules, or clustered microcystic lesions lined by eosinophilic cells.[51] Further studies are necessary to delineate the etiopathogenesis of these tumors.

## DIFFERENTIAL DIAGNOSIS

The differential diagnosis of ACD-associated RCC includes tumors with a prominent cystic appearance and papillary or solid growth patterns. These include papillary RCC, clear-cell RCC, tubulocystic carcinoma, collecting duct carcinoma, and HLRCC-associated renal cancer (see later in this article for the latter). The presence of papillary architecture may raise a differential diagnosis of papillary RCC; however, the presence of other patterns, including solid and sievelike areas, are not classically seen in papillary RCC. Immunohistochemical stains may be helpful in distinguishing papillary RCC from ACD-associated RCC, as the latter stains diffusely positive for racemase, but is negative or only focally positive for CK7; these findings are in contrast to papillary RCC, which is typically positive for CK7 (however, be careful of eosinophilic variants of papillary RCC that may be negative or only focally positive for CK7). Clear-cell RCC tumors display characteristic arborizing or branching vascular septations, are positive for CAIX, and lack intratumoral calcium oxalate crystals. The presence of intracytoplasmic or intercytoplasmic lumina imparting a cribriform/sievelike appearance favors the diagnosis of an ACD-associated RCC.[14,48,50]

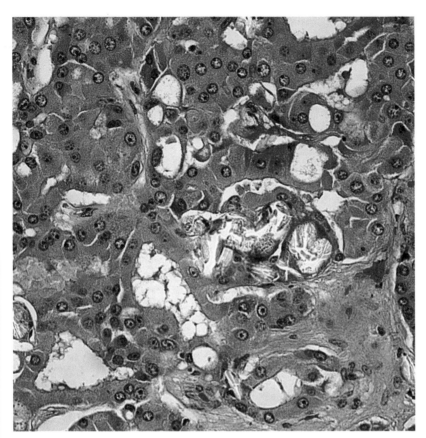

*Fig. 21.* Tumor cells in ACD-associated RCC with abundant granular, eosinophilic cytoplasm and large nuclei with prominent nucleoli. Note the intratumoral oxalate crystals, a relatively specific feature observed in this tumor (H&E, original magnification ×40).

Collecting duct carcinomas and HLRCC-associated RCC are aggressive tumors that demonstrate a multinodular growth pattern with glandular, papillary, and/or solid areas. These tumors are associated with an extensive desmoplastic stromal response and accompanying inflammatory infiltrate, which are not usually encountered in ACD-associated RCC. Of note, IHC stains for detection of loss of fumarate hydratase (FH) and overexpression of S-(2-succino)-cysteine (2SC) are vital tools in the recognition of HLRCC-associated renal carcinomas (see later in this article for more details).[8,14]

## PROGNOSIS

The biological behavior of RCCs in ESRD in general is reported to be less aggressive than that of the RCCs in non-ESRD settings. These tumors often present at a lower stage (confined to the renal parenchyma) and are smaller in size.[52] ACD-associated RCC may have a greater potential for aggressive behavior than other tumor types in ESRD.[14,49]

### Pathologic Key Features

1. ACD-associated RCC is the most common subtype of RCC occurring in end-stage kidneys, including acquired cystic disease.

2. ACD-associated RCCs are usually well circumscribed, often arising within cysts.

3. Microscopically, these tumors demonstrate the presence of multiple small lumina/sieve-like cribriform structures and contain intratumoral oxalate crystals; variable proportions of papillary architecture and clear-cell cytology can be present.

4. Most ACD-associated RCCs are diagnosed at small size with low pT stage and are associated with a relatively favorable outcome; however, a small subset of cases may demonstrate aggressive features.

**Differential Diagnosis**

1. Papillary RCC: these tumors lack solid/sievelike areas and are usually positive for CK7 and AMACR.

2. Clear-cell RCC: distinguished by an arborizing, branching vascular network; IHC stains are helpful, as these tumors are negative for CK7, negative/focally positive for AMACR, and positive for carbonic anhydrase IX.

3. Collecting duct carcinoma: usually exhibit a multinodular infiltrative growth pattern with glandular, papillary, and solid components; prominent desmoplastic stroma and a characteristic inflammatory infiltrate are also often present.

4. HLRCC-associated RCC: has a significant degree of morphologic overlap with collecting duct carcinoma and it can mimic ACD-associated RCC when it contains cystic components; however, IHC stains demonstrate loss of FH and 2SC induction/overexpression. The presence of other diagnostic features, including history of cutaneous and/or uterine leiomyomata is suggestive of this syndromic disorder. Prominent nucleoli with perinucleolar clearing are characteristic, although this may be a focal finding.

## SUCCINATE DEHYDROGENASE–DEFICIENT RENAL CELL CARCINOMA

### INTRODUCTION

An emerging entity in the category of "hereditary RCC" includes tumors demonstrating disruption of the mitochondrial complex II, the succinate dehydrogenase complex. These carcinomas occur as part of familial pheochromocytoma/paraganglioma syndromes, PGL1, PGL3, and PGL4, where affected kindreds harbor germline mutations of the succinate dehydrogenase (SDH) subunit genes SDHD, SDHC, and SDHB, respectively, and are predisposed to development of paragangliomas, gastrointestinal stromal tumors (GISTs), and RCCs.[53] Recent efforts identify that loss of immunohistochemical expression of the SDHB subunit provides a useful, specific means to screen for mutation of the SDHA, SDHB, SDHC, or SDHD subunit, as mutation in any of these subunits seems to destabilize the complex and lead to lack of SDHB expression.[54] Only very recently have larger cohorts been assembled and studied,[55,56] which suggests that SDH-deficient carcinomas are rare (estimated prevalence of 1:500–2000 of renal carcinomas), show predominantly *SDHB* mutations, and show characteristic histomorphology, as described later in this article. SDH-deficient carcinomas show slight male predominance, median age in the fourth to fifth decade, and significant rate of bilaterality (~25%). Syndromically associated GISTs and paragangliomas have been noted among kindreds affected by SDH-deficient RCCs, with significant prevalence (~10%–20%).

### GROSS FEATURES

Given the strong influence of smaller cohort and consultation-based studies of these tumors, relatively little attention has been devoted to their gross features. Between the 2 larger reported cohorts,[55,56] tumor sizes have ranged from subcentimeter to 20 cm, and most have been described grossly as having an unencapsulated solid, red to tan, sometimes hemorrhagic cut surface, sometimes with cystic change. Most all tumors have been confined to the kidney at diagnosis.

### MICROSCOPIC FEATURES, MOLECULAR PATHOGENESIS, IMMUNOHISTOCHEMISTRY, AND DIAGNOSIS

Establishing a diagnosis of SDH-deficient RCC starts with observation of a compatible to suspicious histomorphology, especially in a clinical setting suggestive of syndromic carcinoma. Although the male predominance is weak, the low median age is quite useful, as is the frequent family history of RCC (~20%), paraganglioma (>20%–30%), or GIST (~15%).[55] It is the opinion of the authors that any renal tumor arising in a younger individual merits, minimally, clinician inquiry regarding stigmata of the several syndromes associated with RCC, whereas tumors with compatible morphology arising in a setting of appropriate personal or family history are quite suggestive. Fortunately, these tumors tend to share a reproducible morphology, described by Gill and colleagues[57,58] in 2011, which built on the observations in a case just previously reported.

The characteristic morphology of unencapsulated tumor with compact nests to sheets of eosinophilic polygonal cells with prominently vacuolated cytoplasm (Fig. 22) and distinctive pale eosinophilic cytoplasmic inclusions (Fig. 23) has been validated in 2 larger cohorts.[55,56] The inclusions are thought to represent giant, dysfunctional mitochondria, seen by electron microscopy,[57] although the prospective utility of ultrastructural evaluation has not been validated. The nuclear features of SDH-deficient RCC are unique, with a monotonous neuroendocrinelike morphology (see Fig. 23). Prominent nucleoli are not a common feature. Inclusion of benign tubules within the neoplasm is a common finding (Fig. 24). Lesional encapsulation is infrequent, although metaplastic ossification has been seen.[56] Although less frequent, a significant proportion of cases have shown sarcomatoid transformation.

Loss of expression of SDHB by IHC, particularly when showing its retention in adjacent nonneoplastic renal parenchyma on the same tissue section (ie, serving as an internal positive control), is the best and most specific diagnostic feature. When this occurs, further molecular testing and genetic counseling is warranted for the patient. Other biomarkers are less specific, but have been shown to demonstrate infrequent focal pan-cytokeratin AE1/AE3 expression and an absence of CKIT in tumor cells. Consistent with their renal origin, these tumors show PAX8 expression, and, helpfully, show a pattern of prevalent, intense expression of kidney-specific cadherin (Ksp-Cadherin) in at least one cohort.[56] Certainly, detection of germline mutation of *SDHB* or other succinate deyhydrogenase complex subunit genes remains the gold standard.

## DIFFERENTIAL DIAGNOSIS

Fortunately, given their frequent underrecognition,[58] SDH-deficient RCCs demonstrate relatively reproducible morphologic features, including the aforementioned solid to cystic nodular growths of oncocytic cells, often entrapping perilesional nonneoplastic renal parenchymal elements. The cuboidal cells showing distinctively bubbly cytoplasm and inclusion of eosinophilic or fluidlike material are quite helpful for their identification. Given these features, it is not surprising that the differential diagnosis centers around oncocytic renal neoplasia, which includes oncocytoma, chromophobe RCC, or, in some cases, renal tumors with melanocytic differentiation, including

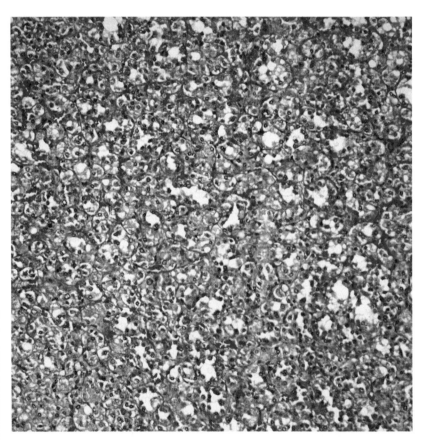

Fig. 22. SDH-deficient RCC composed of small closely packed nests and solid tubules composed of eosinophilic polygonal cells with prominently vacuolated cytoplasm (H&E, original magnification ×20).

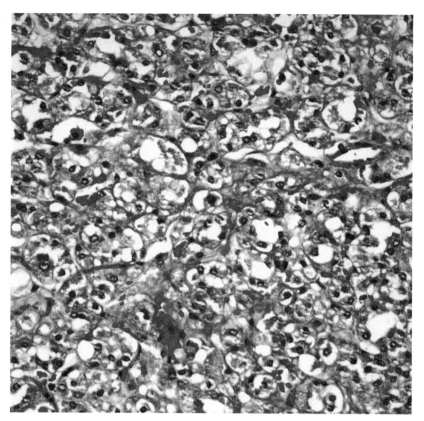

**Fig. 23.** SDH-deficient RCC with distinctive pale eosinophilic cytoplasmic inclusions and low-grade nuclei with round contours and uniform chromatin distribution imparting a neuroendocrinelike appearance (H&E, original magnification ×40).

translocation-associated RCC and EAML (epithelioid PEComas).

First, the degree of solid, confluent growth exhibited by SDH-deficient RCCs is beyond what one might expect in a renal oncocytoma, and this is supported by the published experience of the authors and others.[55,56,58] Conversely, the degree of cytoplasmic vacuolation characteristic of an SDH-deficient carcinoma is beyond that allowable in an oncocytoma. More challenging is the differential with chromophobe RCC, in which perinuclear or cytoplasmic clearing might be confused as the vacuolation seen in SDH-deficient carcinoma. However, the characteristic perinuclear ringlike clearing and prominent cell borders in chromophobe carcinomas differs from the large, bubbly, vacuoles of SDH-deficient carcinoma. Additionally, the telltale raisinoid nuclear atypia of chromophobe is not seen in SDH-deficient carcinoma (which often shows a more neuroendocrinelike "salt and pepper" appearance). Also, SDHB-deficient carcinoma does not show the prevalent KIT (CD117) positivity characteristic of the oncocytoma/chromophobe family of tumors, except in intralesional mast cells. Several features of SDH-deficient carcinomas, including focal keratin positivity, raise consideration of

translocation-associated RCC (especially t[6;11]), whereas the peripheral entrapment of tubules is reminiscent of EAML. Fortunately, melanocytic/perivascular epithelioid cell differentiation markers HMB45 and cathepsin K, which show prevalent positivity in translocation carcinomas and PEComas, have proven consistently negative in cases of SDH-deficient carcinomas studied so far.[56] Similarly, PAX8 expression is quite prevalent in SDH-deficient carcinomas, also contrasting EAMLs.

## PROGNOSIS

Again, given the rarity of SDH-deficient RCC and lack of standardization of treatment, only preliminary conclusions may be made about the prognosis of these tumors, and only then with the caveats and ascertainment biases of consultation-based series. However, evolution of metastatic carcinoma has been noted in approximately 20% of the patients described in the largest series, findings compatible with the 1 in 10 cases described in the authors' experience.[56] Of the 9 total cases with metastasis analyzed by Gill and colleagues, 4 showed disease-specific demise at an average of 18 months after presentation. Of these,

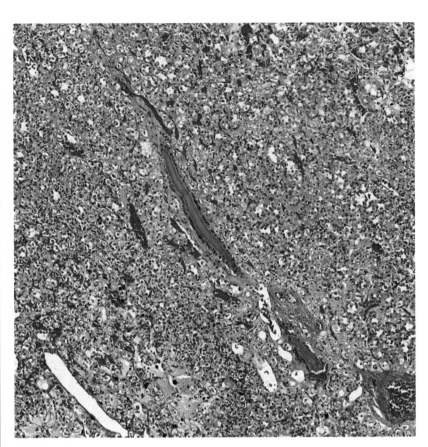

*Fig. 24.* Entrapped perilesional non-neoplastic renal tubules in SDH-deficient RCC (H&E, original magnification ×40); this is a commonly observed feature.

all 4 exhibited grade 3 or 4 nuclei, and 3 showed coagulative necrosis. One additional case showed coagulative necrosis and metastasis, with no further information available, whereas a further 3 cases showed late metastases at 5.5, 9.0, and 30.0 years. Taken together with other reports of these tumors, Gill and colleagues recommend considering tumors with coagulative necrosis, high nuclear grade, sarcomatoid change, or otherwise variant histology as high risk for metastasis, while understanding that such metastasis may occur even after a number of intervening years.

## Pathologic Key Features

1. SDH-deficient RCCs represent a new entity in the spectrum of oncocytic renal tumors, to be suspected especially in younger patients and in those with personal or family history of paragangliomas and GISTs (PGL1, 3, and 4).

2. Grossly, these tumors are unencapsulated and show features similar to other oncocytic neoplasms.

3. Microscopically, SDH-deficient RCCs are solid to partially cystic tumors including sheets and large nests of oncocytic polygonal cells with bubbly cytoplasm, frequent eosinophilic inclusions, and peripheral entrapment of adjacent benign tubules. The nuclei are smooth with even chromatin distribution and inconspicuous nucleoli (neuroendocrinelike).

4. Most affected patients harbor *SDHB* mutations on genetic testing, although mutations of other subunits of the succinate dehydrogenase complex can result in tumorigenesis and loss of SDHB expression by IHC.

5. Metastasis may occur in an infrequent, but distinct minority, of cases.

## Differential Diagnosis

ΔΔ

1. Chromophobe RCC: these tumors show oncocytic features with cytoplasmic flocculence to clearing, with raisinoid "koilocytic" nuclear features, with frequent KIT positivity by IHC.

2. Oncocytoma: these tumors show a nested to microcystic appearance of bland cells with abundant homogeneous cytoplasm and nuclei with fine chromatin, smooth contours, and single central nucleolus.

3. t(6;11) RCC: shows solid or alveolar architecture with variably clear to eosinophilic cells, with usually a "second population" of smaller cells surrounding eosinophilic extracellular deposits of basement membranelike material. These tumors are strongly positive for Melan-A and cathepsin K.

4. Epithelioid angiomyolipomas (PEComas): may show sheets of eosinophilic cells and even perilesional entrapped tubules to microcysts. These tumors are also positive for Melan-A and cathepsin K but negative for PAX-8.

## HEREDITARY LEIOMYOMATOSIS AND RENAL CELL CARCINOMA SYNDROME–ASSOCIATED RENAL CELL CARCINOMA

### INTRODUCTION

Starting in 2001, Launonen and colleagues[59,60] mapped a locus conferring an autosomal dominantly inherited susceptibility to multiple cutaneous and uterine leiomyomas and RCC (Reed syndrome, multiple cutaneous and uterine leiomyomas [MCUL]) to chromosome 1,[60] subsequently determining that the causative gene in affected kindreds was FH.[61] Studies of the clinical features of affected kindreds show a penetrant phenotype of multiple cutaneous leiomyomas (100% of males, >90% of females) with concomitant multiple uterine leiomyomas in approximately 70% of females.[62] The incidence of RCC arising in this setting has been variably estimated in the range of 10% to 30%,[40,62,63] although the syndrome is likely underrecognized. The renal tumors arising in this syndrome, in both males and females, were originally described as high grade and papillary in morphology,[61] although greater morphologic variability has been described more recently, along with frequent aggressive disease course.[64]

### GROSS FEATURES

Experience with this entity is limited; the largest cohort reported describes tumors ranging in size from 2.3 to 20.0 cm, most high stage (perinephric and renal vein or caval extension). Tumors have been described as generally solid, although a significant proportion showed a minor cystic component.[64] Helpful also in understanding the gross appearance of these tumors is a very recent report[65] detailing a rapid autopsy of a patient with HLRCC, wherein the tumor was described as necrotic, multinodular, and infiltrative, with cysts up to 4 cm, involving perinephric and renal sinus fat and the ipsilateral adrenal gland. Metastases were observed, up to 11.5 cm, with fleshy white appearance involving the peritoneum, omentum, spleen, stomach, left and right ovaries, diaphragm, lymph nodes, lung, and liver.

### MICROSCOPIC FEATURES, MOLECULAR PATHOGENESIS, IMMUNOHISTOCHEMISTRY, AND DIAGNOSIS

Although HLRCC-associated RCC has evolved to the point of being recognized as a distinctive entity in the International Society of Urological Pathology Vancouver Classification, the specific criteria for making a prospective diagnosis of HLRCC-associated RCC remain unclear. The main reported cohorts in the surgical pathology literature have focused on study of the features of bona fide cases arising in patients with HLRCC proven to harbor FH mutations.[8,18,64] These studies have uncovered a wealth of variation in the morphology and architecture of these tumors. Originally proposed to be predominantly high-grade RCC with a papillary growth pattern,[61] HLRCC-associated RCCs have been described to show not only papillary but frequent tubulopapillary, cystic, tubulocystic, solid, even prominently tubular areas and may overlap morphologically with collecting duct carcinoma (**Figs. 25** and **26**).[64] One consistent

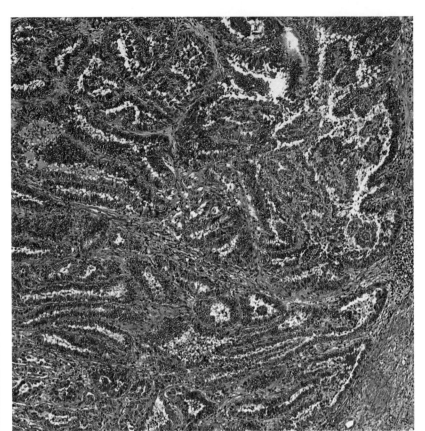

Fig. 25. HLRCC-associated RCC showing a tubulopapillary growth pattern (H&E, original magnification ×10).

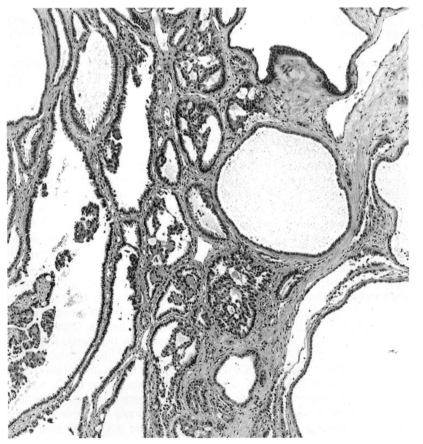

Fig. 26. HLRCC-associated RCC demonstrating a tubulocystic growth pattern. There are areas showing more complex papillations that exceed those seen in tubulocystic carcinoma (H&E, original magnification ×10).

and distinctive feature described has been that of large nuclei with remarkable, "inclusionlike," brightly eosinophilic macronucleolus, often with perinucleolar clearing, apparent at least focally in all of the tumors (**Fig. 27**).[64] Indeed, recently this feature has been even observed among the uterine leiomyomas described in this syndrome.[66]

With the understanding that a number of recognized and unclassified high-grade RCCs in the differential with HLRCC-associated RCC may have prominent nucleoli, quite useful, then, are recent reports that the supraphysiologic fumarate accumulation in *FH*-null carcinoma cells results in induction of aberrant succination of cytosolic and nuclear proteins, specifically S-(2-succino)-cysteine (2SC), which may be detected by IHC. In fact, Chen and colleagues[8] observed that all 9 tumors from patients presenting sporadically but later proven to have HLRCC showed diffuse cytoplasmic and nuclear positivity for 2SC, whereas only minor subsets of high-grade papillary and unclassified carcinomas showed 2SC stain, predominantly cytoplasmic.[18] Thus, they

proposed the stain as a useful diagnostic adjunct. Similarly, very recently IHC for the FH protein (demonstrating loss of FH staining in these tumors) itself has been proposed as a relatively specific, but slightly less sensitive marker for HLRCC-associated RCC (**Fig. 28**).[67] Beyond these features, the immunophenotype for these tumors has not been explored in great detail; in the authors' unpublished experience, most of these tumors show positivity for PAX8, supportive of their arising as a renal primary, which may be quite helpful in the metastatic setting. In our diagnostic and consultative practice, we frequently recommend urologists to specifically elicit family history of skin lesions, multiple uterine myomas, and family history of these features and kidney cancer, with the understanding that uncovering a syndromal case may be of great use for allowing surveillance of affected kindreds. Again, mutation analysis of FH remains the closest approximation to a diagnostic gold standard, while it still remains unclear whether sporadic cases might also occur.

*Fig. 27.* HLRCC-associated RCC demonstrating large tumor cell nuclei with prominent, "inclusionlike," brightly eosinophilic macronucleoli, often with perinucleolar clearing, present at least focally (see inset images on right) (H&E, original magnification ×20, original magnification ×40 in insets).

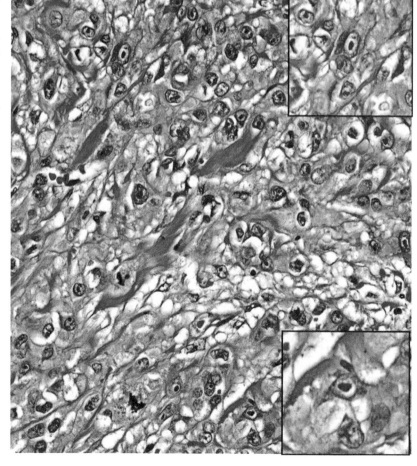

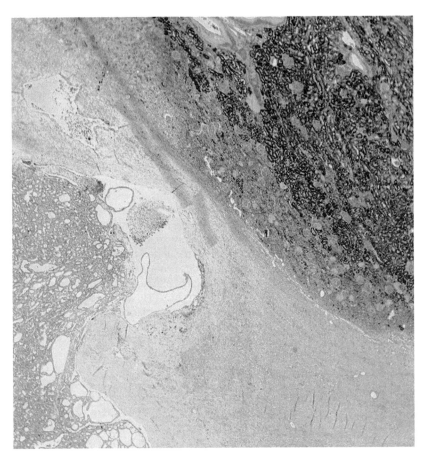

**Fig. 28.** Tumor cells in HLRCC-associated RCC demonstrating loss of FH staining in the tumor cells (*left*). Note that the uninvolved kidney parenchyma shows retained FH staining (*right*) (Immunoperoxidase staining, original magnification ×4).

## DIFFERENTIAL DIAGNOSIS

Given the morphologic variability seen in cases described to this point, the differential diagnosis with several entities presents a pathologic challenge. First, papillary RCC is usually lower nuclear grade, composed of smaller cells, and morphologically more homogeneous than the variable morphology (within and between cases) seen in HLRCC-associated RCC. And, as reported by Chen and colleagues,[8] despite expression of 2-SC in a subset of cases, this marker may have value in this setting. Given the high nuclear grade and the variable papillary and solid and nested morphology frequently seen, MiTF/TFE-family translocation-associated RCC, especially Xp11.2 carcinomas may enter into consideration. Fortunately, translocation carcinomas show melanocytic marker expression in a subset of cases and a scarcity of keratin positivity not seen to this point in HLRCC-associated RCC. Most challenging may be then, is the differential with collecting duct carcinomas (CDCs). These tumors may show significant morphologic overlap with HLRCC-associated RCC (and some previously diagnosed CDCs may represent HLRCC[64]). Prospectively, we recommend that care should be taken to exclude clinical and morphologic features of HLRCC-associated RCC, availing to consultation and genetic counseling and testing, if necessary, before rendering a diagnosis of CDC. We note that the literature is still evolving regarding the relationship between these tumors and hope that emerging biomarkers, such as FH and 2-SC, may help provide clarity in the classification of these tumors.

## PROGNOSIS

Again, only limited experience exists with these tumors; however, in the recent, well-documented series from the pathology literature, a substantial majority of affected patients succumb to metastatic carcinoma within a few years of diagnosis.[8,18,64] Wide dissemination of metastatic disease to a variety of visceral and lymphatic sites has been documented.[64,65] Effective adjuvant therapy has not been established, although promising strategies to target the relative dependence of these tumors on glycolysis are contemplated.[68]

### Pathologic Key Features

1. HLRCC-associated RCC is an emerging entity in the spectrum of high-grade RCCs.

2. Thus far, these tumors have been demonstrated in the setting of the HLRCC syndrome, also known as Reed syndrome or MCUL.

3. Their morphologic spectrum is variable, from papillary to tubular and solid, and may have overlapping features with collecting duct carcinoma.

4. A prominent eosinophilic inclusionlike macronucleolus with perinucleolar clearing is seen at least focally in many cases and should raise the possibility of HLRCC-associated RCC; however, this feature is not entirely specific.

5. These tumors are very aggressive, highlighting the importance of their prospective recognition for genetic counseling and surveillance of affected kindreds.

### Differential Diagnosis

1. High-grade conventional papillary RCC: these tumors tend to be more morphologically uniform than HLRCC-associated RCC; syndromal cases of papillary carcinoma tend to be multiple and lower grade.

2. High-grade MiTF/TFE-family translocation–associated carcinomas: may show similar papillary and high-grade features but demonstrate frequent expression of melanocytic markers (Melan-A, HMB45, and cathepsin K) and either TFE3 or TFEB.

3. Collecting duct carcinoma: may demonstrate significant overlap with HLRCC-associated carcinomas, and hence must be rigorously excluded. The relationship between these entities is in the process of being better elucidated.

## REFERENCES

1. Amin MB, MacLennan GT, Gupta R, et al. Tubulocystic carcinoma of the kidney: clinicopathologic analysis of 31 cases of a distinctive rare subtype of renal cell carcinoma. Am J Surg Pathol 2009;33(3): 384–92.

2. MacLennan GT, Cheng L. Tubulocystic carcinoma of the kidney. J Urol 2011;185(6):2348–9.

3. Gupta R, Billis A, Shah RB, et al. Carcinoma of the collecting ducts of Bellini and renal medullary carcinoma: clinicopathologic analysis of 52 cases of rare aggressive subtypes of renal cell carcinoma with a focus on their interrelationship. Am J Surg Pathol 2012;36(9):1265–78.

4. Argani P, Yonescu R, Morsberger L, et al. Molecular confirmation of t(6;11)(p21;q12) renal cell carcinoma in archival paraffin-embedded material using a break-apart TFEB FISH assay expands its clinicopathologic spectrum. Am J Surg Pathol 2012; 36(10):1516–26.

5. Mosquera JM, Dal Cin P, Mertz KD, et al. Validation of a TFE3 break-apart FISH assay for Xp11.2 translocation renal cell carcinomas. Diagn Mol Pathol 2011;20(3):129–37.

6. Kim SH, Choi Y, Jeong HY, et al. Usefulness of a break-apart FISH assay in the diagnosis of Xp11.2 translocation renal cell carcinoma. Virchows Arch 2011;459(3):299–306.

7. Green WM, Yonescu R, Morsberger L, et al. Utilization of a TFE3 break-apart FISH assay in a renal tumor consultation service. Am J Surg Pathol 2013; 37(8):1150–63.

8. Chen YB, Brannon AR, Toubaji A, et al. Hereditary leiomyomatosis and renal cell carcinoma syndrome-associated renal cancer: recognition of the syndrome by pathologic features and the utility of detecting aberrant succination by immunohistochemistry. Am J Surg Pathol 2014;38(5):627–37.

9. Al-Hussain TO, Cheng L, Zhang S, et al. Tubulocystic carcinoma of the kidney with poorly differentiated foci: a series of 3 cases with fluorescence in situ hybridization analysis. Hum Pathol 2013;44(7): 1406–11.

10. Osunkoya AO, Young AN, Wang W, et al. Comparison of gene expression profiles in tubulocystic carcinoma and collecting duct carcinoma of the kidney. Am J Surg Pathol 2009;33(7):1103–6.

11. Zhou M, Yang XJ, Lopez JI, et al. Renal tubulocystic carcinoma is closely related to papillary renal cell carcinoma: implications for pathologic classification. Am J Surg Pathol 2009;33(12):1840–9.

12. Yang XJ, Zhou M, Hes O, et al. Tubulocystic carcinoma of the kidney: clinicopathologic and molecular characterization. Am J Surg Pathol 2008;32(2): 177–87.

13. Bhullar JS, Thamboo T, Esuvaranathan K. Unique case of tubulocystic carcinoma of the kidney with sarcomatoid features: a new entity. Urology 2011; 78(5):1071–2.

14. Tickoo SK, dePeralta-Venturina MN, Harik LR, et al. Spectrum of epithelial neoplasms in end-stage renal disease: an experience from 66 tumor-bearing kidneys with emphasis on histologic patterns distinct from those in sporadic adult renal neoplasia. Am J Surg Pathol 2006;30(2):141–53.

15. Gobbo S, Eble JN, Grignon DJ, et al. Clear cell papillary renal cell carcinoma: a distinct histopathologic and molecular genetic entity. Am J Surg Pathol 2008;32(8):1239–45.

16. Aron M, Chang E, Herrera L, et al. Clear cell-papillary renal cell carcinoma of the kidney not associated with end-stage renal disease: clinicopathologic correlation with expanded immunophenotypic and molecular characterization of a large cohort with emphasis on relationship with renal angiomyoadenomatous tumor. Am J Surg Pathol 2015;39(7):873–88.

17. Deml KF, Schildhaus HU, Compérat E, et al. Clear cell papillary renal cell carcinoma and renal angiomyoadenomatous tumor: two variants of a morphologic, immunohistochemical, and genetic distinct entity of renal cell carcinoma. Am J Surg Pathol 2015;39(7):889–901.

18. Williamson SR, Cheng L, Eble JN, et al. Renal cell carcinoma with angioleiomyoma-like stroma: clinicopathological, immunohistochemical, and molecular features supporting classification as a distinct entity. Mod Pathol 2015;28(2):279–94.

19. Michal M, Hes O, Havlicek F. Benign renal angiomyoadenomatous tumor: a previously unreported renal tumor. Ann Diagn Pathol 2000;4(5):311–5.

20. Warrick JI, Tsodikov A, Kunju LP, et al. Papillary renal cell carcinoma revisited: a comprehensive histomorphologic study with outcome correlations. Hum Pathol 2014;45(6):1139–46.

21. Hakimi AA, Tickoo SK, Jacobsen A, et al. TCEB1-mutated renal cell carcinoma: a distinct genomic and morphological subtype. Mod Pathol 2015; 28(6):845–53.

22. Hirsch MS, Barletta JA, Gorman M, et al. Renal cell carcinoma with monosomy 8 and CAIX expression: a distinct entity or another member or the clear cell tubulopapillary RCC/RAT family? Mod Pathol 2015; 28(s2):229A.

23. Guo J, Tretiakova MS, Troxell ML, et al. Tuberous sclerosis-associated renal cell carcinoma: a clinicopathologic study of 57 separate carcinomas in 18 patients. Am J Surg Pathol 2014;38(11): 1457–67.

24. Rao P, Monzon F, Jonasch E, et al. Clear cell papillary renal cell carcinoma in patients with von Hippel-Lindau syndrome–clinicopathological features and comparative genomic analysis of 3 cases. Hum Pathol 2014;45(9):1966–72.

25. Williamson SR, Cheng L. Do clear cell papillary renal cell carcinomas occur in patients with von Hippel-Lindau disease? Hum Pathol 2015;46(2):340–1.

26. Williamson SR, Zhang S, Eble JN, et al. Clear cell papillary renal cell carcinoma-like tumors in patients with von Hippel-Lindau disease are unrelated to sporadic clear cell papillary renal cell carcinoma. Am J Surg Pathol 2013;37(8):1131–9.

27. Adam J, Couturier J, Molinié V, et al. Clear-cell papillary renal cell carcinoma: 24 cases of a distinct low-grade renal tumour and a comparative genomic hybridization array study of seven cases. Histopathology 2011;58(7):1064–71.

28. Munari E, Marchionni L, Chitre A, et al. Clear cell papillary renal cell carcinoma: micro-RNA expression profiling and comparison with clear cell renal cell carcinoma and papillary renal cell carcinoma. Hum Pathol 2014;45(6):1130–8.

29. Udager AM, Alva A, Mehra R. Current and proposed molecular diagnostics in a genitourinary service line laboratory at a tertiary clinical institution. Cancer J 2014;20(1):29–42.

30. Amin MB, Gupta R, Ondrej H, et al. Primary thyroid-like follicular carcinoma of the kidney: report of 6 cases of a histologically distinctive adult renal epithelial neoplasm. Am J Surg Pathol 2009;33(3): 393–400.

31. Jung SJ, Chung JI, Park SH, et al. Thyroid follicular carcinoma-like tumor of kidney: a case report with morphologic, immunohistochemical, and genetic analysis. Am J Surg Pathol 2006;30(3):411–5.

32. Dhillon J, Tannir NM, Matin SF, et al. Thyroid-like follicular carcinoma of the kidney with metastases to the lungs and retroperitoneal lymph nodes. Hum Pathol 2011;42(1):146–50.

33. Debelenko LV, Raimondi SC, Daw N, et al. Renal cell carcinoma with novel VCL-ALK fusion: new representative of ALK-associated tumor spectrum. Mod Pathol 2011;24(3):430–42.

34. Marino-Enriquez A, Ou WB, Weldon CB, et al. ALK rearrangement in sickle cell trait-associated renal medullary carcinoma. Genes Chromosomes Cancer 2011;50(3):146–53.

35. Smith NE, Deyrup AT, Mariño-Enriquez A, et al. VCL-ALK renal cell carcinoma in children with sickle-cell trait: the eighth sickle-cell nephropathy? Am J Surg Pathol 2014;38(6):858–63.

36. Sukov WR, Hodge JC, Lohse CM, et al. ALK alterations in adult renal cell carcinoma: frequency, clinicopathologic features and outcome in a large series of consecutively treated patients. Mod Pathol 2012; 25(11):1516–25.

37. Sugawara E, Togashi Y, Kuroda N, et al. Identification of anaplastic lymphoma kinase fusions in renal cancer: large-scale immunohistochemical screening

by the intercalated antibody-enhanced polymer method. Cancer 2012;118(18):4427–36.

38. Ryan C, Mayer N, Cunningham J, et al. Increased ALK1 copy number and renal cell carcinoma—a case report. Virchows Arch 2014;464(2):241–5.

39. Argani P, Hawkins A, Griffin CA, et al. A distinctive pediatric renal neoplasm characterized by epithelioid morphology, basement membrane production, focal HMB45 immunoreactivity, and t(6;11)(p21.1;q12) chromosome translocation. Am J Pathol 2001;158(6):2089–96.

40. Srigley JR, Delahunt B, Eble JN, et al. The International Society of Urological Pathology (ISUP) Vancouver Classification of Renal Neoplasia. Am J Surg Pathol 2013;37(10):1469–89.

41. Argani P, Laé M, Hutchinson B, et al. Renal carcinomas with the t(6;11)(p21;q12): clinicopathologic features and demonstration of the specific alpha-TFEB gene fusion by immunohistochemistry, RT-PCR, and DNA PCR. Am J Surg Pathol 2005;29(2):230–40.

42. Inamura K, Fujiwara M, Togashi Y, et al. Diverse fusion patterns and heterogeneous clinicopathologic features of renal cell carcinoma with t(6;11) translocation. Am J Surg Pathol 2012;36(1):35–42.

43. Rao Q, Liu B, Cheng L, et al. Renal cell carcinomas with t(6;11)(p21;q12): a clinicopathologic study emphasizing unusual morphology, novel alpha-TFEB gene fusion point, immunobiomarkers, and ultrastructural features, as well as detection of the gene fusion by fluorescence in situ hybridization. Am J Surg Pathol 2012;36(9):1327–38.

44. Argani P. MiT family translocation renal cell carcinoma. Semin Diagn Pathol 2015;32(2):103–13.

45. Martignoni G, Pea M, Gobbo S, et al. Cathepsin-K immunoreactivity distinguishes MiTF/TFE family renal translocation carcinomas from other renal carcinomas. Mod Pathol 2009;22(8):1016–22.

46. Smith NE, Illei PB, Allaf M, et al. t(6;11) renal cell carcinoma (RCC): expanded immunohistochemical profile emphasizing novel RCC markers and report of 10 new genetically confirmed cases. Am J Surg Pathol 2014;38(5):604–14.

47. Denton MD, Magee CC, Ovuworie C, et al. Prevalence of renal cell carcinoma in patients with ESRD pre-transplantation: a pathologic analysis. Kidney Int 2002;61(6):2201–9.

48. Sule N, Yakupoglu U, Shen SS, et al. Calcium oxalate deposition in renal cell carcinoma associated with acquired cystic kidney disease: a comprehensive study. Am J Surg Pathol 2005;29(4):443–51.

49. Kuroda N, Tamura M, Taguchi T, et al. Sarcomatoid acquired cystic disease-associated renal cell carcinoma. Histol Histopathol 2008;23(11):1327–31.

50. Pan CC, Chen YJ, Chang LC, et al. Immunohistochemical and molecular genetic profiling of acquired cystic disease-associated renal cell carcinoma. Histopathology 2009;55(2):145–53.

51. Chen YB, Tickoo SK. Spectrum of preneoplastic and neoplastic cystic lesions of the kidney. Arch Pathol Lab Med 2012;136(4):400–9.

52. Ishikawa I, Saito Y, Asaka M, et al. Twenty-year follow-up of acquired renal cystic disease. Clin Nephrol 2003;59(3):153–9.

53. Gill AJ. Succinate dehydrogenase (SDH) and mitochondrial driven neoplasia. Pathology 2012;44(4):285–92.

54. Gill AJ, Pachter NS, Clarkson A, et al. Renal tumors and hereditary pheochromocytoma-paraganglioma syndrome type 4. N Engl J Med 2011;364(9):885–6.

55. Gill AJ, Hes O, Papathomas T, et al. Succinate dehydrogenase (SDH)-deficient renal carcinoma: a morphologically distinct entity: a clinicopathologic series of 36 tumors from 27 patients. Am J Surg Pathol 2014;38(12):1588–602.

56. Williamson SR, Eble JN, Amin MB, et al. Succinate dehydrogenase-deficient renal cell carcinoma: detailed characterization of 11 tumors defining a unique subtype of renal cell carcinoma. Mod Pathol 2015;28(1):80–94.

57. Housley SL, Lindsay RS, Young B, et al. Renal carcinoma with giant mitochondria associated with germ-line mutation and somatic loss of the succinate dehydrogenase B gene. Histopathology 2010;56(3):405–8.

58. Gill AJ, Pachter NS, Chou A, et al. Renal tumors associated with germline SDHB mutation show distinctive morphology. Am J Surg Pathol 2011;35(10):1578–85.

59. Reed WB, Walker R, Horowitz R. Cutaneous leiomyomata with uterine leiomyomata. Acta Derm Venereol 1973;53(5):409–16.

60. Launonen V, Vierimaa O, Kiuru M, et al. Inherited susceptibility to uterine leiomyomas and renal cell cancer. Proc Natl Acad Sci U S A 2001;98(6):3387–92.

61. Tomlinson IP, Alam NA, Rowan AJ, et al. Germline mutations in FH predispose to dominantly inherited uterine fibroids, skin leiomyomata and papillary renal cell cancer. Nat Genet 2002;30(4):406–10.

62. Alam NA, Barclay E, Rowan AJ, et al. Clinical features of multiple cutaneous and uterine leiomyomatosis: an underdiagnosed tumor syndrome. Arch Dermatol 2005;141(2):199–206.

63. Toro JR, Nickerson ML, Wei MH, et al. Mutations in the fumarate hydratase gene cause hereditary leiomyomatosis and renal cell cancer in families in North America. Am J Hum Genet 2003;73(1):95–106.

64. Merino MJ, Torres-Cabala C, Pinto P, et al. The morphologic spectrum of kidney tumors in hereditary leiomyomatosis and renal cell carcinoma (HLRCC) syndrome. Am J Surg Pathol 2007;31(10):1578–85.

65. Udager AM, Alva A, Chen YB, et al. Hereditary leiomyomatosis and renal cell carcinoma (HLRCC): a

rapid autopsy report of metastatic renal cell carcinoma. Am J Surg Pathol 2014;38(4):567–77.

66. Sanz-Ortega J, Vocke C, Stratton P, et al. Morphologic and molecular characteristics of uterine leiomyomas in hereditary leiomyomatosis and renal cancer (HLRCC) syndrome. Am J Surg Pathol 2013;37(1):74–80.

67. Lara Otero K, Linehan MW, Merino MJ. IHC helps to identify renal tumors associated with HLRCC syndrome. Mod Pathol 2014;27(Suppl):243A.

68. Linehan WM, Rouault TA. Molecular pathways: fumarate hydratase-deficient kidney cancer–targeting the Warburg effect in cancer. Clin Cancer Res 2013;19(13):3345–52.

# Diagnosis of Renal Cell Carcinoma
## A Clinician's Perspective

Laurence Albiges, MD, PhD[a], André P. Fay, MD[a], Rana R. McKay, MD[a,b],
Marina D. Kaymakcalan, PharmD[a], Toni K. Choueiri, MD[a,b,*]

## KEYWORDS

• Renal cell carcinoma • Clear cell • Biopsy • Prognosis • Biomarker

## ABSTRACT

Renal cell carcinoma (RCC) is a heterogeneous disease. A rigorous diagnostic assessment by a pathologist with close communication with the clinician provides more accurate prognostication and informed treatment decisions. In the localized setting, an accurate prognostic assessment directs patients to potential adjuvant clinical trials. For patients with advanced disease, the pathologic assessment may have a direct impact on the systemic therapy algorithm. Additionally, it provides the basis for continuous efforts in biomarker development. In rare histologic subtypes, the interaction between clinicians and pathologists provides an opportunity to offer patients specific clinical trials. Molecular characterization platforms may identify targets for therapeutic intervention.

## OVERVIEW

Renal cell carcinoma (RCC) is a relatively common cancer. In 2014, the incidence of RCC in the United States was estimated to be 63,920 cases (kidney and renal pelvic cancers), potentially resulting in 13,860 deaths.[1] Pathologic assessment[2] (see also Hirsch et al, Adult Renal Cell Carcinoma: A Review of Established Entities Form Morphology to Molecular Genetics, Surgical Pathology Clinics, 2015, Volume 8, Issue 4 and Mehra et al, Emerging Entities in Renal Neoplasia, Surgical Pathology Clinics, 2015, Volume 8, Issue 4) plays a crucial role in both localized and metastatic settings where the findings therein define the appropriate management of patients with kidney cancer.

In the localized setting, the pathologist's analysis of the tumor biopsy triggers distinct strategies in the management of small unilateral or bilateral renal masses. After partial or radical nephrectomy, the pathology assessment of the tumor defines the risk of recurrence and aids in determining the monitoring and follow-up plans. In the metastatic setting, the pathologic findings can direct the systemic treatment approach. Non–clear cell RCC (non-ccRCC) deserves special attention given the limited therapeutic agents for this heterogeneous category of disease entities. Over the past decade, new RCC subtypes have been identified for which the clinical outcome may not be fully established.[3] In addition, some specific pathologic features, such as the presence of sarcomatoid differentiation, add major prognostic information that clinicians are likely to use both to refine the overall prognosis estimation and to select treatment options.

This article aims to summarize the clinician's perspective on the pathologic diagnosis of RCC, with a focus on clinicians' expectations of the pathologist to optimize the use of pathologic

Disclosures: All authors have declared no conflict of interest for this work.
[a] Dana-Farber Cancer Institute, Harvard Medical School, 450 Brookline Avenue (DANA 1230), Boston, MA 02215, USA; [b] Brigham and Women's Hospital, Harvard Medical School, Boston, MA, USA
* Corresponding author. Dana-Farber Cancer Institute, 450 Brookline Avenue (DANA 1230), Boston, MA 02215.
E-mail address: toni_choueiri@dfci.harvard.edu

Surgical Pathology 8 (2015) 657–662
http://dx.doi.org/10.1016/j.path.2015.08.001

features, including not only histologic assessment but also immunohistochemistry and cytogenetic and molecular strategies, in the management of kidney cancer.

## RENAL MASS BIOPSY: EXPECTATIONS FROM THE CLINICIANS

### SMALL RENAL MASSES AND LOCALIZED RENAL CELL CARCINOMA

The increasing incidence of small renal masses (SRMs), defined as less than 4 cm,[4] has led to the development of more conservative management strategies to include ablative techniques or active surveillance in select cases. To choose the best strategy, clinicians rely on the biopsy diagnosis provided by pathologists to distinguish from 3 chief groups of lesions: benign tumor, indolent cancer, and aggressive cancer.

Percutaneous biopsy for diagnostic assessment of SRMs has the potential to avoid unnecessary surgeries and support treatment decisions, especially in patients at increased surgical risk.[5] It has been demonstrated that SRM biopsies have both acceptable sensitivity, ranging from 86% to 100%, and specificity for the diagnosis of malignancy.[6] The overall positive predictive value for the diagnosis of malignancy in a report encompassing 2474 renal tumor biopsies was 97.5%, with an overall sensitivity of 92.1% and a specificity of 89.7%.[7] Although these results may be illustrative of high-volume centers, such accuracy is now expected of routine renal mass biopsies, with the understanding that the rate of nondiagnostic biopsy, commonly due to insufficient material, is approximately 22%, according to a large report of 1000 biopsies from a single institution.[8] In addition to differentiating malignant tumors (see also Hirsch et al, Adult Renal Cell Carcinoma: A Review of Established Entities Form Morphology to Molecular Genetics, Surgical Pathology Clinics, 2015, Volume 8, Issue 4 and Mehra et al, Emerging Entities in Renal Neoplasia, Surgical Pathology Clinics, 2015, Volume 8, Issue 4) from benign lesions (see also Arias-Stella and Williamson, Updates in Benign Lesions of the Genitourinary Tract, Surgical Pathology Clinics, 2015, Volume 8, Issue 4) histologic subtype and Fuhrman grade can be assessed on a core biopsy with success rates of 86% to 100%[6] and 64% to 93%, respectively.[9,10]

Molecular analysis performed on renal biopsy specimens may also serve as a diagnostic tool and be part of the decision-making process. Recently, a study attempted to characterize the genetic alterations associated with metanephric adenoma (MA), a rare indolent kidney tumor that may be difficult to differentiate from a small malignant kidney cancer. Because this is a benign tumor, surveillance may be appropriate in most situations, sparing the loss of nephrons. This study identified the v-raf murine sarcoma viral oncogene homolog B1 (BRAF) V600E mutation in 26 of 29 MA cases (approximately 90%). Given that BRAF V600E mutations are present in approximately 90% of all MA cases[11] and BRAF immunohistochemistry is sensitive and specific,[12] this could serve as a potential valuable diagnostic tool in the differential diagnosis of SRMs undergoing a kidney biopsy.

### METASTATIC RENAL CELL CARCINOMA

The use of renal mass biopsy in patients presenting with radiological findings suggestive of metastatic disease is usually more limited. It is commonly restricted to patients not eligible for primary nephrectomy due to comorbidities or to other poor prognostic criteria,[13] which usually drive physicians to offer patients upfront systemic therapy.[14,15] In this specific setting, the role of biopsy is not only to confirm the RCC diagnosis but also to specify the histologic subtype of the tumor, especially if it is of the clear cell subtype where therapeutic options may be available. Conversely, despite the lack of specific systemic therapies for non-ccRCC, identification of such specific histologic tumor subtypes is critical for communicating information about prognosis and potential therapeutic options for patients with metastatic disease, including the potential for clinical trials.

## NEPHRECTOMY SPECIMEN: EXPECTATIONS FROM THE CLINICIANS

Unlike other tumor types where histology can drive distinct therapeutic approaches, RCC is still managed with the same algorithm irrespective of histologic subtype. In patients with localized or locally advanced disease who underwent partial or radical nephrectomy with a curative intent, the pathologist's report encompasses the distinct parameters that define the risk of recurrence.[16] Among these, tumor stage and grade are important features for the prediction of RCC recurrence after nephrectomy. The primary tumor stage, as determined by the latest version of the TNM staging system, is a powerful predictor of cancer-specific survival (CSS).[17,18] According to the 2009 TNM staging system, the 5-year CSS ranges from 94.9% in pT1a to 27.1% in pT4 cancers. In addition, one of the most commonly used postoperative integrated staging system (ISS) models, referred to as Leibovich ISS, integrates several pathologic parameters in addition to the T and N stages: tumor size, Fuhrman grade, and presence or absence of necrosis.[19] Leibovich ISS is restricted to patients with ccRCC and its predictive accuracy was externally validated with a discriminant ability of 78%. Similarly, the prediction of RCC CSS and overall survival in the postoperative setting relies strongly on the pathologic assessment of several features. Both the Karakiewicz nomogram[20] and the University of California, Los Angeles, ISS,[21] use the TNM stage in combination with Fuhrman grade and clinical parameters (Eastern Cooperative Oncology Group performance status or symptoms classification). Therefore, accurate pathologic determination is vital in assessing recurrence risk, RCC-specific mortality, and overall survival.

Although several molecular markers for disease progression have been proposed, currently no biomarkers have been established to assess the risk of recurrence in clinical practice. Recently, Schutz and colleagues[22] investigated the association of single nucleotide polymorphisms in genes implicated in RCC pathogenesis with the likelihood of RCC recurrence after intended curative treatment. In this study, a germline single nucleotide polymorphism in the c-MET gene (rs11762213) was associated with an increased risk of recurrence in patients with localized disease. An external validation set confirmed this association and this germline alteration may be incorporated in future prognostic tools or used to plan further adjuvant clinical trials.[23]

More elaborate approaches to assess recurrence risk, such as gene expression signatures, have been reported, with 3 models already available,[24–26] including a 16-gene signature, recently externally validated in stage I–III ccRCC.[27] These tools, however, are not currently available in clinical practice, and, given the lack of approved adjuvant therapy, the relevance of these signatures is limited to the ability of providing additional prognostic information without direct influence on therapeutic or monitoring guidelines.

In patients with metastatic disease, the impact of nephrectomy pathology reports is similar to that of biopsy reports, with the main information sought by clinicians the confirmation of the histologic subtype and the presence or absence of sarcomatoid/rhabdoid differentiation. First and foremost, the confirmation of RCC is required for administration of systemic therapy or for eligibility of clinical trial participation. Additionally, the histologic subtype, although not integrated in the available prognostic models, may be associated with a distinct prognosis[28] and is a key piece of information needed

to enroll patients in clinical trials given that many of them are restricted to specific histologies. For example, patients with sarcomatoid features or with collecting duct or medullary-type RCC can benefit from cytotoxic platinum-based chemotherapy,[29] which is not used for the conventional type of RCC (ie, ccRCC). Similar to localized disease, pathologic markers have not been included in the prognostic models for patients treated with targeted therapy in the metastatic setting.[13,30–32]

## EVOLVING FIELD OF PROGNOSIS AND PREDICTIVE BIOMARKERS IN RENAL CELL CARCINOMA

Multiple predictive biomarkers have been investigated in ccRCC,[33] but most have fallen short of clinical expectations and none have entered into current clinical practice. New studies, however, continue to show promise. For example, the identification of chromatin remodeling gene mutations as the second most frequent molecular event in ccRCC has led to the identification of distinct molecular subgroups of RCC with distinct phenotypes.[34,35] It is anticipated that once commonly available for diagnostic use, the immunohistochemical staining of BAP1 and PBRM1, which correlates with the mutational profile in these genes, may provide important prognostic information in ccRCC,[36] although therapeutic implications remain unknown.

In the era of immunotherapy, despite robust clinical evidence of activity in a small number of patients, the well-designed SELECT trial failed to identify patients more likely to benefit from high-dose interleukin-2 treatment.[37] The identification of the role of checkpoint blockade in RCC, however, has generated a strong resurgence of interest in identifying biomarkers of response to the programmed cell death 1 (PD-1)/programmed death–ligand 1 (PD-L1) inhibitions.[38] This exciting discovery emphasizes that the role of the pathologist is key in identifying new potential biomarker candidates and standardizing methodologies to assess these biomarkers. Furthermore, the characterization of changes induced by previous therapies may help guide future treatments and clinical research. As an example, the biomarker phase I study of nivolumab in metastatic RCC identified, on sequential biopsies performed prior to PD-1 inhibition and at cycle 2, increased T-cell infiltrates by medians of 70% (CD3$^+$; range 53%–220%) and 88% (CD8$^+$; 61%–257%) respectively.[39] Accordingly, the expression of PD-L1 as a biomarker is being investigated as a pathologic assessment to serve as a predictive biomarker of PD-1 or PD-L1 inhibitors in metastatic RCC. This involves defining the nature of the staining (tumor cells vs infiltrating lymphocytes) as well as the threshold of positivity (any positivity vs 5% for example).[38–41] Callea and colleagues[42] have also reported on the differential PD-L1 expression between primaries and matching metastases, highlighting that PD-L1 expression is mostly observed in areas of highest tumor grade. Pathologists remain the stakeholders of such efforts, and continued translational collaboration is required to make significant progress in such studies.

Unlike other tumor types, few definitive target alterations have been identified in non-ccRCC despite ongoing studies, including the recent molecular characterization of chromophobe tumors.[43] Given the rarity of some of these less common histologic subtypes, increased collaboration among pathologists may prove beneficial, especially in the context of ongoing, large academic or consortia-led programs, such as The Cancer Genome Atlas Network. Additionally, accurate diagnosis of non–clear cell histology also ensures access to dedicated clinical trials, which may offer patients promising drugs in development. As an illustration, MET inhibition in papillary RCC has yielded intriguing results in a phase II trial[44] and an active program investigating this approach in correlation with the status of MET mutation or other specific alterations is ongoing (NCT02127710 and NCT01524926).

Lastly, pathologists may also play a key role in investigating target modulation after systemic therapy.[45] Such findings may ultimately have an impact on treatment sequencing offered to patients or have an impact on the design of clinical trials with combination strategies. Increased expression of the receptor MET after vascular endothelial growth factor (VEGF)/VEGF receptor (VEGFR) inhibition[46] is one of the key features that has led to an ongoing investigation of a dual MET and VEGFR inhibitor (cabozantinib) in a VEGFR tyrosine kinase inhibitor refractory population based on promising results from a phase II study.[47] A phase III clinical trial comparing cabozantinib versus everolimus is currently under way (NCT01865747).

## SUMMARY

In summary, given the constant evolution regarding the classification of RCC,[2,48,49] with the identification of new entities driven by specific molecular alterations (see also Hirsch et al, Adult Renal Cell Carcinoma: A Review of Established Entities Form Morphology to Molecular Genetics, Surgical Pathology Clinics, 2015, Volume 8, Issue 4 and Mehra et al, Emerging Entities in Renal Neoplasia, Surgical Pathology Clinics, 2015, Volume 8, Issue 4), the pathologist's role can include (1) highlighting the differences between newly characterized entities in terms of macroscopic and microscopic features; (2) understanding the underlying biology associated with these entities; (3) recommending the appropriate diagnostic tools (immunohistochemical staining, fluorescence in situ hybridization, sequencing, or other techniques); and (4) reporting appropriate specific prognostic information, if and when available. Ultimately, the close collaboration between clinicians, both urologists and oncologists, with pathologists facilitates optimal management of a patient with kidney cancer. The accurate assessment of tumor histology and extent is key to offering patients the most appropriate plan of care. Moreover, a pathologist's expertise is needed to move the field of biomarker investigation forward, especially in the context of new target identification and new drug development. Finally, non–clear cell histology is a rapidly evolving field. Motivated by the lack of effective systemic therapies available to date, the tremendous effort of molecular characterization may ultimately translate into meaningful clinical information.

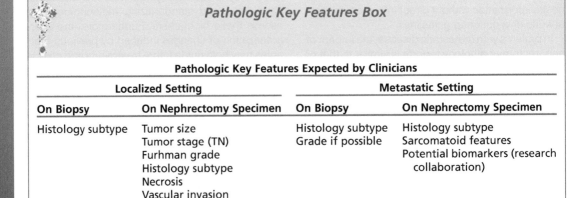

## Pathologic Key Features Box

| Pathologic Key Features Expected by Clinicians | | | |
|---|---|---|---|
| **Localized Setting** | | **Metastatic Setting** | |
| **On Biopsy** | **On Nephrectomy Specimen** | **On Biopsy** | **On Nephrectomy Specimen** |
| Histology subtype | Tumor size<br>Tumor stage (TN)<br>Furhman grade<br>Histology subtype<br>Necrosis<br>Vascular invasion | Histology subtype<br>Grade if possible | Histology subtype<br>Sarcomatoid features<br>Potential biomarkers (research collaboration) |

△△ *Differential Diagnosis*

| Small Renal Masses | Metastatic Disease |
|---|---|
| RCC | RCC |
| Oncocytoma | Urothelial carcinoma |
| Angiomyolipoma | Other carcinoma/ metastatic disease |
| MA | Lymphoma |
| Xanthogranulomatous pyelonephritis | Sarcoma |
| Metastasis from another primary tumor | — |

## REFERENCES

1. Siegel R, Ma J, Zou Z, et al. Cancer statistics, 2014. CA Cancer J Clin 2014;64:9–29.
2. Srigley JR, Delahunt B, Eble JN, et al. The International Society of Urological Pathology (ISUP) vancouver classification of renal neoplasia. Am J Surg Pathol 2013;37(10):1469–89.
3. Deng F-M, Melamed J. Histologic variants of renal cell carcinoma: does tumor type influence outcome? Urol Clin North Am 2012;39:119–32.
4. O'Connor SD, Pickhardt PJ, Kim DH, et al. Incidental finding of renal masses at unenhanced CT: prevalence and analysis of features for guiding management. AJR Am J Roentgenol 2011;197:139–45.
5. Leveridge MJ, Finelli A, Kachura JR, et al. Outcomes of small renal mass needle core biopsy, nondiagnostic percutaneous biopsy, and the role of repeat biopsy. Eur Urol 2011;60:578–84.
6. Volpe A, Finelli A, Gill IS, et al. Rationale for percutaneous biopsy and histologic characterisation of renal tumours. Eur Urol 2012;62:491–504.
7. Lane BR, Samplaski MK, Herts BR, et al. Renal mass biopsy–a renaissance? J Urol 2008;179:20–7.
8. Deshmukh SM, Dhyani M, McGovern FJ, et al. 1065 to biopsy or not to biopsy: results of 1000 renal mass biopsies at a single institution. J Urol 2013; 189:e437.
9. Millet I, Curros F, Serre I, et al. Can renal biopsy accurately predict histological subtype and Fuhrman grade of renal cell carcinoma? J Urol 2012;188:1690–4.
10. Ball MW, Bezerra SM, Gorin MA, et al. Grade heterogeneity in small renal masses: potential implications for renal mass biopsy. J Urol 2015;193(1):36–40.
11. Choueiri TK, Cheville J, Palescandolo E, et al. BRAF mutations in metanephric adenoma of the kidney. Eur Urol 2012;62:917–22.
12. Pinto A, Signoretti S, Hirsch MS, et al. Immunohistochemical staining for BRAF V600E supports the diagnosis of metanephric adenoma. Histopathology 2015;66(6):901–4.
13. Motzer RJ, Bacik J, Schwartz LH, et al. Prognostic factors for survival in previously treated patients with metastatic renal cell carcinoma. J Clin Oncol 2004;22:454–63.
14. National Comprehensive Cancer Network. Kidney cancer (version 3.2014). [Internet]. Available at: http://www.nccn.org/professionals/physician_gls/pdf/kidney.pdf. Accessed June 23, 2014.
15. Leppert JT, Hanley J, Wagner TH, et al. Utilization of renal mass biopsy in patients with renal cell carcinoma. Urology 2014;83:774–9.
16. Meskawi M, Sun M, Trinh Q-D, et al. A review of integrated staging systems for renal cell carcinoma. Eur Urol 2012;62:303–14.
17. Ficarra V, Novara G, Iafrate M, et al. Proposal for reclassification of the tnm staging system in patients with locally advanced (pT3–4) renal cell carcinoma according to the cancer-related outcome. Eur Urol 2007;51:722–31.
18. Novara G, Ficarra V, Antonelli A, et al. Validation of the 2009 TNM version in a large multi-institutional cohort of patients treated for renal cell carcinoma: are further improvements needed? Eur Urol 2010; 58:588–95.
19. Leibovich BC, Blute ML, Cheville JC, et al. Prediction of progression after radical nephrectomy for patients with clear cell renal cell carcinoma: a stratification tool for prospective clinical trials. Cancer 2003;97: 1663–71.
20. Karakiewicz PI, Briganti A, Chun FK-H, et al. Multi-institutional validation of a new renal cancer-specific survival nomogram. J Clin Oncol 2007;25: 1316–22.
21. Zisman A, Pantuck AJ, Dorey F, et al. Improved prognostication of renal cell carcinoma using an integrated staging system. J Clin Oncol 2001;19: 1649–57.
22. Schutz FAB, Pomerantz MM, Gray KP, et al. Single nucleotide polymorphisms and risk of recurrence of renal-cell carcinoma: a cohort study. Lancet Oncol 2013;14:81–7.
23. Hakimi AA, Ostrovnaya I, Jacobsen A, et al. Validation and genomic interrogation of the MET variant rs11762213 as a predictor of adverse outcomes in clear cell renal cell carcinoma [Internet]. J Clin Oncol 2014;32. Available at: http://meetinglibrary.asco.org/content/124087-142. Accessed January 14, 2015.
24. Brooks SA, Brannon AR, Parker JS, et al. ClearCode34: A prognostic risk predictor for localized clear cell renal cell carcinoma. Eur Urol 2014;66:77–84.
25. Choudhury Y, Wei X, Chu Y-H, et al. A multigene assay identifying distinct prognostic subtypes of clear cell renal cell carcinoma with differential

response to tyrosine kinase inhibition. Eur Urol 2015; 67:17–20.

26. Rini BI, Zhou M, Aydin H, et al. Identification of prognostic genomic markers in patients with localized clear cell renal cell carcinoma (ccRCC) [Internet]. J Clin Oncol 2010;28:15s. Available at: http://meetinglibrary.asco.org/content/41897-74. Accessed December 23, 2014.

27. Escudier BJ, Koscielny S, Lopatin M, et al. Validation of a 16-gene signature for prediction of recurrence after nephrectomy in stage I-III clear cell renal cell carcinoma (ccRCC) [Internet]. J Clin Oncol 2014; 32:5s. Available at: http://meetinglibrary.asco.org/content/131088-144. Accessed December 23, 2014.

28. Kroeger N, Xie W, Lee J-L, et al. Metastatic non-clear cell renal cell carcinoma treated with targeted therapy agents: Characterization of survival outcome and application of the International mRCC Database Consortium criteria. Cancer 2013;119: 2999–3006.

29. Pagliaro LC, Tannir N, Sircar K, et al. Systemic therapy for sarcomatoid renal cell carcinoma. Expert Rev Anticancer Ther 2011;11:913–20.

30. Heng DYC, Xie W, Regan MM, et al. Prognostic factors for overall survival in patients with metastatic renal cell carcinoma treated with vascular endothelial growth factor-targeted agents: results from a large, multicenter study. J Clin Oncol 2009;27:5794–9.

31. Manola J, Royston P, Elson P, et al. Prognostic model for survival in patients with metastatic renal cell carcinoma: results from the international kidney cancer working group. Clin Cancer Res 2011;17:5443–50.

32. Heng DYC, Xie W, Regan MM, et al. External validation and comparison with other models of the International Metastatic Renal-Cell Carcinoma Database Consortium prognostic model: a population-based study. Lancet Oncol 2013;14:141–8.

33. Sonpavde G, Choueiri TK. Precision medicine for metastatic renal cell carcinoma. Urol Oncol 2014; 32:5–15.

34. Kapur P, Peña-Llopis S, Christie A, et al. Effects on survival of BAP1 and PBRM1 mutations in sporadic clear-cell renal-cell carcinoma: a retrospective analysis with independent validation. Lancet Oncol 2013;14:159–67.

35. Brugarolas J. Molecular genetics of clear-cell renal cell carcinoma. J Clin Oncol 2014;32:1968–76.

36. Joseph RW, Kapur P, Serie DJ, et al. Loss of BAP1 protein expression is an independent marker of poor prognosis in patients with low-risk clear cell renal cell carcinoma. Cancer 2014;120:1059–67.

37. McDermott DF, Cheng S-C, Signoretti S, et al. The high-dose aldesleukin "select" trial: a trial to prospectively validate predictive models of response

treatment in patients with metastatic renal cell carcinoma. Clin Cancer Res 2014;21(3):561–8.

38. Grosso J, Horak CE, Inzunza D, et al. Association of tumor PD-L1 expression and immune biomarkers with clinical activity in patients (pts) with advanced solid tumors treated with nivolumab (anti-PD-1; BMS-936558; ONO-4538) [Internet]. J Clin Oncol 2013;31. Available at: http://meetinglibrary.asco.org/content/113904-132. Accessed July 18, 2014.

39. Choueiri TK, Fishman MN, Escudier BJ, et al. Immunomodulatory activity of nivolumab in previously treated and untreated metastatic renal cell carcinoma (mRCC): Biomarker-based results from a randomized clinical trial [Internet]. J Clin Oncol 2014;32:5s. Available at: http://meetinglibrary.asco.org/content/125914-144. Accessed June 19, 2014.

40. Motzer RJ, Rini BI, McDermott DF, et al. Nivolumab for Metastatic Renal Cell Carcinoma: Results of a Randomized Phase II Trial. J Clin Oncol 2014;33(13):1430–7.

41. McDermott DF, Sznol M, Sosman JA, et al. Immune correlates and long term follow up of a phase Ia study of MPDL3280A, an engineered PD-L1 antibody, in patients with metastatic renal cell carcinoma (mRCC). Ann Oncol 2014 [abstract: 809O].

42. Callea M, Genega EM, Gupta M, et al. PD-L1 expression in primary clear cell renal cell carcinomas (ccRCCs) and their metastases [Internet]. J Clin Oncol 2014;32. Available at: http://meetinglibrary.asco.org/content/124345-142. Accessed December 22, 2014.

43. Davis CF, Ricketts CJ, Wang M, et al. The somatic genomic landscape of chromophobe renal cell carcinoma. Cancer Cell 2014;26:319–30.

44. Choueiri TK, Vaishampayan U, Rosenberg JE, et al. Phase II and biomarker study of the dual MET/VEGFR2 inhibitor foretinib in patients with papillary renal cell carcinoma. J Clin Oncol 2013;31:181–6.

45. Sharpe K, Stewart GD, Mackay A, et al. The effect of VEGF-targeted therapy on biomarker expression in sequential tissue from patients with metastatic clear cell renal cancer. Clin Cancer Res 2013;19:6924–34.

46. Sennino B, Ishiguro-Oonuma T, Wei Y, et al. Suppression of tumor invasion and metastasis by concurrent inhibition of c-Met and VEGF signaling in pancreatic neuroendocrine tumors. Cancer Discov 2012;2:270–87.

47. Choueiri TK, Pal SK, McDermott DF, et al. A phase I study of cabozantinib (XL184) in patients with renal cell cancer. Ann Oncol 2014;25:1603–8.

48. Lopez-Beltran A, Scarpelli M, Montironi R, et al. 2004 WHO classification of the renal tumors of the adults. Eur Urol 2006;49:798–805.

49. Lopez-Beltran A, Carrasco JC, Cheng L, et al. 2009 update on the classification of renal epithelial tumors in adults. Int J Urol 2009;16:432–43.

# Morphologic and Molecular Characteristics of Bladder Cancer

James P. Solomon, MD, PhD[a], Donna E. Hansel, MD, PhD[b],*

## KEYWORDS

- Bladdder cancer • Urothelial cancers • Molecular alterations • Hematuria

## ABSTRACT

Bladder cancer is the fourth most common cancer in men, and is associated with significant morbidity and mortality. Pathologic evaluation of urothelial cancers relies predominantly on histomorphologic features but can be aided in a small subset of cases by immunohistochemical analyses. Distinction of papillary versus flat lesions, low-grade versus high-grade cytology, and histologic variants and the presence or absence of invasive tumor is important for proper clinical management. Advances in the molecular alterations associated with the various subtypes of urothelial carcinoma have been made but such studies are ongoing.

## OVERVIEW

With more than 74,000 new cases and more than 15,000 deaths each year, urothelial carcinoma of the bladder is one of the most common cancers in the United States. It affects men at a rate 3 times that of women and is the fourth most common cancer diagnosis in men.[1] Hematuria, either gross or microscopic, is the most often presenting symptom, but patients may also experience other nonspecific symptoms, including urinary urgency or dysuria. Smoking is a well-established risk factor for the disease, increasing risk of development by approximately 4-fold.[1] There is no current screening test for urothelial carcinoma, but patients who present with symptoms suspicious for bladder neoplasia undergo a clinical work-up that includes imaging of the upper urinary tracts, urine cytology on voided urine, and white light cystoscopy with bladder biopsy.[2] Once diagnosed, the treatment of urothelial carcinoma depends on the pathologic stage and grade of the tumor (see also Harshman et al, Diagnosis of Bladder Carcinoma: A Clinician's Perspective, Surgical Pathology Clinics, 2015, Volume 8, Issue 4). Surgical excision of tumor burden, either used alone or in combination with intravesicular treatments, such as bacillus Calmette-Guérin, is the mainstay of early-stage cancers. Advanced cancers invasive into the muscularis propria (detrusor muscle) of the bladder are often treated with radical cystectomy, and outcomes are improved with neoadjuvent systemic chemotherapy or radiation treatment.[2] Although the prognosis for noninvasive tumors is good, with a 96% 5-year survival, invasive tumors carry a much worse prognosis, with 70% and 33% 5-year survival rates for localized and regional disease, respectively.[1] Because of the differences in management strategies and prognosis, accurate histopathologic characterization of bladder tumors is of the utmost importance. Great strides have been made in understanding the pathophysiology of urothelial carcinoma; however, the disease seems to have a heterogeneous biology, and various molecular pathways and mutations in many genes are likely involved in tumorigenesis. Nevertheless, the molecular characterization of urothelial carcinoma is currently not performed in routine clinical practice. Additionally, the lack of available predictive biomarkers re-emphasizes

---

[a] Department of Pathology, University of California, San Diego, 9500 Gilman Drive, La Jolla, CA 92093, USA; [b] Division of Anatomic Pathology, Department of Pathology, University of California, San Diego, 9500 Gilman Drive, MC 0612, La Jolla, CA 92093, USA
* Corresponding author.
*E-mail address:* dhansel@ucsd.edu

Surgical Pathology 8 (2015) 663–676
http://dx.doi.org/10.1016/j.path.2015.07.003

the importance of accurate histopathologic staging and grading.

## GROSS FEATURES

There are 2 main growth patterns of urothelial lesions: papillary and flat. The growth patterns are thought to have different molecular mechanisms of growth (discussed later). On cystoscopy or in gross resection specimens, papillary lesions often appear as an exophytic mass with papillary fronds growing outward into the bladder lumen. The lesion may have a cauliflower-like appearance, and there may also be areas of necrosis or ulceration within the lesion. On the other hand, flat, or in situ, lesions, often have a red or velvety gross appearance, contrasting with the smooth tan-gray appearance of normal mucosa, and these areas should be thoroughly sampled.

## MICROSCOPIC FEATURES

### CLASSIFICATION AND GRADING OF UROTHELIAL NEOPLASIA

The classification system of urothelial neoplasia has undergone several revisions since its official inception in 1973. Revisions in 1998 and 1999 preceded the current recommendation established in 2004 by the World Health Organization/International Society of Urologic Pathology

(WHO/ISUP). These classifications determined in 2004 have strict diagnostic criteria, with each of the described lesions having different risks of progression and recurrence.[3] These diagnostic criteria are summarized in **Table 1**.

In general, papillary lesions are classified by their growth pattern and complexity of fibrovascular cores as well as the cytologic features of the overlying epithelium. Urothelial papilloma is a papillary lesion with fine, nonbranching fibrovascular cores and is characterized by a urothelium that is less than 7 cell layers thick with normal polarization with no cellular atypia. These lesions have the lowest risk of recurrence and the lowest risk of progression. A papillary urothelial neoplasm of low malignant potential (PUNLMP) has non-branching fibrovascular cores and an overlying urothelium that may be hyperplastic (**Fig. 1**A, B). The hyperplastic urothelium has an increased number of cell layers but retains its polarity with minimal cellular atypia. There may be a substantial risk of recurrence but a low risk of progression and, therefore, this term was developed so as to not label patients with a cancer diagnosis. Nevertheless, a PUNLMP diagnosis should not represent more than 10% of all papillary urothelial diagnoses. In contrast, low-grade papillary urothelial carcinoma may have branching fibrovascular cores and a urothelium that has lost some cell polarity (see **Fig. 1**C, D). Mild atypia can be seen, including nucleomegaly and irregular nuclear

| Table 1 |
| :--- |
| **Pathologic key features of urothelial carcinoma** |

| | **Pathologic Features** |
| :--- | :--- |
| Normal urothelium | No more than 7 cell layers thick, with polarization from basal layer to overlying superficial layer of umbrella cells |
| **Papillary lesions** | |
| Papilloma | Discrete exophytic lesion with fine, nonbranching fibrovascular cores with overlying normal-appearing urothelium |
| PUNLMP | Nonbranching fibrovascular cores with overlying hyperplastic epithelium with preserved polarity and minimal nuclear atypia |
| Low-grade papillary urothelial carcinoma | Minimal branching of fibrovascular cores and overlying urothelium with loss of polarity and slight variability in nuclear size and shape |
| High-grade papillary urothelial carcinoma | Complex papillary architecture and overlying urothelium with highly atypical cells, including high nuclear-to-cytoplasmic ratio, nuclear pleomorphism, prominent nucleoli, and abundant high-riding mitoses |
| **Flat lesions** | |
| Urothelial hyperplasia | Thickened mucosa with normal polarization and no cytologic atypia |
| Urothelial dysplasia | Slight loss of polarity with mild atypia, including irregular nuclear borders and dense chromatin |
| CIS | Flat lesion with extensive architectural disorder with large, pleomorphic, hyperchromatic nuclei, prominent nucleoli, and abundant high-riding and/or abnormal mitoses |

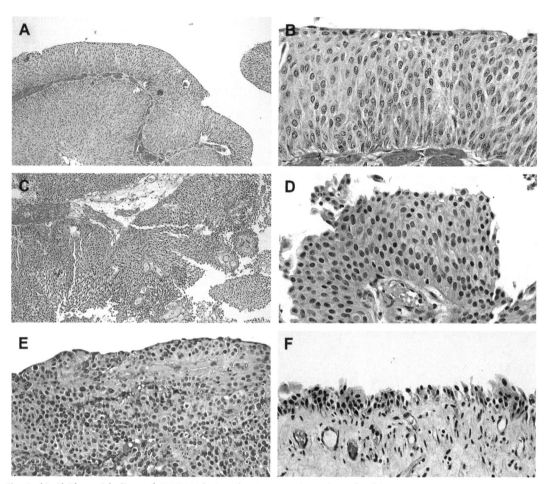

*Fig. 1.* (*A, B*) The epithelium of PUNLMP lesions has increased number of cell layers but retains polarity, and no atypia is seen (H&E, original magnification [*A*] ×100 and [*B*] ×400). (*C, D*) In low-grade papillary urothelial carcinoma, there are loss of polarity and minimal atypia (H&E, original magnification [*C*] ×100 and [*D*] ×400). (*E*) In high-grade papillary urothelial carcinoma, there are complex architecture and atypia (H&E, original magnification ×200). (*F*) Occasionally in high-grade lesions, denudation can occur due to the loss of cell-cell adhesion, and in these cases the clinging cells should be carefully evaluated (H&E, original magnification ×200).

borders, but the nuclear-to-cytoplasmic ratios are typically still low. Mitoses and karyorrhexis may be present but are usually minimal. Finally, high-grade papillary urothelial carcinoma has a complex papillary architecture and a high degree of nuclear atypia, including increased nuclear-to-cytoplasmic ratio, nuclear pleomorphism, presence of nucleoli, and mitoses, especially abnormal mitoses or mitoses high in the urothelium (see **Fig. 1**E, F). The risk of recurrence and progression to invasive disease is highest with high-grade papillary urothelial carcinoma.[3]

Flat lesions also have a distinct classification system. Non-neoplastic urothelium is typically 7 cell layers or less and has normal polarization with maturation from the basal layer to the umbrella layer (**Fig. 2**A). Urothelial hyperplasia is defined by thickening of the mucosa but without any loss of polarization or cytologic atypia. Occasionally, reactive changes can be seen, which are characterized by enlarged nuclei with smooth borders and a single pinpoint nucleolus. These changes are contrasted with flat urothelial dysplasia, in which mild atypia is seen, including irregular nuclear borders, dense chromatin, and some loss of polarity. Occasionally, it can be difficult to distinguish reactive changes from dysplastic changes (see **Fig. 2**B). Lastly, flat urothelial carcinoma in situ (CIS) has extensive disorder (ie, loss of polarity) with large, pleomorphic, hyperchromatic nuclei and prominent nucleoli (see **Fig. 2**C). Typically cells have a high nuclear-to-cytoplasmic ratio, but some have prominent eosinophilic cytoplasm. Mitoses can be close to the surface and may be abnormal.[3]

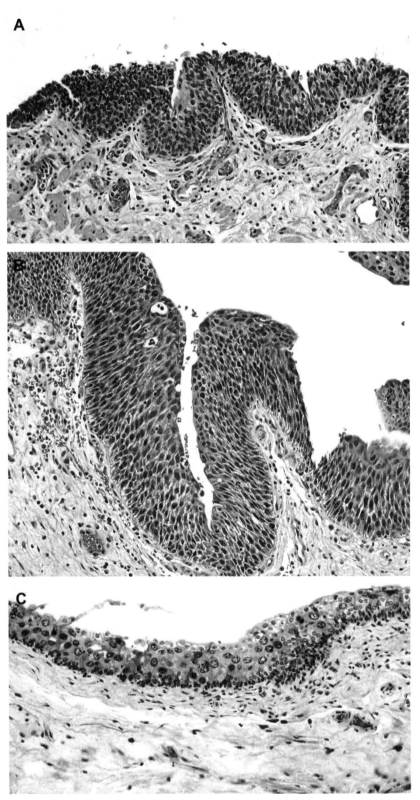

Fig. 2. (A) Normal urothelium is 7 cell layers thick, with maturation from the basal to umbrella layer (H&E, original magnification ×200). (B) It can be difficult to distinguish reactive atypia from urothelial dysplasia, and in these situations, the term, *atypia with uncertain significance*, can be used (H&E, original magnification ×200). (C) Extensive disorder and atypia are seen in urothelial CIS (H&E, original magnification ×200).

In addition to the traditional papillary and flat growth patterns, inverted or endophytic growth patterns are also occasionally seen. These lesions represent growth into and expansion of von Brunn nests by neoplasm, but the intact basement membrane makes these lesions noninvasive. Current recommendations have suggested using the WHO/ISUP system analogous to exophytic papillary lesions to grade inverted lesions: inverted papilloma; inverted PUNLMP; inverted papillary urothelial carcinoma, low grade; and inverted papillary urothelial carcinoma, high grade. The inverted phrasing should be used only if inverted architecture is predominant.[3]

## STAGING

Staging is the most important factor in determining management and prognosis, with the distinction between muscle invasive and non–muscle invasive carcinoma the most critical one (see also Harshman et al, Diagnosis of Bladder Carcinoma: A Clinician's Perspective, Surgical Pathology Clinics, 2015, Volume 8, Issue 4). For this reason, the muscularis propria should always be sampled as part of any endoscopic tumor biopsy or resection, and it is even recommended to perform an immediate deeper biopsy of the tumor bed to ensure that muscularis propria is obtained.[4]

The currently accepted pathologic stages are shown in **Table 2**. Several recent studies have suggested that substaging T1 disease may provide additional prognostic information for clinicians.[5–7] For substaging, some systems often use invasion relative to the muscularis mucosae and the plexus venosus as division points, whereas others have used depth of invasion in millimeters to substage cancers.[6–8] Although substaging may provide prognostic information, there are drawbacks because such systems can be difficult to use. One problem

is that the thickness of the lamina propria and the location and thickness of the muscularis mucosa vary in different areas of the bladder, making it difficult to directly compare and assess invasion.[9] In addition, these systems suffer from a high degree of interobserver variability. Nevertheless, although many of these substaging systems are not standardized and, therefore, currently not widely recommended, the depth of invasion or relationship to muscularis mucosae may be described in a comment, because it seems to correlate with clinical outcome.[3,10]

Although the clinical behavior of urothelial carcinoma correlates best with both the stage and grade of the tumor, several other factors, such as multifocality, tumor size, prior recurrences, and presence of concomitant CIS, also have independent prognostic value. Several scoring systems, such as the European Organisation for Research and Treatment of Cancer risk tables, have been created to include such information and to enable urologists to accurately determine a patient's risk of recurrence and progression.[11,12] For this reason, such information should always be reported.

## DIFFERENTIAL DIAGNOSIS

When classifying noninvasive tumors, the most critical distinction for determining risk of progression and recurrence is between low-grade and high-grade lesions (low-grade vs high-grade papillary urothelial carcinoma and flat urothelial dysplasia vs CIS) Management strategies differ as well, because clinicians are more likely to use intravesicular therapies with the high-grade lesions (see also Harshman et al, Diagnosis of Bladder Carcinoma: A Clinician's Perspective, Surgical Pathology Clinics, 2015, Volume 8, Issue 4). In most cases, this distinction is straightforward compared with the

*Table 2*
Currently accepted stages of urothelial carcinoma

| Stage | Description |
|-------|-------------|
| T0 | No evidence of primary tumor |
| Ta | Noninvasive papillary carcinoma |
| Tis | CIS: flat tumor |
| T1 | Tumor invades subepithelial connective tissue (invasive into lamina propria) |
| T2a | Invasive into superficial (inner half) of the muscularis propria (detrusor muscle) |
| T2b | Invasive into deep (deep half) of the muscularis propria (detrusor muscle) |
| T3a | Microscopically invasive into perivesical tissue |
| T3b | Macroscopically invasive into perivesical tissue |
| T4a | Invasive into adjacent organs: Prostate, seminal vesicles, uterus, vagina |
| T4b | Invasive into pelvic or abdominal wall |

diagnostic separation of the other lower-grade lesions. For example, the PUNLMP category is controversial, because there is often little interobserver reproducibility with discriminating between it and low-grade papillary urothelial carcinoma.[13] A study demonstrated that removing it from the grading system greatly improves agreement between pathologists,[14] and as a result some alternative grading schemes have been suggested.[15]

Another distinction that is difficult to make is that of severe reactive atypia from urothelial dysplasia and CIS. Reactive changes are typically characterized by enlarged cells with large, smooth nuclei and a single pinpoint nucleolus, whereas dysplastic changes are characterized by irregular nuclear borders and clumped chromatin. The difficulty lies in that in practice these entities can often look similar. In addition, in both reactive change and low-grade dysplasia, basally located mitoses can often be identified.[16] In these situations, immunohistochemistry can aid in the diagnosis. Cytokeratin 20 (CK20) expression shows diffuse, full-thickness staining in urothelial CIS but only stains the superficial umbrella cell layer in normal urothelium. Sensitivity and specificity for CK20 have been shown greater than 70% and greater than 90%, respectively.[3] Immunohistochemistry for p53 may also useful, because it typically shows strong and diffuse nuclear reactivity in urothelial CIS and only scattered cells positive in reactive lesions; however, the overall sensitivity of p53 is relatively low. CD44 may be useful because it is positively expressed under normal conditions in the basal cell layer and is absent in full-thickness urothelial CIS. Finally, HER2/neu staining is often positive in urothelial dysplasia and may be a useful adjunct marker as well. Multiple studies have demonstrated that using these markers in combination often helps distinguish reactive atypia from urothelial dysplasia.[17–19] If no consensus can be reached, especially after the use of immunohistochemical stains, the grade of "atypia of unknown significance" can be reported, which signals clinicians to follow the patient more closely and procure additional tissue if clinically indicated.[20]

Heterogeneity in nuclear morphology/cytology is common, and several studies have examined criteria, such as grading the tumor based on the highest area identified in the tumor or ignoring areas that make up less than 5% of the total tumor. Regardless, heterogeneity seems most relevant in noninvasive papillary carcinomas that have a mixture of low-grade and high-grade cytology. In general, 5% or greater of high-grade urothelial carcinoma is enough to increase the diagnostic grade to high grade. In areas that show less than 5% high-grade morphology, however, a variety of

terms have been applied, including "high-grade papillary urothelial carcinoma in a background of low-grade papillary urothelial carcinoma" and "low-grade papillary urothelial carcinoma with focal high-grade features." Including factors such as prior diagnosed urothelial neoplasia, size of the lesion, multifocality, concurrent CIS, or positive cytology specimens can assist in the diagnosis and management of challenging cases. On the whole, these distinctions remain largely a morphologic diagnosis, and there are no current immunohistochemical or molecular ancillary tests for grading lesions.[3,21]

Another point is that any lesion with invasion should be graded as high grade. This recommendation is made for multiple reasons. First, grading has been shown less of a prognostic factor compared with stage in invasive urothelial carcinoma, because the recurrence rates, progression rates, and clinical outcomes do not differ significantly between low-grade and high-grade invasive lesions.[22,23] In addition, up to 96% of invasive cancers show at least some portion of high-grade histology.[22] Therefore, all invasive urothelial carcinomas should be called high grade, because the high-grade features may be deceptive, there is a sampling issue, or the tumor may have a variant low-grade morphology (ie, as seen with the nested variant of urothelial carcinoma), discussed later.[3]

Distinguishing the presence and depth of invasion to determine the stage of the tumor can also be difficult. The presence of inverted papillary growth patterns or involvement of von Brunn nests by in situ neoplasia can mimic invasion. At the same time, artifacts, such as cautery and crush effects, can make assessment even more difficult. In these situations, again, immunohistochemistry can be used. Pankeratins, such as AE1/AE3, can be used to highlight urothelial carcinoma cells and to determine if they are infiltrating through a stroma that may be obscured by inflammation or to highlight invasive carcinoma cells in cauterized sections.[3] In more bona fide areas of invasion, the true depth of invasion is often difficult to determine because the muscularis mucosae has variable thickness in different areas of the bladder and can be confused with the muscularis propria, especially if tangentially sectioned or if the location of the biopsy is not known. Several studies have assessed immunohistochemical markers in distinguishing muscularis mucosae from muscularis propria. Smoothelin shows strong, intense staining of the muscularis propria but weak to absent staining of the muscularis mucosae.[24] Utility of this antibody has been limited, however, due to challenges with standardization between laboratories and variable staining patterns.[25] At minimum, a fragment of muscularis propria uninvolved by tumor should be present on the tissue section to use as a positive internal control. Another study has suggested that use of a panel of stains, including desmin, vimentin, and smoothelin, is useful in assessing true depth of invasion, because desmin stains smooth muscle cells and vimentin has a staining pattern opposite to that of smoothelin – strongly positive in muscularis mucosa and weak to negative in the muscularis propria.[26] Pending further studies, such markers may be useful to distinguish the muscularis mucosae from muscularis propria and to potentially distinguish invasion into the detrusor muscle from a desmoplastic stromal reaction.[27] Overall, because staging of invasive tumors is such a critical decision and greatly affects management, great care should be taken to be as accurate as possible.

Several diagnostic pitfalls should be considered when diagnosing urothelial carcinoma. For flat lesions, an often troublesome occurrence is urothelial denudation of a papillary lesion, mimicking CIS. For example, instrumentation, intravesicular therapy, or prior radiation treatment (ie, for prostatic adenocarcinoma) can cause denudation of the epithelium. The shoulder (ie, lateral extension of a papillary urothelial carcinoma along the mucosa) or the base of a papillary lesion in a secondary deep biopsy can be misinterpreted as coexisting CIS. In addition, high-grade papillary urothelial carcinoma like urothelial CIS, although to a lesser extent, can also be associated with denudation due to the discohesion of the neoplastic cells. Therefore, extra vigilance is needed to examine and compare the cytomorphology of the neoplastic cells that remain clinging to the surface of a tissue fragment or are present with other lesional papillary tissues to identify high-grade non-CIS lesions, because misdiagnosing the CIS can have significant clinical implications (see also Harshman et al, Diagnosis of Bladder Carcinoma: A Clinician's Perspective, Surgical Pathology Clinics, 2015, Volume 8, Issue 4). Complete urothelial denudation should be reported, and correlation with cytology results is especially crucial in patients with such specimens.[3]

Patients who have undergone prior treatment of urothelial carcinoma and are currently under surveillance present another set of problems. Treatments of bladder cancer may include intravesicular therapy, systemic chemotherapy, radiation therapy, and photodynamic and laser therapy in addition to surgical resection, and many of these may result in reactive changes to the urothelium in subsequent surveillance biopsies. Other urologic conditions, such as renal calculi, catheterization, trauma, or infection, can also cause reactive changes. Reactive changes can include pseudocarcinomatous epithelial hyperplasia and can mimic neoplastic changes.[28] Therefore, knowledge of prior therapy is of utmost important for pathologists. In addition, after treatment with resection and/or intravesicular treatments, residual disease may present as small, multifocal lesions that may show hyperplasia or treatment effect. Although the presence of fibrovascular cores suggests neoplasia and should be reported as such, flat dysplastic lesions/CIS can be more difficult, especially distinguishing from treatment effect. Molecular or immunohistochemical studies can sometimes help distinguish these lesions, but results are often difficult to interpret. Overall, the clinical impression and cystoscopic findings should be correlated with histologic findings.[3]

## Pitfalls
### IN THE DIAGNOSIS OF UROTHELIAL CARCINOMA

| Pitfalls | Recommendations |
|---|---|
| High-grade lesions can have denuded epithelium due to discohesion of the neoplastic cells. | Thorough examination of any clinging cells for atypia should be performed. Correlation with clinical history and cytology results |
| Reactive changes are difficult to distinguish from urothelial dysplasia. | Immunohistochemistry for CK20, p53, CD44, and/or HER2/neu can be performed. |
| Morphologic heterogeneity is seen within a single tumor. | Quantify and/or describe all morphologies seen, including any variant morphologies, such as micropapillary, and correlate with clinical information and cystoscopic findings. |
| Cautery artifact or tangential sectioning | Highlighting neoplastic cells with a pankeratin and smooth muscle cells with desmin or smoothelin can aid in evaluation and staging of invasion. |

## VARIANT MORPHOLOGIES

Many variants of urothelial carcinoma have been described, and the current recommendations emphasize reporting such urothelial carcinoma variants, which currently seem under-reported.[3] In addition, multiple variants may be present in the same patient, and, when encountered, should be reported as a percentage of each subtype. The most common variant morphologies seen are urothelial carcinomas with squamous or glandular differentiation, which seem to have outcomes similar to those of conventional urothelial carcinomas.[29,30] Other variant morphologies seem to have much more aggressive clinical behavior, which may affect clinical management (see also Harshman et al, Diagnosis of Bladder Carcinoma: A Clinician's Perspective, Surgical Pathology Clinics, 2015, Volume 8, Issue 4).

The nested variants of urothelial carcinoma, including the large and small nested variants, have a deceptively bland appearance and often mimic von Brunn nest proliferation or a noninvasive inverted growth pattern, despite being invasive carcinoma.[31] Deep biopsies may show invasion into muscularis propria, which would signal invasive carcinoma, but more superficial biopsies are often difficult to interpret as carcinoma. This variant often carries a poor prognosis, although the poor prognosis could be attributed to late diagnosis due to its bland appearance.[32]

Urothelial carcinoma with small tubules is a rare lesion that also has a bland appearance and it is characterized by small tubules mixed with solid small nests of tumor cells. The cytology is often bland and low-grade appearing, and these lesions are often mistaken for nephrogenic adenoma or cystitis cystica and glandularis. The prognosis of this lesion is not well understood, because sufficient cases have not been reported.[3,33]

Urothelial carcinoma with rhabdoid features is an aggressive variant and is often present in high-grade and poorly differentiated urothelial carcinoma. Histologically, it is composed of discohesive sheets of rhabdoid cells with vesicular nuclei. The presence of these features are associated with an aggressive clinical course, similar to the plasmacytoid variant of urothelial carcinoma (discussed later) and should be reported.[3]

Urothelial carcinoma with chordoid features is characterized by cords of cells in an abundant myxoid matrix. The differential diagnosis often includes chordoma, myxoid chondrosarcoma, myoepithelioma, and yolk sac tumor. In diagnosing these tumors, immunohistochemistry is helpful because staining for p63 and other high-molecular-weight cytokeratins is positive in the tumor, whereas markers for the other tumors in the differential are negative. These tumors have an aggressive clinical course, and patients often present with deeply invasive tumors and nodal or distant metastases.[34]

Plasmacytoid urothelial carcinoma is another rare aggressive variant so named because it is characterized by loosely cohesive ovoid cells with abundant eosinophilic cytoplasm mimicking sheets of plasma cells. Many patients present at an advanced stage with metastases, and although it is sensitive to neoadjuvant chemotherapy, the disease often recurs and the long-term survival rate is low.[35]

Micropapillary urothelial carcinoma is one of the more widely prevalent and most frequently described variants and is associated with an aggressive clinical course and late-stage disease (Fig. 3A). Some studies have demonstrated that the proportion or quantity of micropapillary differentiation should be reported, because it has been correlated with stage-specific and disease-specific survival.[36,37] Noninvasive micropapillary urothelial carcinoma is characterized by small slender clusters of cells without true vascular cores. Interobserver reproducibility for diagnosing invasive micropapillary morphology includes using the following morphologic features: multiple nests in the same lacuna, intracytoplasmic vacuolization, and epithelial ring forms.[38] The differential diagnosis may include metastatic müllerian papillary serous adenocarcinoma and micropapillary adenocarcinomas from the breast or other sites. Lymphovascular invasion in this variant is often present and should be sought. Because of the aggressive nature of micropapillary urothelial carcinomas, some have recommended early cystectomy,[39] although a more conservative approach may be taken if only focal micropapillary areas are seen.[37] Therefore, the percentage of micropapillary morphology, lymphovascular invasion, and concomitant CIS should always be reported when present.

Finally, urothelial carcinoma with sarcomatoid differentiation is a rare variant associated with very aggressive behavior (see Fig. 3B, C). Grossly, tumors can form large polypoid intraluminal masses. Microscopically, tumors are often biphasic, with an epithelial component of traditional urothelial carcinoma, squamous cell carcinoma, or adenocarcinoma and a mesenchymal component resembling a high-grade spindle cell neoplasm. Heterologous elements may also be present. The tumor cells of the mesenchymal component are often large bizarre cells with highly atypical features. If sarcomatoid features are present, aggressive treatment with cystectomy and adjuvant chemotherapy and radiation should be considered[40,41] (see also Harshman et al, Diagnosis of Bladder Carcinoma: A Clinician's

*Fig.* 3. Many variant morphologies of urothelial carcinoma exist, some of which have worse prognoses. (*A*) Micropapillary urothelial carcinoma (H&E, original magnification ×200). (*B, C*) Urothelial carcinoma with sarcomatoid differentiation (H&E, original magnification [*B*] ×100 and [*C*] ×400).

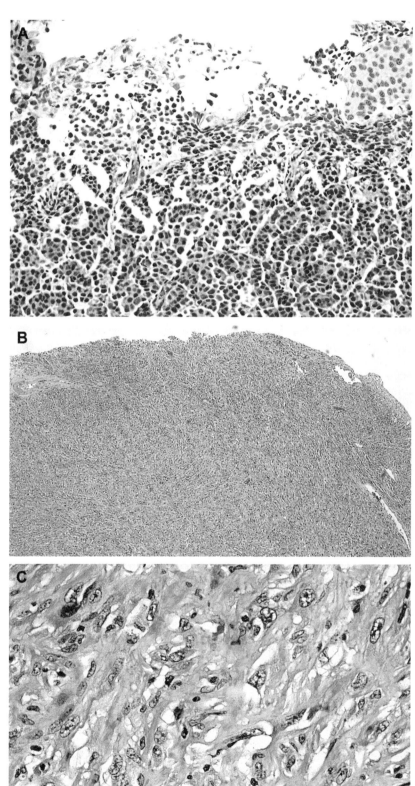

Perspective, Surgical Pathology Clinics, 2015, Volume 8, Issue 4).

## MOLECULAR PATHOLOGY OF UROTHELIAL CARCINOMA

As discussed previously and by Harshman and colleagues (Diagnosis of Bladder Carcinoma: A Clinician's Perspective, Surgical Pathology Clinics, 2015, Volume 8, Issue 4), many of the management decisions and prognostic information are based primarily on histologic features of urothelial carcinoma. In contrast to many other solid tumors, where molecular diagnostics are a vital part of management paradigms, the understanding of the molecular and genetic features of urothelial carcinoma has lagged behind. The molecular landscape of urothelial carcinoma is not as well defined, and similar molecular tests are not clinically in widespread use. The reason for this is that in most epithelial-derived tumors, the pathways affecting cell growth and proliferation that seem to be affected are relatively conserved. The molecular pathogenesis of urothelial carcinoma seems, however, much more heterogeneous, and alterations in several different pathways are thought to contribute to urothelial carcinoma tumorigenesis. It is hypothesized that the different growth patterns and different clinical behaviors of various urothelial tumors that are seen may be the result of different molecular pathways being affected. Even low-grade noninvasive papillary tumors and high-grade invasive tumors may be completely different at the molecular and biologic level, thus partially explaining their different clinical outcomes.

In general, alterations in chromosome 9 seem to be an early event in the development of urothelial neoplasia. Loss of heterozygosity in this chromosome is prevalent in a high percentage of bladder cancer, and it is thought that mutations in genes located here may give rise to genetic instability to cause further changes genetic changes. One gene that is located in a region of chromosome 9 that is often affected is the tuberous sclerosis gene *TSC1*, a tumor suppressor gene that is important in regulating the mammalian target of rapamycin pathway (mTOR). Mutations in *TSC1* are found in a high proportion of bladder cancers, suggesting an important role for this gene in urothelial neoplasia.

Low-grade papillary urothelial carcinoma seems associated with pathways that are important in cell growth and proliferation, including the mitogen-activated protein kinase (MAPK) and phosphoinositide 3-kinase (PI3K) pathways. Mutations in *HRAS*, a Ras GTPase proto-oncogene, were the first to be discovered. These mutations affect the protein's GTPase activity, constitutively activating it and resulting in activation of MAPK and PI3K, ultimately leading to increased cell growth and survival. In addition to activating *HRAS* itself, mutations in genes upstream to *HRAS*, such as fibroblast growth factor receptor 3 (*FGFR3*), a tyrosine kinase receptor, also constitutively activate these pathways. In urothelial cancer, mutations in *FGFR3* and *HRAS* are mutually exclusive and, therefore, functionally equivalent.[42] Mutations in *FGFR3* are identified in noninvasive papillary tumors at a much higher rate than in flat CIS or in invasive tumors, suggesting that its presence may be a favorable prognostic factor.[43,44] Also associated with low-grade noninvasive carcinoma are mutations in *PIK3CA*, which encodes the catalytic subunit of PI3K. Mutations in *PIK3CA* have been demonstrated to be associated with low-grade noninvasive lesions and recurrence-free survival.[45,46]

In contrast, high-grade flat and invasive lesions are associated with mutations in tumor suppressor proteins that affect regulation of the cell cycle. One such mutation that is often seen in high-grade lesions is in *TP53*. Mutations in both alleles of *TP53* result in loss of the p53 activity that is necessary for regulating the G1/S transition of the cell cycle. Histologically this correlates with an increase in p53 protein expression. Mutations are also often seen in genes encoding other cell-cycle regulating proteins downstream of *TP53*, including *p16*, *p21*, *p27*, *cyclin D1*, *cyclin D3*, and retinoblastoma (*RB*).[47] In addition, it is thought that mutations in these proteins can occur in superficial lesions, which may be a second-hit event that causes low-grade lesions to become invasive. Several studies have been performed to examine whether the presence of mutations in these genes held clinical significance. Although mutations in *TP53* have been shown to add independent prognostic information in some studies,[48,49] many of the results on the other individual cell-cycle regulating proteins have been mixed, likely due to the multiple roles of many of these proteins and the complexity and interaction of the affected biologic pathways. Using some of these markers in combination, however, has been shown to occasionally improve survival prognostication.[50–52]

Examining many of these markers in parallel seems to correlate with the histologic and clinical characteristics of the tumor. In a recent study,[53] the molecular signature of urothelial cancer was examined using gene expression analysis for multiple genes, including *FGFR3*, *PIK3CA*, *KRAS*, *HRAS*, *NRAS*, *TP53*, *CDKN2A*, and *TSC1*. Two distinct molecular signatures were identified, one of which was characterized by increased genomic instability. Using these signatures, the investigators were able to classify bladder cancer into low-grade and high-grade tumors and nonmuscle invasive and muscle invasive cancers with good accuracy. In addition, the molecular signature provided independent prognostic information for metastasis and disease-specific survival, suggesting that these molecular signatures could be used as an adjunct to histopathologic characteristics.[53]

Although the biological differences between low-grade papillary superficial tumors and flat high-grade invasive tumors are the best described and understood, there may be many additional biologic subdivisions with different molecular characteristics. A recent study examined a meta-dataset of gene expression and identified 2 distinct molecular subtypes of high-grade bladder cancer. Drawing a parallel to breast cancer, the 2 subtypes were termed *luminal* and *basal-like*. The luminal tumors had a molecular signature more similar to superficial umbrella cells, expressing high levels of uroplakin and CK20, whereas the basal-like tumors expressed cytokeratin 5,14, 6B, and CD44, which are more characteristic of urothelial basal cells. In addition, they found that the luminal subtype had a significantly better prognosis than the basal-like subtype.[54] Another recent study confirmed this result, defining additional markers that may be able to distinguish luminal and basal urothelial carcinomas, while adding another subtype, the p53-like bladder cancer, that is more resistant to chemotherapy.[55]

Probably the most comprehensive molecular subclassification study has been performed by the Cancer Genome Atlas project.[56] In this landmark study that examined 131 cases of muscle-invasive urothelial carcinoma, the investigators examined data on whole-genome sequencing, whole-exome sequencing, DNA copy number, complete mRNA and microRNA expression, DNA methylation, and protein expression and phosphorylation. They found consistent mutations in many genes previously identified, including *TP53*, *PIK3CA*, *RB1*, *FGFR3*, and *TSC1*, confirming many prior studies. In addition, they were able to subclassify muscle-invasive urothelial carcinoma into 4 different molecular types based on expression of specific mRNAs and proteins. Integrating all of the data, they were able to identify a few pathways that are consistently dysregulated in bladder cancer, including the p53/RB tumor suppressor pathway and the PI3K/AKT/mTOR and the RTK/RAS pathways, that affect cell proliferation and survival and pathways that affect epigenetic changes, such as chromatin remodeling and histone modification. These latter pathways, which affect epigenetic pathways, were seen in 89% of bladder tumors, more than in any other cancer studied, suggesting that there may be many subtle epigenetic causes of urothelial neoplasia that are still poorly understood.[56]

Although many of the biomarkers discussed in this article may have prognostic and treatment implications, testing for them is not currently routinely recommended in clinical practice, and histopathologic grading and staging remain the most important information. Nonetheless, many studies have been examining the clinical relevance of genetic and immunohistochemical markers either individually or in combination to potentially aid in prognostic evaluation of bladder cancer. Tumor proliferation index as measured by Ki-67 has been shown to have independent prognostic information, because it correlates with tumor grade and stage.[57,58] It has also been linked to decreased progression-free survival and disease-specific survival rates.[57,58] Another study examined its use in combination with CK20 expression in pT1 tumors and found that both are associated with increased recurrence and decreased cancer-specific survival, and therefore Ki-67 and CK20 may be useful for risk stratification.[59] Another study proposed a molecular grade based on the combination of *FGFR3* mutation status and Ki-67 expression. The molecular grade was found to have independent prognostic information for progression and disease-specific survival and increased the accuracy of a predictive model over that of just using the histologic features described earlier.[60,61]

Finally, several other receptor tyrosine kinases have been examined in urothelial cancer. The receptor kinases epidermal growth factor receptor, human epidermal growth factor receptor 2 (HER2), and vascular endothelial growth factor are prognostic factors in many other cancers that have available targeted molecular therapies. Mutations and/or overexpression in these markers have been shown associated with worse clinical outcome, including increased recurrence and progression and decreased survival.[62–65]

Overall, although great strides have been taken in understanding the biology of urothelial cancer, much work is still necessary to understand clinical relevance and to define the role of the pathologist in evaluating these markers. Nevertheless, although the understanding for urothelial carcinoma may not be as robust in some other cancers, there are still several molecular biomarkers that have prognostic value and targeted therapeutics that are currently in development. In the near future, the authors are hopeful that reporting a diagnosis of bladder cancer will combine clinical patient information, histopathologic characteristics, immunohistochemical markers, and molecular alterations to provide a personalized diagnosis and optimizing management for patients.

## REFERENCES

1. American Cancer Society. Cancer facts and figures: 2014. Atlanta (GA): American Cancer Society; 2014.
2. Morgan TM, Cookson MS, Netto G, et al. Bladder cancer overview and staging. In: Hansel DE, McKenney JK, Stephenson AJ, et al, editors. The urinary tract: a comprehensive guide to patient diagnosis and management. New York: Springer Science and Business Media; 2012. p. 83–112.
3. Soloway M, Khoury S, editors. Bladder cancer, ed. 2. 2nd edition. Bristol (United Kingdom): International Consultation on Urological Disease; 2012. 2nd International Consultation On Bladder Cancer – Vienna.
4. Kim W, Song C, Park S, et al. Value of immediate second resection of the tumor bed to improve the effectiveness of transurethral resection of bladder tumor. J Endourol 2012;26(8):1059–64.
5. Amin MB, McKenney JK, Paner GP, et al. Icud-eau international consultation on bladder cancer 2012: pathology. Eur Urol 2013;63(1):16–35.
6. van Rhijn BWG, van der Kwast TH, Alkhateeb SS, et al. A new and highly prognostic system to discern t1 bladder cancer substage. Eur Urol 2012;61(2): 378–84.
7. Chang WC, Chang YH, Pan CC. Prognostic significance in substaging of t1 urinary bladder urothelial carcinoma on transurethral resection. Am J Surg Pathol 2012;36(3):454–61.
8. Brimo F, Wu CB, Zeizafoun N, et al. Prognostic factors in t1 bladder urothelial carcinoma: the value of recording millimetric depth of invasion, diameter of invasive carcinoma, and muscularis mucosa invasion. Hum Pathol 2013;44(1):95–102.
9. Paner GP, Ro JY, Wojcik EM, et al. Further characterization of the muscle layers and lamina propria of the urinary bladder by systematic histologic mapping - implications for pathologic staging of invasive urothelial carcinoma. Am J Surg Pathol 2007;31(9): 1420–9.
10. Hansel DE, Amin MB, Comperat E, et al. A contemporary update on pathology standards for bladder cancer: transurethral resection and radical cystectomy specimens. Eur Urol 2013;63(2):321–32.
11. Sylvester RJ, van der Meijden APM, Oosterlinck W, et al. Predicting recurrence and progression in individual patients with stage ta t1 bladder cancer using eortc risk tables: a combined analysis of 2596 patients from seven eortc trials. Eur Urol 2006;49(3): 466–77.
12. Altieri VM, Castellucci R, Palumbo P, et al. Recurrence and progression in non-muscle-invasive bladder cancer using eortc risk tables. Urol Int 2012;89(1):61–6.
13. Murphy WM, Takezawa K, Maruniak NA. Interobserver discrepancy using the 1998 world health organization/international society of urologic pathology classification of urothelial neoplasms: practical choices for patient care. J Urol 2002;168(3):968–72.
14. Tuna B, Yorukoglu K, Duzcan E, et al. Histologic grading of urothelial papillary neoplasms: impact of combined grading (two-numbered grading system) on reproducibility. Virchows Arch 2011;458(6): 659–64.
15. Cheng L, MacLennan GT, Lopez-Beltran A. Histologic grading of urothelial carcinoma: a reappraisal. Hum Pathol 2012;43(12):2097–108.
16. Eble JN, Sauter G, Epstein JI, et al. Tumors of the urinary system, in World health organization classification of tumours: pathology and genetics of tumours of the urinary system and male genital organs. Lyon (France): IARC Press; 2004.
17. Harnden P, Eardley I, Joyce AD, et al. Cytokeratin 20 as an objective marker of urothelial dysplasia. Br J Urol 1996;78(6):870–5.
18. Jung S, Wu CB, Eslami Z, et al. The role of immunohistochemistry in the diagnosis of flat urothelial lesions: a study using ck20, ck5/6, p53, cd138, and her2/neu. Ann Diagn Pathol 2014;18(1):27–32.
19. Yildiz IZ, Recavarren R, Armah HB, et al. Utility of a dual immunostain cocktail comprising of p53 and ck20 to aid in the diagnosis of non-neoplastic and neoplastic bladder biopsies. Diagn Pathol 2009;(4):35.
20. Jackson R, Al-Ahmadie H, Reuter VE, et al. Bladder cancer overview and staging. In: Hansel DE, McKenney JK, Stephenson AJ, et al, editors. The urinary tract: a comprehensive guide to patient diagnosis and management. New York: Springer Science and Business Media; 2012. p. 83–112.
21. Amin MB, Smith S, Reuter VE, et al. Update for the practicing pathologist: the international consultation on urologic disease – european association of urology consultation on bladder cancer. Mod Pathol 2015;28(5):612–30.
22. Otto W, Denzinger S, Fritsche HM, et al. The who classification of 1973 is more suitable than the who classification of 2004 for predicting survival in pt1 urothelial bladder cancer. BJU Int 2011;107(3): 404–8.
23. Watts KE, Montironi R, Mazzucchelli R, et al. Clinicopathologic characteristics of 23 cases of invasive low-grade papillary urothelial carcinoma. Urology 2012;80(2):361–6.
24. Paner GP, Shen SS, Lapetino S, et al. Diagnostic utility of antibody to smoothelin in the distinction of muscularis propria from muscularis mucosae of the urinary bladder a potential ancillary tool in the pathologic staging of invasive urothelial carcinoma. Am J Surg Pathol 2009;33(1):91–8.
25. Miyamoto H, Sharma RB, Illei PB, et al. Pitfalls in the use of smoothelin to identify muscularis propria

invasion by urothelial carcinoma. Am J Surg Pathol 2010;34(3):418–22.

26. Council L, Hameed O. Differential expression of immunohistochemical markers in bladder smooth muscle and myofibroblasts, and the potential utility of desmin, smoothelin, and vimentin in staging of bladder carcinoma. Mod Pathol 2009;22(5):639–50.

27. Roberts JA, Waters L, Ro JY, et al. Smoothelin and caldesmon are reliable markers for distinguishing muscularis propria from desmoplasia: a critical distinction for accurate staging colorectal adenocarcinoma. Int J Clin Exp Pathol 2014;7(2):792–6.

28. Lane Z, Epstein JI. Polypoid/papillary cystitis: a series of 41 cases misdiagnosed as papillary urothelial neoplasia. Am J Surg Pathol 2008;32(5):758–64.

29. Blacks PC, Brown GA, Dinney CPN. The impact of variant histology on the outcome of bladder cancer treated with curative intent. Urol Oncol 2009;27(1):3–7.

30. Taylor JM, Bochner B, Mahul BA, et al. Muscle-invasive urothelial carcinoma: conventional and variant subtypes. In: Hansel DE, McKenney JK, Stephenson AJ, et al, editors. The urinary tract: a comprehensive guide to patient diagnosis and management. New York: Springer Science and Business Media; 2012. p. 143–63.

31. Volmar KE, Chan TY, De Marzo AM, et al. Florid von brunn nests mimicking urothelial carcinoma - a morphologic and immunohistochemical comparison to the nested variant of urothelial carcinoma. Am J Surg Pathol 2003;27(9):1243–52.

32. Dhall D, Al-Ahmadie H, Olgac S. Nested variant of urothelial carcinoma. Arch Pathol Lab Med 2007;131(11):1725–7.

33. Amin MB. Histological variants of urothelial carcinoma: diagnostic, therapeutic and prognostic implications. Mod Pathol 2009;22:S96–118.

34. Cox RM, Schneider AG, Sangoi AR, et al. Invasive urothelial carcinoma with chordoid features a report of 12 distinct cases characterized by prominent myxoid stroma and cordlike epithelial architecture. Am J Surg Pathol 2009;33(8):1213–9.

35. Dayyani F, Czerniak BA, Sircar K, et al. Plasmacytoid urothelial carcinoma, a chemosensitive cancer with poor prognosis, and peritoneal carcinomatosis. J Urol 2013;189(5):1656–61.

36. Comperat E, Roupret M, Yaxley J, et al. Micropapillary urothelial carcinoma of the urinary bladder: a clinicopathological analysis of 72 cases. Pathology 2010;42(7):650–4.

37. Gaya JM, Palou J, Algaba F, et al. The case for conservative management in the treatment of patients with non-muscle-invasive micropapillary bladder carcinoma without carcinoma in situ. Can J Urol 2010;17(5):5370–6.

38. Sangoi AR, Beck AH, Amin MB, et al. Interobserver reproducibility in the diagnosis of invasive micropapillary carcinoma of the urinary tract among urologic pathologists. Am J Surg Pathol 2010;34(9):1367–76.

39. Ghoneim IA, Miocinovic R, Stephenson AJ, et al. Neoadjuvant systemic therapy or early cystectomy? Single-center analysis of outcomes after therapy for patients with clinically localized micropapillary urothelial carcinoma of the bladder. Urology 2011;77(4):867–70.

40. Venyo AK-G, Titi S. Sarcomatoid variant of urothelial carcinoma (carcinosarcoma, spindle cell carcinoma): a review of the literature. ISRN Urol 2014;2014:794563.

41. Bansal A, Kumar N, Sharma SC. Sarcomatoid variant of urothelial carcinoma of the urinary bladder. J Cancer Res Ther 2013;9(4):571–3.

42. Jebar AH, Hurst CD, Tomlinson DC, et al. Fgfr3 and ras gene mutations are mutually exclusive genetic events in urothelial cell carcinoma. Oncogene 2005;24(33):5218–25.

43. Billerey C, Chopin D, Aubriot-Lorton MH, et al. Frequent fgfr3 mutations in papillary non-invasive bladder (pta) tumors. Am J Pathol 2001;158(6):1955–9.

44. van Rhijn BWG, Lurkin I, Radvanyi F, et al. The fibroblast growth factor receptor 3 (fgfr3) mutation is a strong indicator of superficial bladder cancer with low recurrence rate. Cancer Res 2001;61(4):1265–8.

45. Dueñas M, Martínez-Fernández M, García-Escudero R, et al. Pik3ca gene alterations in bladder cancer are frequent and associate with reduced recurrence in non-muscle invasive tumors. Mol Carcinog 2015;54(7):566–76.

46. Lopez-Knowles E, Hernandez S, Malats N, et al. Pik3ca mutations are an early genetic alteration associated with fgfr3 mutations in superficial papillary bladder tumors. Cancer Res 2006;66(15):7401–4.

47. Wu XR. Urothelial tumorigenesis: a tale of divergent pathways. Nat Rev Cancer 2005;5(9):713–25.

48. Malats W, Bustos A, Nascimento CM, et al. P53 as a prognostic marker for bladder cancer: a meta-analysis and review. Lancet Oncol 2005;6(9):678–86.

49. George B, Datar RH, Wu L, et al. P53 gene and protein status: the role of p53 alterations in predicting outcome in patients with bladder cancer. J Clin Oncol 2007;25(34):5352–8.

50. Shariat SF, Ashfaq R, Sagalowsky AI, et al. Predictive value of cell cycle biomarkers in nonmuscle invasive bladder transitional cell carcinoma. J Urol 2007;177(2):481–7.

51. Shariat SF, Bolenz C, Godoy G, et al. Predictive value of combined immunohistochemical markers in patients with pt1 urothelial carcinoma at radical cystectomy. J Urol 2009;182(1):78–84.

52. Shariat SF, Chade DC, Karakiewicz PI, et al. Combination of multiple molecular markers can improve

prognostication in patients with locally advanced and lymph node positive bladder cancer. J Urol 2010;183(1):68–75.

53. Lindgren D, Frigyesi A, Gudjonsson S, et al. Combined gene expression and genomic profiling define two intrinsic molecular subtypes of urothelial carcinoma and gene signatures for molecular grading and outcome. Cancer Res 2010;70(9):3463–72.

54. Demrauer JS, Hoadley KA, Chism DD, et al. Intrinsic subtypes of high-grade blader cancer reflect the hallmarks of breast cancer biology. Proc Natl Acad Sci U S A 2014;111(8):3110–5.

55. Choi W, Porten S, Kim S, et al. Identification of distinct basal and luminal subtypes of muscle-invasive bladder cancer with different sensitivities to frontline chemotherapy. Cancer Cell 2014;25(2):152–65.

56. Weinstein JN, Akbani R, Broom BM, et al. Comprehensive molecular characterization of urothelial bladder carcinoma. Nature 2014;507(7492):315–22.

57. Quintero A, Alvarez-Kindelan J, Luque RJ, et al. Ki-67 mib1 labelling index and the prognosis of primary tat1 urothelial cell carcinoma of the bladder. J Clin Pathol 2006;59(1):83–8.

58. Margulis V, Lotan Y, Karakiewicz PI, et al. Multi-institutional validation of the predictive value of ki-67 labeling index in patients with urinary bladder cancer. J Natl Cancer Inst 2009;101(2):114–9.

59. Bertz S, Otto W, Denzinger S, et al. Combination of ck20 and ki-67 immunostaining analysis predicts recurrence, progression, and cancer-specific survival in pt1 urothelial bladder cancer. Eur Urol 2014;65(1):218–26.

60. van Rhijn BWG, Vis AN, van der Kwast TH, et al. Molecular grading of urothelial cell carcinoma with fibroblast growth factor receptor 3 and mib-1 is superior to pathologic grade for the prediction of clinical outcome. J Clin Oncol 2003;21(10):1912–21.

61. van Rhijn BWG, Zuiverloon TCM, Vis AN, et al. Molecular grade (fgfr3/mib-1) and eortc risk scores are predictive in primary non-muscle-invasive bladder cancer. Eur Urol 2010;58(3):433–41.

62. Bolenz C, Shariat SF, Karakiewicz PI, et al. Human epidermal growth factor receptor 2 expression status provides independent prognostic information in patients with urothelial carcinoma of the urinary bladder. BJU Int 2010;106(8):1216–22.

63. Chaux A, Cohen JS, Schultz L, et al. High epidermal growth factor receptor immunohistochemical expression in urothelial carcinoma of the bladder is not associated with egfr mutations in exons 19 and 21: a study using formalin-fixed, paraffin-embedded archival tissues. Hum Pathol 2012;43(10):1590–5.

64. Chen PCH, Yu HJ, Chang YH, et al. Her2 amplification distinguishes a subset of non-muscle-invasive bladder cancers with a high risk of progression. J Clin Pathol 2013;66(2):113–9.

65. Kopparapu PK, Boorjian SA, Robinson BD, et al. Expression of vegf and its receptors vegfr1/vegfr2 is associated with invasiveness of bladder cancer. Anticancer Res 2013;33(6):2381–90.

# Diagnosis of Bladder Carcinoma
## A Clinician's Perspective

Lauren C. Harshman, MD[a],[*],[1], Mark A. Preston, MD, MPH[b],[1],
Joaquim Bellmunt, MD, PhD[a], Clair Beard, MD[c]

**KEYWORDS**
- Bladder cancer • Nonmetastatic muscle-invasive bladder cancer
- Non–muscle-invasive bladder cancer • Histologic variants

## ABSTRACT

In 2014, more than 74,000 new cases and 15,000 deaths from bladder cancer were estimated to occur. The most reliable prognostic factors for survival are pathologic stage and histologic grade. Accordingly, a good understanding of the pathologic features of these cancers is essential to guide optimal clinical treatment, which requires a multidisciplinary team of pathologists, urologists, radiation oncologists, and medical oncologists. This review highlights several clinical scenarios in which detailed pathologic evaluation and accurate reporting impact clinical management.

## OVERVIEW

Optimizing the treatment of bladder cancer requires accurate staging and precise pathologic evaluation. Bladder cancer encompasses a spectrum of disease states from superficial, non-invasive tumors to advanced localized muscle invasive cancer to metastatic spread. Identifying the extent of disease and characterizing the histology is critical to tailoring the treatment for the patient with the overall objectives of minimizing the degree of therapy administered and maintaining quality of life. Close multidisciplinary collaborations between clinicians and pathologists is essential to enhanced clinical outcomes for our patients.

## NON–MUSCLE-INVASIVE BLADDER CANCER

Approximately 75% of patients with bladder cancer present with disease confined to the mucosa (noninvasive papillary urothelial carcinoma, stage Ta or urothelial carcinoma in situ [CIS], stage Tis) or submucosa (superficially invasive urothelial carcinoma, stage T1) (**Fig. 1**).[1] Although these cancers have been called "superficial" in the past, the more accurate terminology is non–muscle-invasive bladder cancer (NMIBC), as the highest form of NMIBC is T1 disease, which is invasive into the lamina propria (see **Fig. 1**) and has the potential for aggressive distant spread. Because of its high prevalence and the more than 500,000 people in the United States living with NMIBC, it is one of the most expensive cancers to manage on a per-patient basis.[2] Clinical and pathologic factors that contribute to the risks of recurrence and progression include number of tumors, tumor size, prior recurrence, T-stage (see **Fig. 1**), concurrent CIS, and tumor grade (see also Solomon and Hansel, Morphology and Molecular Characteristics of Bladder Cancer, Surgical Pathology Clinics, 2015, Volume 8, Issue 4). Depending on the presence of these risk factors, 5-year rates of recurrence and progression can range from 31% to 78% and 0.8% to 45%, respectively.[3] The high risk of recurrence with NMIBC requires frequent and long-term monitoring with close cystoscopic surveillance as well as consideration of intravesical

[a] Lank Center for Genitourinary Oncology, Dana-Farber Cancer Institute, Harvard Medical School, 1230 DANA, 450 Brookline Ave, Boston, MA 02215, USA; [b] Division of Urology, Brigham and Women's Hospital, Harvard Medical School, 45, Francis street, Boston, MA 02115, USA; [c] Department of Radiation Oncology, Brigham and Women's Hospital, Harvard Medical School, Boston, MA 02115, USA
[1] Contributed equally.
* Corresponding author.
*E-mail address:* LaurenC_Harshman@DFCI.HARVARD.EDU

Surgical Pathology 8 (2015) 677–685
http://dx.doi.org/10.1016/j.path.2015.07.004
1875-9181/15/$ – see front matter © 2015 Elsevier Inc. All rights reserved.

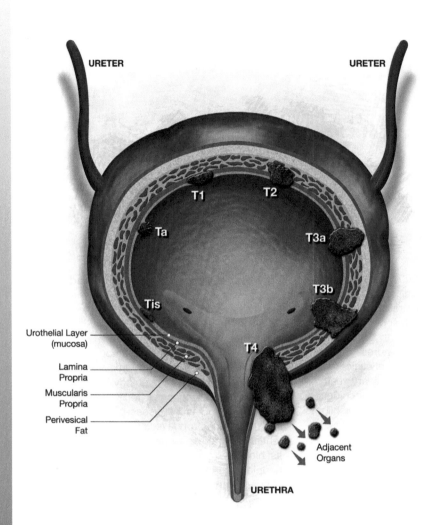

*Fig. 1.* Bladder cancer staging (TNM).

instillations of bacillus Calmette-Guerin (BCG) or chemotherapeutics aimed at preventing or delaying recurrence and progression.

Patients with NMIBC commonly present with gross or microscopic hematuria or lower urinary tract symptoms, such as urinary frequency or dysuria. Evaluation includes a thorough history and physical, urinalysis, urine cytology, cystoscopy, and upper tract imaging with computed tomography scan. To evaluate the urethra and bladder, the urologist will perform a cystoscopy. If tumor or erythema is visualized, the site, size, number of lesions, and appearance, whether papillary or solid, should be noted. If a suspicious area is seen, the patient should be taken to the operating room for biopsy and fulguration. If actual tumor is found, a transurethral resection of a bladder tumor (TURBT) should be performed. The goal of endoscopic treatment is full assessment of the bladder mucosa and urethra so as to make the correct diagnosis with regard to

subtype, grade, and extent (stage) (see also Solomon and Hansel, Morphology and Molecular Characteristics of Bladder Cancer, Surgical Pathology Clinics, 2015, Volume 8, Issue 4), and to remove all visible lesions. If done correctly, the procedure may be curative in addition to diagnostic. It is critical to evaluate whether there is deep detrusor muscle (muscularis propria) invasion present and, thus, additional biopsies taken from the tumor base should be performed.

Important components of the pathology summary include the histologic subtype (eg, urothelial carcinoma, small cell, squamous cell, adenocarcinoma), location of the evaluated sample, grade of each lesion, depth of tumor invasion (stage), presence of CIS, presence of detrusor muscle in the specimen, presence of lymphovascular invasion (LVI), and presence of aberrant variants (eg, micropapillary, plasmacytoid) (see also Solomon and Hansel, Morphology and Molecular Characteristics of Bladder Cancer, Surgical Pathology Clinics,

2015, Volume 8, Issue 4). All of these factors are critical to optimizing the clinical plan for the patient with newly diagnosed or recurrent NMIBC.

Arguably, the most important component in deciding treatment is the depth of tumor invasion and whether or not detrusor muscle invasion is present. If such muscle invasion is present, the patient needs definitive treatment with a radical cystectomy, bilateral pelvic node dissection, and urinary diversion as standard of care.[4] Alternatively, bladder-sparing protocols of chemoradiation also can be considered.[5] With the exception of grade 1 Ta tumors and potentially primary CIS, if there is no muscle in the specimen after initial resection, a repeat resection must be conducted for definitive diagnosis. In all T1 and high-grade (former World Health Organization grade 3/3) tumors, repeat TURBT is recommended after initial resection. The importance of this process is evidenced by the presence of residual tumor in 33% to 53% of cases and the upstaging of upward of 25% on repeat evaluation.[3] In fact, upstaging to muscle invasion on re-resection is even more likely in pT1 tumors without muscle present in the initial specimen.[3,6]

In patients with NMIBC, the grade of tumor and presence of CIS strongly influence whether serial cystoscopic surveillance or intravesical treatment with BCG or mitomycin is recommended to reduce the odds of recurrence or progression to a higher stage of bladder cancer. BCG is the gold standard intravesical treatment for high-grade Ta or T1 urothelial cell carcinoma and CIS.[7,8] In meta-analysis, BCG has been shown to decrease risk of progression by approximately 27% (odds ratio 0.73, $P = .001$) compared with control groups.[7] Significant variability in staging and grading of bladder cancer among pathologists is common,[3,9] which may have important treatment implications. This issue is especially notable for the diagnosis of CIS where agreement is present in only 70% to 78% of cases and may be in part due to the change in World Health Organization grading schemes between 1973 and 2004.[3,10,11] Alternatively, the overuse of a CIS diagnosis in the "shoulder" or base of papillary lesions is noted (per communication with Dr Michelle Hirsch, Brigham and Women's Hospital Pathologist, 2015).

Other pathologic findings that have important prognostic and treatment implications include the presence of lymphovascular invasion[12] or micropapillary histologic variants,[13] (see also Solomon and Hansel, Morphology and Molecular Characteristics of Bladder Cancer, Surgical Pathology Clinics, 2015, Volume 8, Issue 4) both of which portend a worse prognosis. Furthermore, detailed characterization of the T1 invasion in terms of proximity to the muscularis mucosae[14] or whether there is microscopic versus extensive invasion[15] is very helpful from a clinical perspective. Early cystectomy despite absence of muscle invasion is commonly advised in cases with adverse pathologic features, such as micropapillary variant, refractory CIS, or extensive T1 disease.[16]

Another important scenario to consider is tumor that presents in a bladder diverticulum, which poses unique challenges to the urologist performing the resection. Often, the location of the diverticulum, a narrow diverticular neck, or concern for bladder perforation results in a "sampling" or incomplete resection of the bladder tumor. Whereas Ta disease can be safely removed when feasible, one should be wary of a diagnosis of high-grade T1 disease, which may be understaged and actually be a stage T3 (ie, into perivesicular adipose tissue) lesion due to the absence of the muscle layer in a diverticulum.[3] Given these challenges, if the tumor is isolated, early consideration of partial cystectomy may be warranted if technically feasible. As part of surgical planning and completion of staging, random biopsies should be performed to ensure the absence of tumor or CIS elsewhere in the bladder. If the diverticulum is very posterior or near the trigone, a radical cystectomy may be required due to the inability to completely resect or optimally treat with intravesical agents.

In summary, NMIBC is the most frequent type of bladder cancer. Although having high recurrence rates, it also has high cure rates if managed with close surveillance, complete transurethral resection, and intravesical treatments. Early radical cystectomy, even in the absence of muscle invasion, should be considered in patients whose tumors have concerning pathologic features. Strong indications for definitive surgical management include T1 disease with variant histology (small cell, glandular, micropapillary), T1 disease with LVI, concomitant CIS, high-volume tumor at presentation, BCG refractory disease, or CIS of prostatic ducts. Accurate pathologic description with sufficient detail is vital for managing patients with NMIBC.

## IDENTIFICATION OF BLADDER CANCER VARIANTS

Urothelial carcinoma is the most common type of bladder cancer, comprising approximately 90% of cases in the United States. Less frequent subtypes include squamous cell carcinoma (5%) or adenocarcinoma (2%), along with rarer tumors such as small cell carcinoma, rhabdomyosarcoma, lymphoma, pheochromocytoma, or even metastases to the bladder.[1,2,17] However, within the urothelial carcinoma subclass, bladder cancer variants are increasingly being identified on pathologic assessment, which is likely due to heightened awareness of the histologic variance coupled with increasing recognition of the importance variants play in clinical management and outcome. The World Health Organization recently identified 13 urothelial carcinoma histologic variants (Box 1).[17] Common variants included micropapillary, squamous differentiation, glandular differentiation, sarcomatoid, and plasmacytoid (see also Solomon and Hansel, Morphology and Molecular Characteristics of Bladder Cancer, Surgical Pathology Clinics, 2015, Volume 8, Issue 4).

Certain bladder cancer variants, such as micropapillary, glandular, and plasmacytoid, often portend a worse prognosis and, thus, even T1 high-grade tumors are more likely to benefit from early cystectomy than ongoing management with BCG or other intravesical agents.[3,16] These variants are commonly more aggressive and resistant to BCG even if the tumor is not invasive into the detrusor muscle at initial diagnosis.[18] They also carry an increased risk of early spread to regional lymph nodes or distant sites.[13,18] Using surveillance, epidemiology, and end results data, a recent study identified 120 patients with micropapillary bladder cancer between 2001 and 2008, which

accounted for 0.1% of the bladder cancer cases during that time frame.[19] Compared with nonvariant urothelial carcinoma, the micropapillary subtype presented with more high-grade (86.1% vs 38.7%, $P<.0001$) and higher-stage disease (NMIBC: 40.8% vs 90.4%, $P<.0001$). For non–muscle-invasive micropapillary (n = 49), only 4 patients underwent definitive therapy in the form of radical cystectomy; none of these patients died of their disease, whereas in the patients who did not receive definitive therapy (n = 45), 7 cancer-specific deaths occurred (15.6%). The investigators concluded that regardless of grade, all micropapillary bladder cancer should be managed as high-grade disease, and that cystectomy should be strongly considered in all cases.

In summary, pathologic identification of variants of bladder cancer contributes greatly to decision-making regarding intravesical treatments, chemotherapy, and timing of radical cystectomy and urinary diversion.

## NONMETASTATIC MUSCLE-INVASIVE BLADDER CANCER

Despite being one of the most widely studied diseases, the management of nonmetastatic muscle-invasive bladder cancer (stage pT2; see **Fig. 1**) remains controversial. The patient and physician have several treatment decision points for this potentially curative disease with radical cystectomy versus bladder preservation with radiation therapy being the primary choices. Chemotherapy is generally recommended with both approaches to improve outcomes. The pathologic features of the tumor (see also Solomon and Hansel, Morphology and Molecular Characteristics of Bladder Cancer, Surgical Pathology Clinics, 2015, Volume 8, Issue 4) play an important role in the decision for either local approach.

Radical cystectomy with pelvic lymph node dissection can achieve recurrence-free and overall survival rates of 68% and 66% at 5 years, and prognosis significantly correlates with pathologic stage and lymph node involvement.[4] If extirpation is chosen, the role of perioperative chemotherapy, given either in the neoadjuvant or adjuvant setting, must be considered. The rationale for preoperative chemotherapy includes (1) rapid treatment of microscopic metastases; (2) in vivo evaluation of chemosensitivity; (3) downstaging or shrinkage of the primary tumor, which can facilitate surgical removal; (4) preserved renal function permitting optimal drug delivery with cisplatin; and, perhaps most importantly, (5) a more precise endpoint of treatment that can be measured both

---

**Box 1**
**Variants of invasive urothelial carcinoma**

Squamous differentiation

Glandular differentiation

Nested pattern

Microcystic

Micropapillary

Plasmacytoid and lymphoma-like

Sarcomatoid/carcinosarcoma

Giant cell

Lymphoepithelioma-like

Trophoblastic differentiation

Clear cell

Lipid cell

Undifferentiated

*Adapted from* Eble J, Sauter G, Epstein JI, et al. World Health Organization classification of tumours. Pathology and genetics of tumours of the urinary system and male genital organs. Lyon (France): IARC Press; 2004.

radiologically and pathologically. The most definitive evidence on improving clinical outcomes with neoadjuvant chemotherapy comes from 2 phase III studies, which is further bolstered by meta-analysis data.[20–22] Collectively, these studies demonstrate the ability of neoadjuvant cisplatin-based chemotherapy to increase disease-specific survival (DSS) by approximately 10% and overall survival by 5% to 14%. The phase III SWOG trial evaluated 3 doses of preoperative MVAC (methotrexate, vinblastine, Adriamycin, cisplatin) followed by surgery compared with resection alone in patients with T2-4N0M0 disease.[22] The investigators observed a 14% increase in 5-year overall survival and a clinically significant 31-month increase in median overall survival (46 vs 77 months, $P = .06$). Whether this approach should be considered in clinical T2 disease is controversial. However, subset analysis of this trial highlights that the benefit was not limited to T3 or greater disease. A significant increase in median survival from 75 to 105 months was observed in patients with T2 disease, whereas T3-T4a disease had a more than 40-month increase from 24 to 65 months with the addition of chemotherapy.

The SWOG study also highlighted the importance of achieving a pathologic disease-free state (pT0, pathologic complete response [pCR]). In the MVAC arm, 38% of patients achieved a pT0 state compared with 15% in the cystectomy arm ($P<.001$). At the time of reporting, the median overall survival had not been reached in the pT0 patients compared with 3.8 years in the patients who had residual disease despite the combination therapy. pCR has consistently been shown to be a biomarker of increased survival in several studies.[23–25]

The optimal neoadjuvant cisplatin-based treatment has not been determined. No trial has directly compared the regimens proven effective in the metastatic setting: MVAC, gemcitabine/cisplatin (GC), and dose-dense MVAC. Many physicians extrapolate from phase 3 data in the metastatic setting where GC and MVAC have been shown to be essentially equally effective with GC generally being more tolerable.[26,27] Similarly, attempts to enhance the tolerability of MVAC and shorten the administration time from 12 to 8 weeks have driven the investigation of "dose-dense" (dd) or "accelerated" MVAC. In the metastatic setting, ddMVAC has equivalent efficacy to traditional MVAC with a significantly increased rate of complete responses and enhanced progression-free survival (PFS).[28] Two prospective single-arm studies of neoadjuvant ddMVAC in urothelial carcinoma have demonstrated pCR rates of 26% to

38% and significant radiologic responses in 62%.[24,29]

Retrospective analyses support the general equivalence of GC to MVAC regimens in the neoadjuvant setting as well.[25,30,31] In a consecutive patient series from 28 international centers including ours, the Retrospective International Study of Cancers of the Urothelium (RISC) consortium observed pCR rates in 31% of the 146 patients on GC and 29% of the 66 patients on MVAC.[30] Most (77%) MVAC patients received the dose-dense schedule. No differences were seen in overall survival between the 2 groups (hazard ratio [HR] 0.64, confidence interval [CI] 0.34–1.22, $P = .17$).

The phase 2 COXEN trial is an ongoing biomarker validation and discovery study that is randomizing patients to either GC or ddMVAC and will provide the first direct comparison of these 2 regimens in terms of pT0 rate and toxicity in the neoadjuvant setting (NCT02177695). Planned gene expression sequencing analyses may afford additional predictive information, which is desperately needed.

The goal of adjuvant cisplatin-based therapy is to eliminate persistent local and or micrometastatic disease. Advantages of this approach compared with neoadjuvant chemotherapy are that it permits the most accurate staging and decreases overtreatment. Adjuvant therapy ensures that the surgery occurs quickly. Drawbacks to postsurgical administration are that chemotherapy administration may not occur or may be delayed due to postoperative complications, renal insufficiency, or decreased performance status making the patient ineligible for cisplatin. Pathologic evaluation plays a critical role in determining whether adjuvant chemotherapy is indicated. Adjuvant therapy is generally considered when there is evidence of extravesicular extension (stage pT3, pT4; see **Fig. 1**), node-positive disease, or angiolymphatic invasion; features that portend a recurrence rate of 75% to 80% by 5 years.[4,32]

Prospective trial data supporting adjuvant administration have been less definitive due to poor accrual to phase 3 studies, but the overall consensus from meta-analyses and most prospective studies is that there is likely clinical benefit in terms of reducing the risk of both recurrence and death and increasing survival.[33,34] The difficulty in interpreting these trials is because they often used nonstandard cisplatin regimens and/or were underpowered due to early closure for poor accrual. Meta-analyses have revealed that cisplatin-based therapy likely reduces the risk of recurrence (HR 0.68, $P<.001$, 12% absolute reduction), increases DSS (pooled HR 0.66, 95%

CI 0.45–0.91, $P$ = .014), reduces the risk of death (RR 0.75, $P$ = .001), and increases overall survival (HR 0.74–0.77, ~10% absolute increase).[33,34]

Three recently reported trials have asked the question of timing of postoperative therapy in terms of immediate versus delayed administration at the time of recurrence in patients with pT3-T4 or N+M0 disease.[35–37] Although all were closed early for poor accrual and thus underpowered, 2 of the 3 appeared to demonstrate clinical benefit with early administration. In the Spanish Oncology Genitourinary Group trial, patients were randomized either to the triplet regimen of paclitaxel, gemcitabine, and cisplatin for 4 cycles or observation with therapy only at relapse.[36] At a median follow-up of 30 months, the triplet regimen appeared to significantly increase disease free survival (DFS), time to progression (TTP), and DSS with a 5-year overall survival rate of 60% versus 30% ($P$<.0009). Median overall survival had not been reached in the treated arm compared with 26 months in the control arm. In a second study, European Organization for Research and Treatment of Cancer investigators asked the question of whether use of any of the most frequently administered regimens (GC, MVAC, or ddMVAC) for 4 cycles improved survival compared with deferred therapy with 6 cycles at relapse.[37] Keeping in mind that it was underpowered, at median follow-up of 7 years, the primary endpoint of median overall survival was not significantly different. However, they did observe a significant increase in PFS at 5 years (47.6% vs 31.8%, HR 0.54, $P$<.0001) with median PFS of 3.1 versus 0.99 years. In terms of overall survival, there was a trend to improvement in 5-year rate at 53.6% versus 47.7%, with a nonsignificant 22% reduction in risk of death with a median survival of 6.7 versus 3.9 years (HR 0.78, $P$ = .13). The third study was an Italian multicenter trial that randomized patients to adjuvant GC versus surveillance, with chemotherapy at relapse.[35] With only 194 of 610 patients accrued over a 6-year period, there appeared to be a suggestion of benefit to treating at relapse over immediate therapy with median DFS of 42.3% versus 37.2% (HR 1.08, 95% CI 0.73–1.59, $P$ = .7). The median 5-year overall survival was 48.5% with no significant difference between the 2 arms (HR 1.29, 95% CI 0.84–1.99, $P$ = .24). Ultimately given the underpowered nature, the data from these 3 studies will add to meta-analyses but are insufficient to reliably base treatment recommendations.

In summary, all of the phase 3 adjuvant chemotherapy studies in urothelial cancer closed to poor accrual. Although there are some conflicting results, most prospective trials and meta-analyses suggest that adjuvant administration of cisplatin-based regimens achieve clinical benefits in terms of reducing recurrence rates, increasing PFS, and improving disease-specific and overall survival. Thus, in patients who do not receive neoadjuvant chemotherapy, we recommend adjuvant cisplatin-based therapy in patients who have high-risk pathologic features such as extravesicular extension, nodal involvement, or evidence of LVI.[4,32]

Pathology may also influence the choice of urinary diversion, which is typically in the form of either an ileal conduit or an orthotopic ileal neobladder. If the disease is known to be locally advanced based on preoperative imaging or due to intraoperative findings (eg, gross extravesical extension, involved nodes, or positive margins on frozen section), it is usually prudent to proceed with an ileal conduit to allow for the possibility of postoperative radiation to the surgical bed that is unencumbered by the presence of an ileal neobladder in the radiation field.

In patients unfit or unwilling to undergo radical cystectomy, bladder preservation therapy is a potentially curative alternative that allows the patient to retain a functional bladder. This strategy, which is also known as trimodality therapy, involves maximal debulking TURBT to remove any visible tumor followed by radiation with concurrent chemotherapy. If the patient is eligible and willing to have salvage cystectomy for residual muscle-invasive disease, a repeat TURBT should be performed near the end or after radiation is complete. Although many can be cured with bladder preservation therapy, approximately 20% to 30% of patients require immediate or eventual salvage cystectomy for persistent disease.[38,39]

Pathology and imaging play a critical role in determining eligibility for bladder preservation therapy. Optimal candidates for this approach have solitary lesions smaller than 5 cm, T2 or T3 disease without evidence of hydronephrosis, ability to perform a complete TURBT, and minimal to no CIS.[5] Multifocal disease or CIS raises upfront concerns as to whether radiation and chemotherapy can completely eradicate disease. Persistent CIS may also lead to a higher chance of recurrence in the remaining bladder. Close communication with the pathologist is critical to confirm whether CIS after a previous biopsy or TURBT is real or actually just a "shoulder lesion"; that is, the edge or stalk of a current or previously resected papillary tumor, as the former may be overused and have significant clinical implications. Hydronephrosis reflects the tumor involvement at the level of the ureterovesicular junction. It is often cited as a contraindication, given concerns over the ability to do a complete TURBT and has been associated with worse clinical outcomes with bladder preservation approaches.[38] Several studies have shown a significant or trend to significant benefit in outcomes including overall survival in patients who have had a visibly complete TURBT.[38,39] The updated series from the Massachusetts General Hospital of patients treated with various bladder preservation protocols from 1986 to 2002 showed statistically significant benefits on univariate analysis in pCRs, overall survival, DSS, and need for subsequent cystectomy in patients who had visibly complete TURBTs.[39] On multivariate analysis, clinical T-stage and complete response to induction therapy remained the most important predicators of improved DSS and overall survival.

Radiation for invasive bladder cancer delivers 64 to 65 Gy to the bladder and 44 to 45 Gy to the adjacent pelvic nodes. Multiple studies have shown an improvement in local control and recurrence-free survival in patients treated with both chemotherapy and radiotherapy compared with patients treated with radiotherapy alone.[5] The optimal chemotherapy regimen has not yet been determined. Given that cisplatin is radiosensitizing and the most effective agent in the metastatic setting, it forms the backbone of many chemoradiation regimens. Concurrent cisplatin-based therapies have been proven to augment the effect of radiation and have the potential to eradicate micrometastases as well.[40,41] Non–cisplatin-based regimens, such as fluorouracil (5-FU)/mitomycin-C (MMC) have also proven effective.[42] Compared with no chemotherapy, a phase 3 study demonstrated that the addition of 5-FU/MMC to radiation significantly decreased the incidence of local recurrence at 2 years (67% vs 54%, HR 0.68, 95% CI 0.48–0.96; $P = .03$). There was a trend to improved overall survival at 5 years: 48% versus 35% (HR: 0.82; 95% CI 0.63–1.09; $P = .16$). This trial also highlighted that we may not need to radiate pelvic lymph nodes in all patients, as it was not mandated in the trial and the rates of pelvic nodal recurrences were low. Alternative radiosensitizing options for cisplatin-ineligible patients include regimens effective in other cancers, such as carboplatin/paclitaxel or low doses of gemcitabine.[43,44] Unlike with surgery, neoadjuvant chemotherapy has not been proven to enhance survival in addition to concurrent chemoradiation[39,41] and, thus, our practice generally does not administer induction doses or adjuvant chemotherapy after bladder preservation.

No randomized studies have directly compared cystectomy to bladder preservation approaches.

Although fraught with selection bias, 5-year overall survival outcomes in combined analyses of patients with T2-T4a disease appear comparable at 45% to 57%.[4,22,38,39,41,42] A recent pooled analysis of 6 Radiation Therapy Oncology Group bladder preservation trials demonstrated good 5-year and 10-year DSS at 71% and 65%, respectively, with 5-year and 10-year overall survival rates of 57% and 36%.[38] Only 14% experienced a recurrence of muscle-invasive tumors and 20% underwent eventual cystectomy. If bladder preservation therapy is chosen, close surveillance for local recurrence is required, with serial cystoscopies, urine cytologies, and imaging.

In summary, definitive therapy in the form of radical cystectomy or bladder preservation therapy with chemoradiation can achieve cures and improve outcomes in nonmetastatic muscle-invasive bladder cancer. Two randomized phase 3 trials and several meta-analyses demonstrate that cisplatin-based chemotherapy before cystectomy significantly improves overall survival, pathologic response, and DFS. Unfortunately, neoadjuvant administration is often underused due to physician acceptance regarding the perceived modest clinical benefits, but it remains the gold standard if patients can receive cisplatin-based therapy and plan to undergo radical cystectomy. If upfront chemotherapy is not given, adjuvant cisplatin-based therapy should be considered in patients whose tumors exhibit extravesicular extension, nodal involvement, or evidence of lymphovascular invasion. Alternatively, a trimodality regimen of aggressive completion TURBT combined with chemoradiation has also demonstrated similar 5-year outcomes with the added benefit of enhanced quality of life given bladder preservation. All approaches require close communication between the patient and a multidisciplinary team of surgeons, radiation oncologists, and medical oncologists. Any issues regarding reported pathologic findings should be discussed with the pathologist for clarification.

## SUMMARY

The treatment and outcomes of bladder cancer depend on accurate staging and precise pathologic evaluation. NMIBC is the most frequent form of bladder cancer and has high recurrence rates requiring long-term management. Early identification of aggressive variants and pathologic features, such as recurrent high-grade CIS, micropapillary disease, or extensive high-grade T1 disease, is critical, as these patients may warrant early cystectomy. The management of nonmetastatic muscle-invasive disease is more heterogeneous, but cure is possible with definitive therapy in the form of radical cystectomy with pelvic lymph node dissection combined with perioperative cisplatin-based chemotherapy or aggressive bladder preservation protocols with chemoradiation. Ultimately, the treatment of bladder cancer is a multidisciplinary effort requiring close collaboration with clinicians and their pathologists. Understanding of the implications of the various histologic findings and their implications for clinical management will optimize the clinical outcomes of our patients.

## REFERENCES

1. Burger M, Catto JW, Dalbagni G, et al. Epidemiology and risk factors of urothelial bladder cancer. Eur Urol 2013;63(2):234–41.
2. Siegel R, Ma J, Zou Z, et al. Cancer statistics, 2014. CA Cancer J Clin 2014;64(1):9–29.
3. Babjuk M, Burger M, Zigeuner R, et al. EAU guidelines on non-muscle-invasive urothelial carcinoma of the bladder: update 2013. Eur Urol 2013;64(4):639–53.
4. Stein JP, Lieskovsky G, Cote R, et al. Radical cystectomy in the treatment of invasive bladder cancer: long-term results in 1,054 patients. J Clin Oncol 2001;19(3):666–75.
5. Ploussard G, Daneshmand S, Efstathiou JA, et al. Critical analysis of bladder sparing with trimodal therapy in muscle-invasive bladder cancer: a systematic review. Eur Urol 2014;66(1):120–37.
6. Dalbagni G, Vora K, Kaag M, et al. Clinical outcome in a contemporary series of restaged patients with clinical T1 bladder cancer. Eur Urol 2009;56(6):903–10.
7. Sylvester RJ, van der MA, Lamm DL. Intravesical bacillus Calmette-Guerin reduces the risk of progression in patients with superficial bladder cancer: a meta-analysis of the published results of randomized clinical trials. J Urol 2002;168(5):1964–70.
8. Lamm DL. Preventing progression and improving survival with BCG maintenance. Eur Urol 2000;37(Suppl 1):9–15.
9. May M, Brookman-Amissah S, Roigas J, et al. Prognostic accuracy of individual uropathologists in noninvasive urinary bladder carcinoma: a multicentre study comparing the 1973 and 2004 World Health Organisation classifications. Eur Urol 2010;57(5):850–8.
10. Witjes JA, Moonen PM, van der Heijden AG. Review pathology in a diagnostic bladder cancer trial: effect of patient risk category. Urology 2006;67(4):751–5.
11. Murphy WM, Takezawa K, Maruniak NA. Interobserver discrepancy using the 1998 World Health Organization/International Society of Urologic Pathology classification of urothelial neoplasms: practical choices for patient care. J Urol 2002;168(3):968–72.
12. Cho KS, Seo HK, Joung JY, et al. Lymphovascular invasion in transurethral resection specimens as predictor of progression and metastasis in patients with newly diagnosed T1 bladder urothelial cancer. J Urol 2009;182(6):2625–30.
13. Kamat AM, Dinney CP, Gee JR, et al. Micropapillary bladder cancer: a review of the University of Texas M. D. Anderson Cancer Center experience with 100 consecutive patients. Cancer 2007;110(1):62–7.
14. Orsola A, Trias I, Raventos CX, et al. Initial high-grade T1 urothelial cell carcinoma: feasibility and prognostic significance of lamina propria invasion microstaging (T1a/b/c) in BCG-treated and BCG-non-treated patients. Eur Urol 2005;48(2):231–8 [discussion: 238].
15. van Rhijn BW, van der Kwast TH, Alkhateeb SS, et al. A new and highly prognostic system to discern T1 bladder cancer substage. Eur Urol 2012;61(2):378–84.
16. Herr HW, Sogani PC. Does early cystectomy improve the survival of patients with high risk superficial bladder tumors? J Urol 2001;166(4):1296–9.
17. Chalasani V, Chin JL, Izawa JI. Histologic variants of urothelial bladder cancer and nonurothelial histology in bladder cancer. Can Urol Assoc J 2009;3(6 Suppl 4):S193–8.
18. Kamat AM, Gee JR, Dinney CP, et al. The case for early cystectomy in the treatment of nonmuscle invasive micropapillary bladder carcinoma. J Urol 2006;175(3 Pt 1):881–5.
19. Vourganti S, Harbin A, Singer EA, et al. Low grade micropapillary urothelial carcinoma, does it exist? Analysis of management and outcomes from the surveillance, epidemiology and end results (SEER) database. J Cancer 2013;4(4):336–42.
20. Neoadjuvant chemotherapy in invasive bladder cancer: update of a systematic review and meta-analysis of individual patient data advanced bladder cancer (ABC) meta-analysis collaboration. Eur Urol 2005;48(2):202–5 [discussion: 205–6].
21. Griffiths G, Hall R, Sylvester R, et al. International phase III trial assessing neoadjuvant cisplatin, methotrexate, and vinblastine chemotherapy for muscle-invasive bladder cancer: long-term results of the BA06 30894 trial. J Clin Oncol 2011;29(16):2171–7.
22. Grossman HB, Natale RB, Tangen CM, et al. Neoadjuvant chemotherapy plus cystectomy compared with cystectomy alone for locally advanced bladder cancer. N Engl J Med 2003;349(9):859–66.
23. Neoadjuvant cisplatin, methotrexate, and vinblastine chemotherapy for muscle-invasive bladder cancer: a randomised controlled trial. International collaboration of trialists. Lancet 1999;354(9178):533–40.
24. Choueiri TK, Jacobus S, Bellmunt J, et al. Neoadjuvant dose-dense methotrexate, vinblastine, doxorubicin, and cisplatin with pegfilgrastim support in muscle-invasive urothelial cancer: pathologic, radiologic, and

biomarker correlates. J Clin Oncol 2014;32(18):1889–94.

25. Dash A, Pettus JA, Herr HW, et al. A role for neoadjuvant gemcitabine plus cisplatin in muscle-invasive urothelial carcinoma of the bladder: a retrospective experience. Cancer 2008;113(9):2471–7.

26. von der Maase H, Hansen SW, Roberts JT, et al. Gemcitabine and cisplatin versus methotrexate, vinblastine, doxorubicin, and cisplatin in advanced or metastatic bladder cancer: results of a large, randomized, multinational, multicenter, phase III study. J Clin Oncol 2000;18(17):3068–77.

27. von der Maase H, Sengelov L, Roberts JT, et al. Long-term survival results of a randomized trial comparing gemcitabine plus cisplatin, with methotrexate, vinblastine, doxorubicin, plus cisplatin in patients with bladder cancer. J Clin Oncol 2005;23(21):4602–8.

28. Sternberg CN, de Mulder PH, Schornagel JH, et al. Randomized phase III trial of high-dose-intensity methotrexate, vinblastine, doxorubicin, and cisplatin (MVAC) chemotherapy and recombinant human granulocyte colony-stimulating factor versus classic MVAC in advanced urothelial tract tumors: European Organization for Research and Treatment of Cancer protocol no. 30924. J Clin Oncol 2001;19(10):2638–46.

29. Plimack ER, Hoffman-Censits JH, Viterbo R, et al. Accelerated methotrexate, vinblastine, doxorubicin, and cisplatin is safe, effective, and efficient neoadjuvant treatment for muscle-invasive bladder cancer: results of a multicenter phase II study with molecular correlates of response and toxicity. J Clin Oncol 2014;32(18):1895–901.

30. Galsky MD, Harshman LC, Crabb SJ, et al, RISC Investigators. Comparative effectiveness of gemcitabine plus cisplatin (GC) versus methotrexate, vinblastine, doxorubicin, plus cisplatin (MVAC) as neoadjuvant therapy for muscle-invasive bladder cancer (MIBC). J Clin Oncol 2014;32(5s):4512.

31. Yuh BE, Ruel N, Wilson TG, et al. Pooled analysis of clinical outcomes with neoadjuvant cisplatin and gemcitabine chemotherapy for muscle invasive bladder cancer. J Urol 2013;189(5):1682–6.

32. Dorff TB, Tsao-Wei D, Miranda G, et al. Adjuvant chemotherapy for locally advanced urothelial carcinoma: an overview of the USC experience. World J Urol 2009;27(1):39–44.

33. Adjuvant chemotherapy in invasive bladder cancer: a systematic review and meta-analysis of individual patient data advanced bladder cancer (ABC) meta-analysis collaboration. Eur Urol 2005;48(2):189–99 [discussion: 199–201].

34. Leow JJ, Martin-Doyle W, Rajagopal PS, et al. Adjuvant chemotherapy for invasive bladder cancer: a 2013 updated systematic review and meta-analysis of randomized trials. Eur Urol 2013;66(1):42–54.

35. Cognetti F, Ruggeri EM, Felici A, et al. Adjuvant chemotherapy with cisplatin and gemcitabine versus chemotherapy at relapse in patients with muscle-invasive bladder cancer submitted to radical cystectomy: an Italian, multicenter, randomized phase III trial. Ann Oncol 2012;23(3):695–700.

36. Paz-Ares LG, Solsona E, Esteban E, et al. Randomized phase III trial comparing adjuvant paclitaxel/gemcitabine/cisplatin (PGC) to observation in patients with resected invasive bladder cancer: results of the Spanish Oncology Genitourinary Group (SOGUG) 99/01 study. J Clin Oncol 2010;28(18s):LBA4518.

37. Sternberg CN, Skoneczna I, Kerst JM, et al. Immediate versus deferred chemotherapy after radical cystectomy in patients with pT3-pT4 or N+ M0 urothelial carcinoma of the bladder (EORTC 30994): an intergroup, open-label, randomised phase 3 trial. Lancet Oncol 2014;16(1):76–86.

38. Mak RH, Hunt D, Shipley WU, et al. Long-term outcomes in patients with muscle-invasive bladder cancer after selective bladder-preserving combined-modality therapy: a pooled analysis of Radiation Therapy Oncology Group protocols 8802, 8903, 9506, 9706, 9906, and 0233. J Clin Oncol 2014;32(34):3801–9.

39. Efstathiou JA, Spiegel DY, Shipley WU, et al. Long-term outcomes of selective bladder preservation by combined-modality therapy for invasive bladder cancer: the MGH experience. Eur Urol 2012;61(4):705–11.

40. Coppin CM, Gospodarowicz MK, James K, et al. Improved local control of invasive bladder cancer by concurrent cisplatin and preoperative or definitive radiation. The National Cancer Institute of Canada Clinical Trials Group. J Clin Oncol 1996;14(11):2901–7.

41. Shipley WU, Winter KA, Kaufman DS, et al. Phase III trial of neoadjuvant chemotherapy in patients with invasive bladder cancer treated with selective bladder preservation by combined radiation therapy and chemotherapy: initial results of Radiation Therapy Oncology Group 89-03. J Clin Oncol 1998;16(11):3576–83.

42. James ND, Hussain SA, Hall E, et al. Radiotherapy with or without chemotherapy in muscle-invasive bladder cancer. N Engl J Med 2012;366(16):1477–88.

43. Oh KS, Soto DE, Smith DC, et al. Combined-modality therapy with gemcitabine and radiation therapy as a bladder preservation strategy: long-term results of a phase I trial. Int J Radiat Oncol Biol Phys 2009;74(2):511–7.

44. van Hagen P, Hulshof MC, van Lanschot JJ, et al. Preoperative chemoradiotherapy for esophageal or junctional cancer. N Engl J Med 2012;366(22):2074–84.

# Tumors of the Testis
## Morphologic Features and Molecular Alterations

Brooke E. Howitt, MD[a], Daniel M. Berney, FRCPath[b],*

## KEYWORDS

- Testis • Seminoma • Embryonal • Yolk-sac tumor • Teratoma • Germ cell tumor • i12p

## ABSTRACT

This article reviews the most frequently encountered tumor of the testis; pure and mixed malignant testicular germ cell tumors (TGCT), with emphasis on adult (postpubertal) TGCTs and their differential diagnoses. We additionally review TGCT in the postchemotherapy setting, and findings to be integrated into the surgical pathology report, including staging of testicular tumors and other problematic issues. The clinical features, gross pathologic findings, key histologic features, common differential diagnoses, the use of immunohistochemistry, and molecular alterations in TGCTs are discussed.

## OVERVIEW

Germ cell tumors are the most common testicular tumors. This chapter has an emphasis on adult (postpubertal) TGCTs and their differential diagnoses. The article is divided into 3 parts: primary TGCT, TGCT in the postchemotherapy setting, and the pathology report: staging of testicular tumors and other problematic issues. The clinical features, gross pathologic findings, key histologic features, common differential diagnoses, and the use of immunohistochemistry are discussed. Molecular alterations, including the use of cytogenetic tests for isochromosome 12p, are also covered.

## GERM CELL TUMORS AND THE DIFFERENTIAL DIAGNOSIS

### INTRODUCTION

TGCTs account for approximately 95% of all testicular tumors, and overall have a more than 90% 5-year survival rate,[1-3] with fatal cases almost always related to higher clinical stage at presentation, late tumor recurrences, the development of somatic-type malignancy in recurrent tumors, or treatment-related toxicity. The importance of TGCT classification relates to the many options for treatment in the vast spectrum of these neoplasms, avoiding common mimickers of different malignant potential, and increasingly refined classification to avoid overtreatment of indolent lesions. In few other areas of pathology can the Hippocratic maxim "Do no harm" be better applied. Accurate diagnosis of testicular neoplasms can not only save the lives of young men, but also prevent potential overtreatment by surgery, chemotherapy, or radiotherapy (see also Bernard and Sweeney, Diagnosis and Treatment of Testicular Cancer: A Clinician's Perspective, Surgical Pathology Clinics, 2015, Volume 8, Issue 4).

TGCTs are currently classified by the 2004 World Health Organization (WHO)[4] into seminoma (including classic and spermatocytic types) and nonseminomatous germ cell tumors (NSGCT), although one-third of TGCTs are mixed seminomas/NSGCTs. Of note, in the upcoming 2015 WHO classification (in press), spermatocytic seminoma is renamed (herein referred to as "spermatocytic tumor") to reflect its indolent behavior and its

[a] Department of Pathology, Brigham and Women's Hospital, Harvard Medical School, 75 Francis Street, Boston, MA 02115, USA; [b] Orchid Tissue Laboratory, St. Bartholomew's Hospital, Barts Cancer Institute, Queen Mary University of London, Charterhouse Square, London EC1A 7BE, UK
* Corresponding author.
E-mail address: D.Berney@bartsandthelondon.nhs.uk

surgpath.theclinics.com

biologic distinction from conventional-type semi-noma. Although the range of patient age at diagnosis for TGCT is wide (infants to >75 years), young men (age 20–40 years) are the most common age group affected by TGCT and relative frequencies of TGCT subtypes change with age.[5,6] Pure seminoma is the most common TGCT, followed by mixed germ cell tumors. Pure embryonal carcinomas are only occasionally encountered, whereas postpubertal pure yolk-sac tumors and choriocarcinoma are rare in the testis. The vast majority of TGCTs (>80%) have the cytogenetic aberration of increased copies ("isochromosome") of the short arm of chromosome 12 (i12p) and also are typically associated with intratubular germ cell neoplasia of unclassified type (IGCNU); the latter is also renamed in the upcoming 2015 WHO (in press) and is herein referred to by the new name, "germ cell neoplasia in situ" (GCNIS). However, there are some notable exceptions to this, including spermatocytic tumor and some teratomatous tumors. It has been suggested that the WHO 2015 classification be based on tumor association with GCNIS and genetic changes. These possible changes are mentioned in the specific entities described. A summary of immunohistochemistry (IHC) in TGCT and formal recommendations in the use of IHC in the diagnosis of testicular tumors were recently reported.[7] Because of the overlap in IHC profiles, biomarkers are discussed for individual TGCT types, instead, they are discussed with regard to differential diagnoses (see later in this article) and when exceptions to a rule occur. Isochromosome 12p, other alterations involving 12p, as well as non-12p aberrations in TGCT, are covered herein.

## GROSS FEATURES OF TESTIS, PURE AND MIXED MALIGNANT GERM CELL TUMORS

The initial handling of the gross specimen on the cutting bench is of crucial importance for accurate histotyping and staging of the tumor. In general, timely and proper fixation protocols are imperative for optimal histologic assessment. All testicular tumors, regardless of histotype, can be treated similarly on the cutting bench with few exceptions. Sections to be submitted for routine evaluation are included in **Table 1**. Examination and evaluation of the tunica vaginalis (ie, is it easily movable or fixed?) is best done on gross examination and confirmed histologically. Care should be taken to use clean tools to avoid transposition of tumor cells into vascular spaces, onto specimen surfaces, or into tissue crevices, all of which could affect staging if interpreted microscopically to represent true vascular invasion or tumor spread.

*Table 1*
**Sections to be submitted on a radical orchiectomy**

| | |
|---|---|
| Spermatic cord | 1. Spermatic cord resection margin |
| | 2. Sampling of gross involvement of tumor in spermatic cord OR Sections from the middle and distal spermatic cord if grossly unremarkable |
| Tumor | 3. Generous sampling of tumor, including areas of different coloration, consistency, necrosis, hemorrhage, and scarring (at least 1 block per cm of tumor) |
| | 4. Sampling of tumor interface with normal parenchyma |
| | 5. Tumor to rete/hilar area |
| | 6. Tumor to closest approach to tunica albuginea and vaginalis |
| Other structures to sample | 7. Uninvolved testis |
| | 8. Epididymis |

The gross characteristics of TGCT are generally similar regardless of subtype, present as solid, fleshy nodules, often well-circumscribed, and associated with varying amounts of hemorrhage and/or necrosis. Classic seminoma is typically a tan to pale yellow solid, fleshy, and well-circumscribed mass with frequent small foci of hemorrhage and necrosis (**Fig. 1A**). In intertubular seminoma, a distinct mass may not be apparent and instead occasional irregularities in texture or color are seen.[8] The gross features of spermatocytic tumor are similar to that seen in classic seminoma, but the cut surface may be slightly more gelatinous rather than fleshy.[9]

Yolk-sac tumors are typically well-circumscribed, white to tan/gray or yellow nodule(s) with a glistening cut surface (see **Fig. 1B**) and cystic change may be present. Necrosis and hemorrhage may be focal or extensive. In the mixed NSGCT, extensive sampling to identify the yolk-sac tumor (YST) component should be undertaken in the setting of elevated serum alpha-fetoprotein (AFP). In embryonal carcinoma (EC), extensive necrosis and hemorrhage are common (see **Fig. 1C**). Local extension beyond the testis is present in approximately one-quarter of cases of pure EC, requiring thorough gross evaluation and

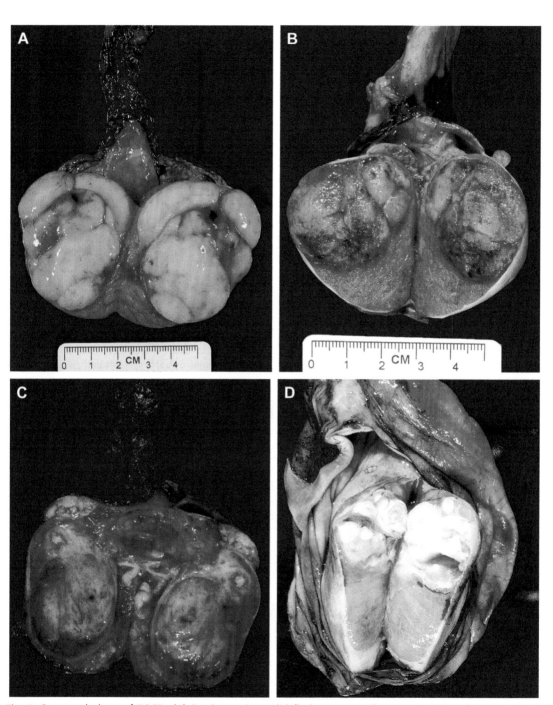

*Fig. 1.* Gross pathology of TGCTs. (*A*) Seminoma is a solid fleshy tan to yellow mass which is frequently well-circumscribed and may have small foci of hemorrhage or necrosis. (*B*) YST is a solid mass with more heterogeneity and a rough cut surface with frequent foci of hemorrhage. (*C*) EC is similar to YST, has a variegated cut surface with frequent and sometimes extensive necrosis and hemorrhage. (*D*) Teratoma is easiest to recognize on gross examination when cartilaginous tissue and cystic spaces are present, as shown here.

sampling.[10,11] Teratoma in the testis is typically a solid mass with a heterogeneous cut surface (see **Fig. 1**D), which may contain cysts of various sizes, and bone and cartilage may be grossly visible. Dermoid cysts of the testis are grossly similar to that

seen in the ovary, with a predominantly cystic structure filled with hair and sebaceous material and may be difficult to distinguish grossly from teratoma. Choriocarcinoma may present as a solitary or multifocal mass in the testis, with extensive necrosis and hemorrhage, and macroscopic evidence of vascular invasion often readily appreciated on gross examination.

## SEMINOMATOUS GERM CELL TUMORS

### Classic Seminoma

#### Clinical features

Seminoma is the most common germ cell tumor, accounting for approximately 50% of all TGCTs.[12] Seminoma occurs in older men when compared with NSGCT with a mean age of 40 years, and more than 80% occurring after the age of 30.[12] Additionally, most TGCTs in men older than 60 are seminoma.[13] Patients typically present with a painless or vaguely painful mass, and bilateral disease is rare (<2%). The outcome for pure seminoma is extremely good, with greater than 95% survival at 5 years due to its radiosensitive and chemosensitive nature.

#### Microscopic features

Although classic seminoma may be an easy and straightforward diagnosis, it can also show great variation, leading to misdiagnosis. Usually, seminoma grows in nests and sheets of cells, with thin fibrous septa separating nests and lobules of tumor cells. Within the septa are variably prominent lymphocytes (Fig. 2A–C). When properly fixed and processed, the cell borders are distinct. Seminoma tends to have a rather monotonous appearance of cells with clear to pale to eosinophilic cytoplasm. Nuclei are typically large (but generally not pleomorphic) and contain very prominent often smudged nucleoli. The nuclear contours are mostly rounded but often at least one edge has a squared-off corner (see Fig. 2A, inset). In addition to lymphocytic inflammation, granulomatous inflammation is common, and may be extensive (see Fig. 2D). The inflammation is so extensive in rare cases that it almost obliterates the tumor cells. Away from the main mass, intertubular seminoma is common (Fig. 3A), and frequently associated with GCNIS. Pure intertubular seminoma is rare but much easier to miss in cases of widespread GCNIS. Tubular (see Fig. 3B), signet ring (see Fig. 3C), and rhabdoid (see Fig. 3D) variants of seminoma have been described. The tubular variant retains the basic

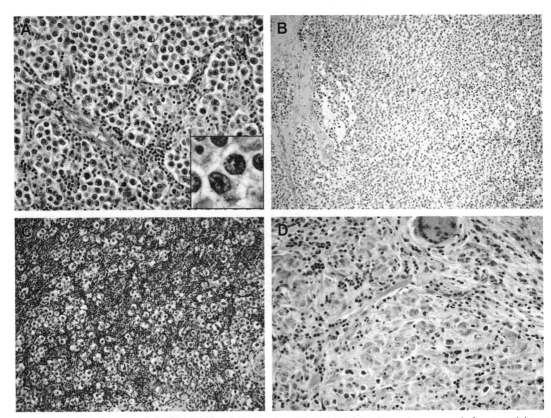

Fig. 2. Microscopic features of classic seminoma: inflammatory infiltrates. (A) Seminoma is composed of nests and sheets of tumor cells with characteristic "squared-off" nuclei. Seminoma may lack a prominent lymphocytic infiltrate (B) or be associated with an extremely prominent lymphocytic infiltration (C). (D) Granulomatous inflammation is common and may be more abundant than the tumor cells (hematoxylin-eosin, original magnification [A, D] ×400; [B, C] ×200).

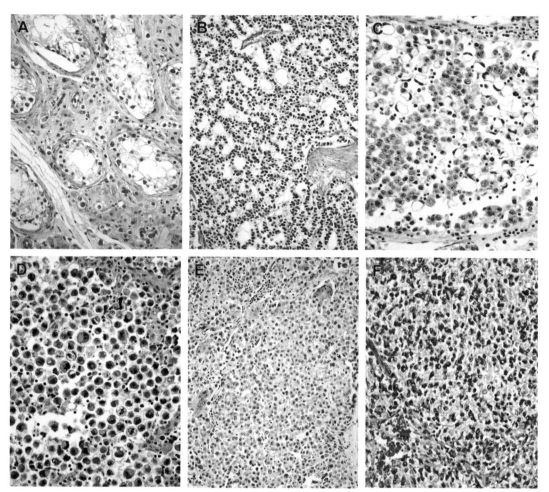

*Fig. 3.* Microscopic features of seminoma. (*A*) Intertubular seminoma is a pattern that may be missed due to the subtle infiltrative growth pattern between tubules, typically near germ cell neoplasia in situ (previously "intratubular germ cell neoplasia, unclassified type"). (*B*) Uncommonly seminoma may show a "tubular" or pseudoglandular pattern of growth, although areas of more classic seminoma are usually present elsewhere in the tumor. (*C*) Signet ring cell morphology may be seen in seminoma, but has no prognostic significance. (*D*) Rhabdoidlike morphology in seminoma may be secondary to suboptimal fixation or as a form of increased atypia. Similar to other morphologic variants of seminoma, there is no clinical significance. (*E*) Seminoma may be associated with syncytiotrophoblast, and a mildly elevated serum B-HCG. (*F*) Improperly fixed seminoma lacks the well-formed cell borders and nuclear morphology characteristic of seminoma (hematoxylin-eosin, original magnification ×400).

cytomorphometry, and the tubules often contain macrophages. Signet ring change is usually mixed with more typical appearances.[14] Syncytiotrophoblast (synT) may be present, dispersed throughout the tumor randomly (see **Fig. 3**E), and can be associated with mild elevation of serum Beta-hCG. Morphologic features of seminoma may be less readily apparent with improper fixation (see **Fig. 3**F).

## Spermatocytic Tumor (Previously Called Spermatocytic Seminoma)

### Clinical features

In 2015, the WHO classification (in press) renamed spermatocytic seminoma as "spermatocytic tumor" (ST) to reflect its indolent to benign behavior (in contrast to classic seminoma), and thereby avoiding clinical confusion and the potential for inappropriate therapy. ST is uncommon, representing approximately 1% of all TGCTs and typically occurs in older men and is more commonly bilateral than other TGCTs; however, these tumors have been reported in males as young as 19 years of age.[15] STs are typically pure, clinically indolent, and rarely if ever metastasize, even in the presence of lymphovascular invasion. The exception for aggressive behavior includes cases containing coexisting sarcoma, in which metastasis has been documented.[16,17] For this reason, no therapy beyond the initial orchiectomy is required.

## Microscopic features

ST is composed of 3 types of admixed tumor cells: small, medium/intermediate, and large/giant (**Fig. 4**). The medium-sized cells usually predominate and may mimic so-called "anaplastic" seminoma, as the latter also show a preponderance of intermediate-sized cells.[18] The giant cells are often multinucleate and demonstrate conspicuous pleomorphism with "spirene" chromatin, but they may represent a minority of tumor cells. Apoptosis is a frequent finding in ST.[19] The tumor cells tend to lack the glycogenation seen in typical seminoma, and the small cells of ST may even be mistaken for lymphocytes due to the scant cytoplasm. Unlike classic seminoma, thin fibrous septa with accompanying lymphocytes and/or granulomatous inflammation are uncommon. Atypical mitoses are very common in ST, which is one of the few "benign" tumors to show this feature. Also in contrast to classic seminoma, ST has no association with GCNIS but may demonstrate intratubular growth.

## Immunohistochemistry and molecular

ST lacks immunoreactivity seen in classic seminoma (ie, ST is typically negative for OCT3/4[20,21]; however, they are positive for SALL4,[22,23] and in approximately 50% of cases, c-kit[24,25]). NUT, GAGE7, and NY-ESO-1 have recently been suggested as more specific and sensitive markers.[26] Keratin (Cam5.2) may be positive in some cases.[27] Unlike classic seminoma and other NSGCTs, ST lacks i12p,[28] but rather has recurrent gains of chromosome 9, and may be diploid or tetraploid.[28]

> ### Key Points
> #### SEMINOMA
>
> - Older men compared with nonseminomatous germ cell tumors
> - Solid, tan, fleshy mass ± necrosis/hemorrhage
> - Sheets and nests separated by fibrous septa containing lymphocytes
> - Granulomatous inflammation common
> - "Squared-off" nuclei
> - Distinct cell borders
> - SALL4, OCT3/4, CKIT, D2-40, SOX17 positive
> - LCA, CD30, SOX2, GPC3, AFP, Beta-hCG negative
> - Isochromosome 12p in most cases

## NONSEMINOMATOUS GERM CELL TUMORS

### Embryonal Carcinoma

#### Clinical features

EC affects young men, with a mean age of 32 years.[5] Although pure EC of the testis is not common, EC is commonly encountered as a component of mixed NSGCT.[5,10,12,29] The proportion of EC in a mixed TGCT can influence treatment decisions in some settings (adjuvant treatment vs surveillance)[30,31] (see also Bernard and Sweeney, Diagnosis and Treatment of Testicular Cancer: A Clinician's Perspective, Surgical Pathology Clinics, 2015, Volume 8, Issue 4).

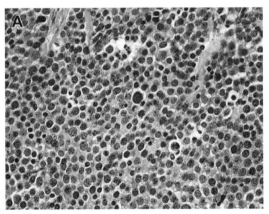
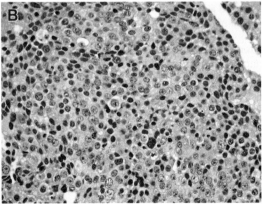

*Fig. 4.* Spermatocytic tumor (previously called "spermatocytic seminoma"). (*A*) Spermatocytic tumor is composed of 3 main tumor cell morphologies: large, intermediate, and small, all of which are evident here. (*B*) In some spermatocytic tumors, the large or giant cells are sparse and the small cells may mimic lymphocytes, potentially causing diagnostic confusion with classic seminoma (hematoxylin-eosin, original magnification ×400).

## Microscopic features

EC can display a variety of growth patterns, including solid, papillary, tubular, and glandular. Solid growth is most common, but is usually accompanied by other architectural patterns.[32] The tumor cells of EC are large with a moderate amount of amphophilic cytoplasm and indistinct cell borders (Fig. 5A). Nuclei are large and exhibit pleomorphism, one or more prominent nucleoli, and abundant mitoses are present. Extensive necrosis is common in EC (see Fig. 5B). Occasionally, EC can display cleared cytoplasm and well-visualized cell borders, possibly raising confusion with seminoma. Like seminoma, scattered syncytiotrophoblasts are common in EC and are associated with mildly elevated serum Beta-human chorionic gonadotropin (hCG). Although the identification of EC in a mixed TGCT is generally straightforward, the percentage of EC component may guide patient management (60% is a frequent cutoff), thus recognizing less common variant morphology is critical. Immunohistochemistry can be extremely helpful in this regard, guided by morphologic differential diagnosis.

### Yolk-Sac Tumor

#### Clinical features

YST is the most common TGCT in children, occurring predominantly in boys younger than 2 years[33,34]; pure YST in the postpubertal setting is exceedingly rare, although YST is a common component of mixed NSGCT. YST is almost always associated with elevated serum AFP[35–38] and in many cases the elevation is very high (>10,000 ng/mL).

#### Microscopic features

YST has a very wide variety of histologic morphologies, which can have significant overlap with

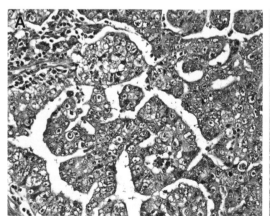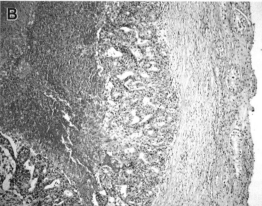

*Fig. 5.* Microscopic features of EC. (*A*) EC is characterized by significant cytologic atypia, frequent mitoses, amphophilic cytoplasm, and indistinct cell borders. (*B*) Necrosis, which may be extensive, is often seen with embryonal carcinoma (hematoxylin-eosin, original magnification [*A*] ×400; [*B*] ×200).

other subtypes of TGCT; thus, YST components can be easily overlooked or underestimated in mixed TGCT. The most common pattern in YST is reticular or microcystic (Fig. 6A). Myxoid stroma is frequently associated with YST (see Fig. 6B). Schiller-Duval bodies are common and consist of a ring of YST surrounding a blood vessel, typically within a cystic space (see Fig. 6C). Intracytoplasmic hyaline globules and extracellular dense eosinophilic material (so-called "parietal" differentiation) are also common, but often a focal finding (see Fig. 6D). YST may be difficult to recognize when the tumor has myxoid or microcystic features (Fig. 7A), predominantly solid (see Fig. 7B) or glandular (see Fig. 7C) growth, and hepatoid or pleomorphic cytology; some of these features (ie, glandular growth and pleomorphic cytology) may be present in EC, making the distinction difficult. Hepatoid YST is composed of sheets of large polygonal cells with abundant eosinophilic cytoplasm, centrally placed nuclei with prominent

nucleoli (see Fig. 7D),[39] and is rarely the only pattern of YST present in a mixed TGCT. Because YST occurs almost exclusively in mixed TGCT and demonstrates varied morphologies, the presence and volume estimation of YST in a mixed TGCT can be challenging.

## Teratoma (Postpubertal)

### Clinical features

Pure teratoma is uncommon in the testis in the postpubertal setting, accounting for fewer than 5% of all TGCTs; however, in children, prepubertal pure teratoma comprises nearly one-third of the testicular tumors. Additionally, teratoma (present as mature or immature elements or both) is frequently present as a component of mixed TGCT. Postpubertal teratoma may be associated with metastasis in approximately one-third of cases, and is typically composed of teratoma plus or minus other TGCT components.[11,40]

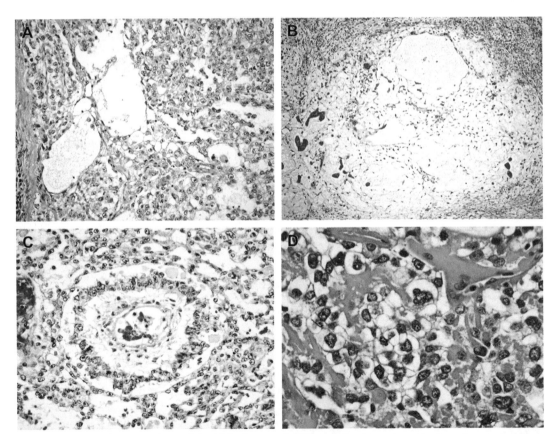

Fig. 6. Microscopic features of YST. (A) YST is characterized by moderate nuclear atypia, a frequent reticular growth pattern, and microcyst formation. (B) Myxoid and spindled stroma is another common but underappreciated pattern of YST, which frequently accompanies more classic morphologies. (C) Schiller-Duval bodies, composed of neoplastic YST cells forming a ring around a blood vessel, are common but not always present. (D) Parietal differentiation (dense eosinophilic basement membrane material) is a helpful diagnostic finding in YST (hematoxylin-eosin, original magnification [A, C] ×400; [B] ×200; [D] ×600).

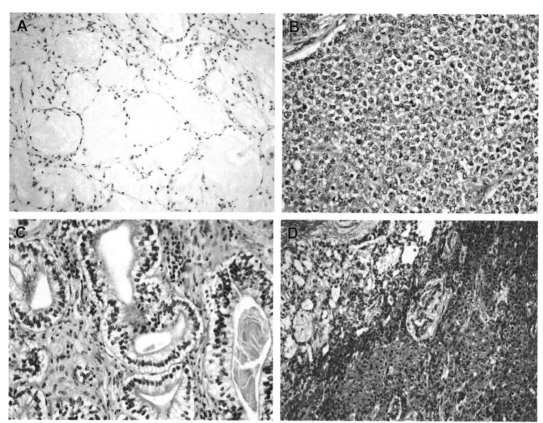

*Fig. 7.* Microscopic features of YST: less common patterns. (*A*) YST may show minimal cytologic atypia with extensive microcystic architecture and attenuated tumor cells. (*B*) Solid YST is a less typical pattern, thus more prone to diagnostic confusion. (*C*) Glandular YST typically resembles secretory endometrium with columnar cells and prominent cytoplasmic vacuoles. (*D*) Hepatoid YST cells contain more abundant and eosinophilic cytoplasm and very prominent nucleoli (lower right hand corner) but are almost always admixed with classic YST (upper left) (hematoxylin-eosin, original magnification ×200).

Some studies have shown a favorable prognosis for mixed TGCT that are predominantly composed of teratoma. It has become apparent that occasionally there may be teratomas in adults that show all the features of prepubertal teratomas and have a favorable benign prognosis (see later in this article for more detail). It has been suggested that these "prepubertal-type teratomas" together with dermoid cysts and epidermoid cysts be classified separately.[41,42]

## Microscopic features

Teratoma is composed of a wide variety of structures derived from ectodermal, endodermal, and mesodermal elements. Epithelia, both squamous and glandular, are common, as are foci of cartilage. Immature teratomatous elements are frequently seen admixed with the mature teratoma elements (**Fig. 8**A), and this finding has no additional bearing on classification or prognostication; therefore, distinction of immature elements in a final pathology report is not necessary and can

simply be referred to as "teratoma." The primary differential diagnosis to consider when immature elements are present is primitive neuroectodermal tumor (PNET); the presence of the latter does have prognostic significance, especially if present following chemotherapy and/or in metastatic sites.

## Prepubertal-Type Teratoma, Dermoid and Epidermoid Cysts

### Clinical features

Some forms of mature teratoma are benign and it has been long recognized that those that occur in the prepubertal setting do not metastasize. However, even in the postpubertal setting it is being increasingly recognized that some rare cases can also have a benign clinical course. These include dermoid and epidermoid cysts that are akin to similar counterparts commonly seen in the ovary. Occasionally there are also tumors that show all the features of a prepubertal teratoma, but in the postpubertal setting (determined

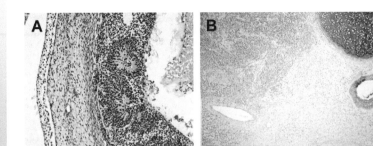
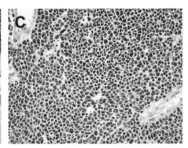

*Fig. 8.* Microscopic features of teratoma and PNET. (*A*) In teratoma, immature elements, including immature neuroepithelial elements, are frequently present. (*B*) PNET forms a discrete nodule (left), typically associated with teratoma (right). The significance of PNET limited to the primary testicular tumor is unclear. (*C*) On higher magnification, PNET is characterized by confluent sheets of very primitive appearing nuclei (hematoxylin-eosin, original magnification [*A*] ×200; [*B*] ×100; [*C*] ×400).

by the presence of spermatogenesis), and behave in a benign manner. It has been suggested to call these lesions "prepubertal type teratomas."[41] These tumors are important to recognize, as the uniformly benign clinical behavior is drastically different from that seen in typical postpubertal mature teratoma of the testis.

### Microscopic features
Epidermoid cysts display a simple epidermal (squamous) lined cyst, whereas dermoid cysts have associated pilosebaceous units. In prepubertal-type teratomas, other mature elements may be present, similar to those seen in ovarian mature cystic teratoma. Cytologic atypia, mitoses, and immature elements are not present. The absence of GCNIS and lack of evidence for a regressed TGCT is requisite for the diagnosis of these tumors; when possible demonstrating a lack of i12p also can be helpful. The seminiferous tubules should show normal spermatogenesis in the adult setting.

### *Primitive Neuroectodermal Tumor*

#### Clinical features
PNET, typically associated with teratoma or mixed TGCT, portends a worse prognosis,[43,44] but only after it is seen in the metastatic setting when it tends to be resistant to standard TGCT chemotherapy regimens. Accordingly, a PNET-specific regimen may be suitable in unresectable cases. PNET primary in the testis should be noted and quantified, but probably treated in a similar fashion to standard NSGCT. Occasionally pure PNET is seen in the testis, but metastases will present as other germ cell elements. The treatment for this is uncertain.

#### Microscopic features
PNET is characterized by discrete, expansile nodule(s) of immature neuroepithelium, typically present as back-to-back or confluent tubules, or as sheets of primitive-appearing cells (see **Fig. 8**B,

C). Fibrillary neuropil is often apparent. Minor PNET elements in TGCT carry no clinical significance, and if PNET is mentioned, it is important to emphasize it is of limited significance in primary tumors, although one article suggests, when extensive, there may be a higher risk of extratesticular spread. Immature renal epithelium, akin to that seen in nephroblastoma/Wilms tumor, can mimic PNET. Immunohistochemistry can be helpful in this regard, as WT-1 is positive in nephroblastomalike areas, whereas PNET is negative for nuclear WT-1.[45] There is no specific immunohistochemical stain for PNET, although they are generally positive for cytokeratin, vimentin, synaptophysin, and neuron-specific enolase. PNET morphologically resembles pediatric-type posterior fossa tumors (central PNET), and likewise lacks the chromosome 22 rearrangements frequently seen in peripheral PNET.[44,45]

### *Choriocarcinoma*

#### Clinical features
Choriocarcinoma is exceedingly rare in pure form in the testis,[12,46] but can be seen as a component of a mixed germ cell tumor. In contrast to other TGCTs, most patients with pure choriocarcinoma present with symptoms related to metastatic disease, rather than a palpable testicular mass. Serum Beta-hCG levels are markedly elevated, and gynecomastia may be present in a subset of patients. Testicular choriocarcinoma is rapidly fatal if untreated; however, even after widespread dissemination, cure is now possible with combination chemotherapy (see also Bernard and Sweeney, Diagnosis and Treatment of Testicular Cancer: A Clinician's Perspective, Surgical Pathology Clinics, 2015, Volume 8, Issue 4).

#### Microscopic features
Choriocarcinoma is associated with extensive hemorrhage and necrosis and is composed of 2

types of trophoblast cells, mononucleated tropho-blast and syncytiotrophoblast (synT), which may be present in varying amounts (Fig. 9). The mono-nucleated trophoblast cells are characterized by medium-sized cells with a moderate amount of clear to pale eosinophilic cytoplasm, and nuclei with irregular contours, coarse chromatin, and one or more nucleoli. The cell borders are typically distinct. The synT cells are characterized by a much larger cell size, frequent multinucleation, densely eosinophilic to slightly amphophilic cyto-plasm, and markedly hyperchromatic, irregular nuclei. The synT cells may show large intracyto-plasmic vacuolization, imparting a microcystic appearance. Lymphovascular invasion is easily identified in virtually 100% of cases.

**Immunohistochemistry and molecular features**

Choriocarcinoma is positive for SALL4 in most cases (~70%) although frequently in a patchy manner, and is entirely negative for OCT3/4. Like almost all tumors with trophoblastic differentiation, keratins, including CK7, are strongly positive in choriocarcinoma. Beta-hCG is strongly expressed in the synT cells; however, this marker can be

difficult to use and interpret due to high back-ground staining. GATA3 has also recently been shown to be expressed in trophoblastic tu-mors.[47,48] The mononucleated trophoblastic component appears to comprise a mixture of var-iably differentiated trophoblast cells; that is, cyto-trophoblast and intermediate trophoblast cells based on p63 expression (positive and negative, respectively).[46]

**The Most Common Differential Diagnoses in Testicular Germ Cell Tumors**

**Seminoma versus embryonal carcinoma**

Seminoma may occasionally show increased cyto-logic atypia, bordering on that of EC (Fig. 10A). Oc-casionally seminoma also may be associated with extensive necrosis (see Fig. 10B). When atypia and necrosis are present in seminoma, the differen-tial diagnosis of EC is often raised. Furthermore, when seminoma is poorly fixed, the cytoplasm may appear denser and cell borders indistinct. Likewise, when EC contains foci of solid growth with clear cytoplasm, the morphologic distinction can be difficult and is clinically relevant (see also Bernard and Sweeney, Diagnosis and Treatment

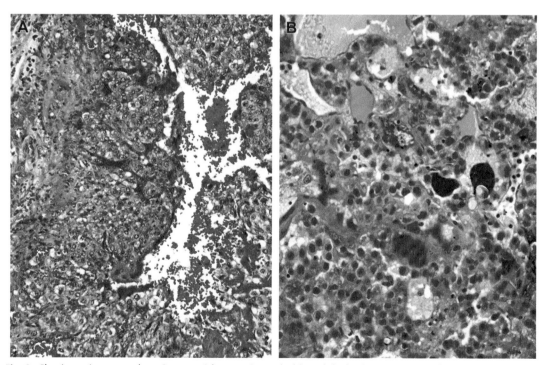

*Fig. 9.* Choriocarcinoma and seminoma with syncytiotrophoblast. (*A*) Choriocarcinoma is always associated with hemorrhage, and is composed of 2 cell types: mononuclear trophoblasts, which are often "capped" by the multi-nucleated syncytiotrophoblast. (*B*) Syncytiotrophoblast may also be seen in seminoma (shown here) as well as other germ cell tumors, and alone do not represent a separate component of choriocarcinoma. Unlike choriocar-cinoma with its fairly uniform capping, in seminoma the syncytiotrophoblast cells are randomly admixed within the tumor cells (hematoxylin-eosin, original magnification [*A*] ×200; [*B*] ×400).

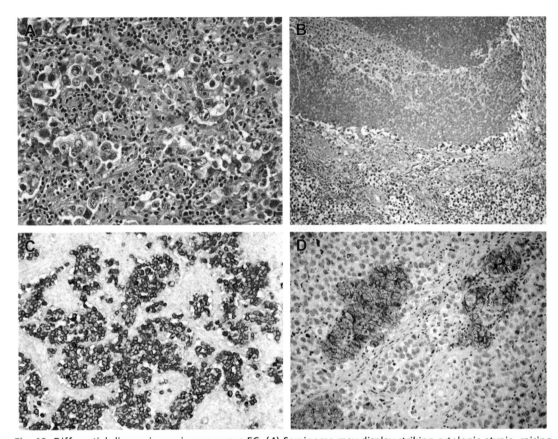

*Fig. 10.* Differential diagnosis: seminoma versus EC. (*A*) Seminoma may display striking cytologic atypia, raising the possibility of EC. (*B*) Seminoma may uncommonly be associated with extensive necrosis mimicking EC. Immunohistochemical stains are very helpful in this differential, and c-kit (*C*) and CD30 (*D*) are highly sensitive and specific markers of seminoma and embryonal carcinoma, respectively. Note the absence of CD30 in surrounding seminoma cells (*D*) ([*A, B*] hematoxylin-eosin, original magnification [*A*] ×400; [*B*] ×200; [*C*] c-kit immunohistochemical stain, original magnification ×200; [*D*] CD30 immunohistochemical stain, original magnification ×200).

of Testicular Cancer: A Clinician's Perspective, Surgical Pathology Clinics, 2015, Volume 8, Issue 4). Seminoma with only borderline changes suggestive of EC is occasionally seen and should not be overinterpreted when the focus is adjacent to necrosis.[19] A limited panel of IHC can reliably distinguish between seminoma (SOX2 and CD30 negative/c-kit and D240+; see **Fig. 10**C) and EC (SOX2 and CD30+ and c-kit/D2-40 negative; see **Fig. 10**D, **Table 2**).[49,50]

**Table 2**
Immunohistochemistry in testicular germ cell tumors

| Tumor Type | SALL4 | OCT4 | CD30 | GPC3 | AFP | Keratin | c-kit | D2-40 | Sox2 | hCG | GATA3 |
|---|---|---|---|---|---|---|---|---|---|---|---|
| Classic/typical seminoma | + | + | − | −[c] | − | − | + | + | − | −[c] | −[c] |
| Spermatocytic tumor[a] | + | − | − | − | − | − | −/+ | − | − | − | − |
| Embryonal carcinoma | + | + | + | −/+[c] | − | −/+ | − | − | + | −[c] | −[c] |
| Yolk-sac tumor | + | − | − | + | + | + | −/+ | − | − | − | +/− |
| Teratoma[b] | +/− | −/+ | − | − | − | + | − | − | +/− | − | −/+ |
| Choriocarcinoma | +/− | − | − | + | −/+ | + | − | −/+ | − | + | + |

−, negative; +, positive.
[a] Previously called "spermatocytic seminoma."
[b] Staining patterns depend on the teratomatous elements present.
[c] Individual syncytiotrophoblast present in GCTs may be positive for Beta-hCG, GPC3, and GATA3.

## Seminoma versus yolk-sac tumor

Seminoma can uncommonly display microcystic (Fig. 11A) or alveolar (see Fig. 11B) growth patterns, likely due to edema, mimicking that of YST; although in microcystic YST the cells lining the cystic spaces are typically flattened and attenuated.[51] Likewise, solid growth of YST may be mistaken for seminoma (see Fig. 11C). Like seminoma, YST has distinct cell borders and pale to clear cytoplasm, although nuclear atypia is generally more notable in YST. A small percentage of solid YSTs may also have fibrous septa with or without lymphocytic infiltrates, mimicking seminoma.[39] Immunohistochemistry is helpful, as OCT3/4 is positive in seminoma but never in YST, and glypican 3 (GPC3) is positive in YST but not in seminoma (see Fig. 11D). GATA3 is often positive at least focally in YST and is always negative in seminoma.[47,52] It is important to be aware that solid patterns of YST can display c-kit reactivity, and seminoma can be (focally) keratin positive; thus these 2 markers are not always helpful in the differential diagnosis.

## Classic seminoma versus spermatocytic tumor

So-called "anaplastic" ST with a preponderance of intermediate cells may raise the possibility of seminoma. ST tends to have denser cytoplasm and less-distinct cell borders (Fig. 12A). Classic seminoma may also display some pleomorphism (see Fig. 12B), raising the possibility of ST. The lack of prominent lymphocytes as well as OCT3/4 negativity distinguishes ST from typical seminoma. C-kit is not as helpful because it can be positive in both tumor types.[25]

## Embryonal carcinoma versus yolk-sac tumor

YST can cause diagnostic confusion with EC, particularly the glandular pattern, as glandular EC can show vacuolization[32] similar to glandular

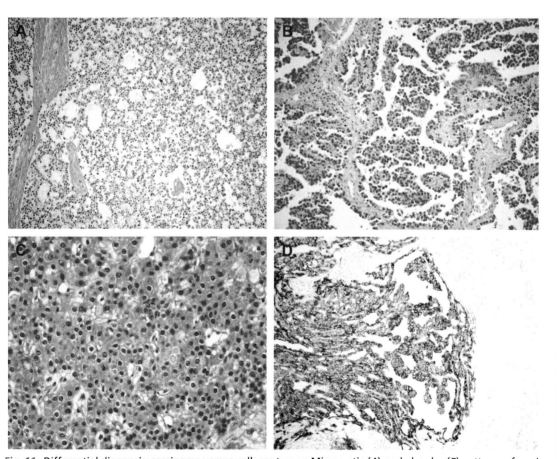

*Fig. 11.* Differential diagnosis: seminoma versus yolk-sac tumor. Microcystic (*A*) and alveolar (*B*) patterns of seminoma may be mistaken for YST. (*C*) Solid YST, which has a more eosinophilic appearance and prominent nucleoli, may be confused with seminoma, but still lacks prominent cell borders. Immunohistochemistry, particularly OCT3/4 (positive in seminoma, negative in YST; not shown) and Glypican3 (*D*) (positive in yolk-sac tumor) are helpful in this distinction ([*A, B, C*] hematoxylin-eosin, original magnification [*A*] ×100; [*B*] ×200; [*C*] ×400; [*C*] glypican3 immunohistochemical stain, original magnification ×200).

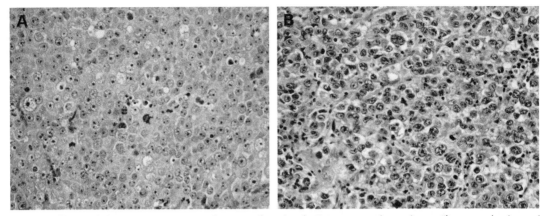

*Fig. 12.* Differential diagnosis: spermatocytic tumor (previously "spermatocytic seminoma") versus classic seminoma. (*A*) Spermatocytic tumor lacks the well-delineated cell borders and lymphocytic infiltrate seen in classic seminoma. (*B*) Occasionally classic seminoma may demonstrate variation in cell size and nuclear atypia mimicking a spermatocytic tumor, but the presence of fibrous septa with lymphocytes is a helpful diagnostic clue to the diagnosis (lymphocytes best seen upper right) (hematoxylin-eosin, original magnification ×400).

YST, both of which mimic early secretory endometrium. However, in EC the cytoplasm is generally more basophilic compared with the cleared or eosinophilic cytoplasm of YST. The polyembryoma pattern (**Fig. 13**A) may be overlooked, resulting in misclassification of a mixed TGCT as pure EC. Polyembryoma has an immature-appearing mesenchyme and closely associated thin linear strips of YST are surrounded by EC (see **Fig. 13**A). EC may grow around blood vessels, mimicking Schiller-Duval bodies seen in YST (see **Fig. 13**B). A small IHC panel, particularly OCT3/4, GPC3, SOX2, and CD30, aids in this distinction. Additionally, GATA3 has been shown to stain YST at least focally and is negative in EC.[47,52]

## Choriocarcinoma versus other testicular germ cell tumors

In choriocarcinoma, syncytiotrophoblast (synT) cells seem to wrap around or "cap" the mononuclear trophoblast cells (see **Fig. 9**A), but both seminoma and EC may have synT cells randomly scattered throughout the tumor (see **Fig. 9**B). Rarely, choriocarcinoma may be almost entirely composed of cytotrophoblast cells with only infrequent syncytiotrophoblast cells. In this case, EC might be mistaken for the cytotrophoblastic population of choriocarcinoma. Morphologic clues include the basophilic cytoplasm and significant pleomorphism in EC, and the notable syncytial growth in EC, which is in direct contrast to the well-defined cell

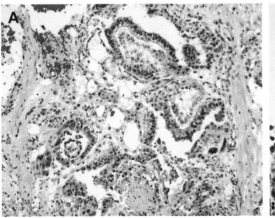
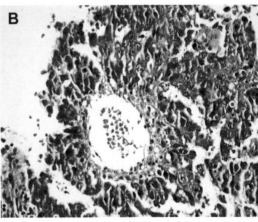

*Fig. 13.* Differential diagnosis: EC versus YST. (*A*) EC frequently occurs with YST, as shown here with strips or rings of columnar EC surrounding smaller and more attenuated strips of YST, consistent with the polyembryoma pattern. (*B*) EC may also grow around blood vessels, mimicking the Schiller-Duval bodies of YST. The more severe cytologic atypia and denser cytoplasm favors EC over YST, but these features are not entirely specific (hematoxylin-eosin, original magnification [*A*] ×200; [*B*] ×400).

borders of choriocarcinoma. Immunohistochemistry is also helpful in this regard, as a limited panel of OCT3/4, CK7, and GATA3 able to reliably distinguish seminoma or EC (OCT3/4+; CK7/GATA3−) from choriocarcinoma (OCT3/4−; CK7/GATA3+).[47,48,52] SALL4 is frequently positive in choriocarcinoma, thus it is not helpful in the differential diagnosis.

## Yolk-sac tumor versus teratoma

Teratomatous stroma can share some morphologic features with myxoid YST. Similarly, glandular YST can easily be mistaken for a component of teratoma. SALL4 and GPC3 are most helpful in this distinction, although SALL4 may also be positive in teratomatous elements. Epithelial membrane antigen (EMA) may be positive in carcinomas arising from teratomatous epithelium. The finding of keratin positivity would support a myxoid/spindled YST over teratomatous stroma.[53]

## Postpubertal teratoma versus epidermoid/dermoid cysts and "prepubertal-type teratoma"

Teratoma is often associated with other TGCT elements, but when pure, the possibility of a "prepubertal-type teratoma" or dermoid cyst might be raised. Dermoid cysts show only skin appendage-like mixed elements. If there is any cytologic atypia or significant mitoses in the teratomatous elements, then the tumor is best classified as a typical teratoma. Likewise, the presence of GCNIS and scarring or atrophy in the surrounding testis (ie, regressed tumor) precludes the diagnosis. It has been suggested that "postpubertal teratomas" be classified based on the presence or absence GCNIS, that is, with other malignant GCTs or with epidermoid/dermoid cysts and prepubertal teratoma, respectively,[42] as the latter appear to have more in common with benign mature ovarian cystic teratomas. i(12p) has been shown to be absent in cases devoid of GCNIS, and may be diagnostically helpful by use of fluorescence in situ hybridization (FISH).[54]

## Postpubertal teratoma versus carcinoma/sarcoma

Somatic-type malignancies may occasionally arise in primary, untreated TGCTs; however, as the vast majority of these are recognized in the postchemotherapy setting, they will be discussed in detail in a later section.

## Seminoma versus lymphoma/plasmacytoma

Seminoma, when poorly fixed, may lack distinct cell borders, and in some cases appears plasmacytoid (Fig. 14A). Hematopoietic neoplasms, particularly lymphomas and plasmacytic (see Fig. 14B) tumors, may occur as primary or secondary neoplasms in the testis, and morphologically may be mistaken for seminoma (see Fig. 14C).[55,56] Lymphomas (see Fig. 14D) lack well-defined cell borders, are often discohesive, and tumor nuclei are folded and convoluted. Although granulomatous inflammation is common in seminoma (see Fig. 14E), a significant histiocytic population, mimicking granulomatous inflammation, also may be present in lymphoma (see Fig. 14F); so this morphologic feature is not specific for seminoma. If a hematopoietic neoplasm is suspected or considered, immunohistochemistry is helpful; SALL4 and OCT3/4 to identify seminoma, and CD45, CD20, and CD3 to recognize most lymphomas. CD138 is helpful if a plasmacytic neoplasm is suspected.

## Testicular germ cell tumor versus sex-cord stromal tumors

TGCTs, particularly seminoma, show varying architectural growth patterns that may overlap with sex-cord stromal tumors (Fig. 15A–C). The most common difficulty is with malignant Sertoli cell tumor (SCT), which may demonstrate predominantly solid and/or nested growth patterns. SCTs typically have clear to very pale cytoplasm, and some have intracellular glycogen[57] and rarely prominent nucleoli, thereby closely resembling the appearance of seminoma when solid or nested growth is present (see Fig. 15D, E). However, in many cases, associated tubular growth of SCT is present, aiding in the diagnosis (see Fig. 15F). In general, nuclei of SCT are smaller and more uniform than those of seminoma, and seminoma is frequently accompanied by GCNIS. YST, particularly the solid and hepatic variants with interspersed cystic spaces, can mimic the architecture of juvenile granulosa cell tumor (not shown), although this differential is typically encountered in the prepubertal setting. Rarely, other sex-cord stromal tumors, such as Leydig cell tumors, may display microcystic architecture, thus raising the possibility of YST.[58] Immunohistochemical markers for seminoma (SALL4, OCT3/4) are negative in SCT, whereas a sensitive and specific marker of sex-cord differentiation, SF-1, is negative in TGCT. Inhibin, synaptophysin, calretinin, and WT1 may be positive in sex-cord stromal tumors, but extent of staining can vary and will depend on the subtype of SCT. In contrast, GCTs are negative for these biomarkers.

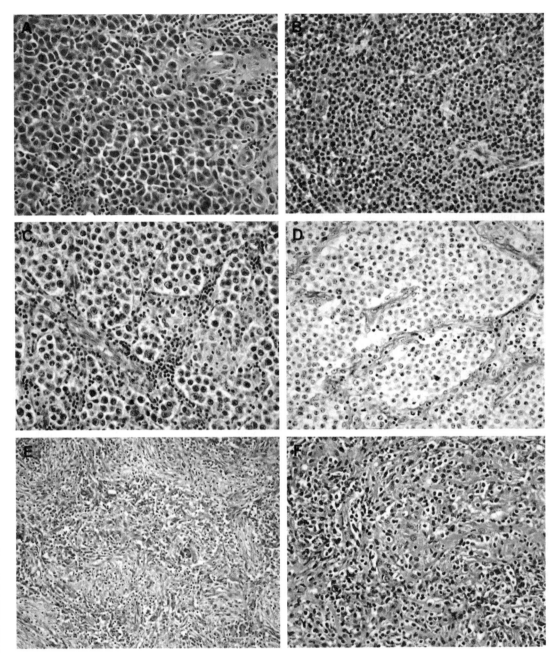

**Fig. 14.** Differential diagnosis: seminoma versus hematopoietic neoplasms. Plasmacytoid seminoma (*A*) is morphologically similar to plasmacytoma (*B*); however, both clinical setting and immunohistochemistry are sufficient to distinguish between these 2 entities. Seminoma (*C*) may be morphologically confused with lymphoma (*D*) involving the testis, but immunohistochemistry is helpful in ambiguous cases. Granulomatous inflammation is common in seminoma (*E*) but may also be seen in lymphomas (*F*) (hematoxylin-eosin, original magnification [*A, C, D, F*] ×400; [*B, E*] ×200).

## Metastatic carcinoma versus testicular germ cell tumor

The younger age of the patient and presence of other GCT components makes this an infrequent diagnostic problem, but a large subset of nonincidental metastatic carcinoma to the testis do not have a known history of other malignancy, and many of the carcinomas contain clear cytoplasm (**Fig. 16**A) and display intratubular growth (see **Fig. 16**B),[59] thus rarely mimicking seminoma (see **Fig. 16**C), EC, or YST. If the possibility of secondary carcinoma is considered and

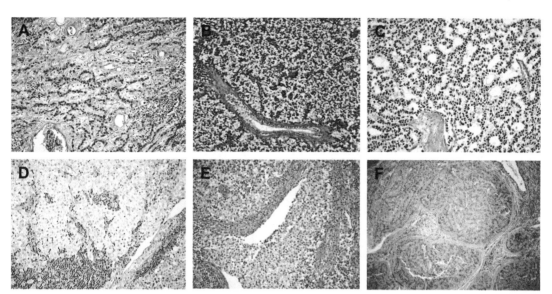

*Fig. 15.* Differential diagnosis: germ cell tumor versus sex-cord stromal tumors. Seminoma (*A–C*) is the most common germ cell tumor to be confused with sex-cord stromal tumors. Conversely, Sertoli cell tumors (*D–F*) are the most common sex-cord stromal tumor to be mistaken for a germ cell tumor. Corded growth (*A*) is a pattern seen in both seminoma and Sertoli cell tumors. Tubular variants of seminoma, with palisading nuclei and abundant cytoplasm (*B*), and well-formed tubules (*C*) are unusual but well described. Sertoli cell tumors (*D–F*) may have plump cells with abundant cytoplasm and distinct cell borders. Lymphocytic infiltrates may also be present (*D*). The morphologic overlap with seminoma is evident, and immunohistochemistry quickly resolves this differential diagnosis (see text for more detail) (hematoxylin-eosin, original magnification [*A, C, D, E*] ×200; [*B, F*] ×100).

immunohistochemistry is performed, then the diagnosis is usually straightforward; the presence of SALL4 (see **Fig. 16**D) and/or OCT3/4 staining supports a diagnosis of TGCT, whereas EMA positivity and SALL4 and OCT3/4 negativity would support metastatic carcinoma. An additional panel of biomarkers would then be used to determine primary site. This distinction is critical for appropriate management of the patient (see also Bernard and Sweeney, Diagnosis and Treatment of Testicular Cancer: A Clinician's Perspective, Surgical Pathology Clinics, 2015, Volume 8, Issue 4).

## Cytogenetic Aberrations Involving Chromosome 12p

The vast majority of postpubertal TGCTs have increased copies of all or partial segments of the short arm (p) of chromosome 12. Most commonly, this is manifest as isochromosome 12p; or "i(12p)," in which there is simultaneous loss of 12q and gain of 12p (**Fig. 17**). The remaining cases contain extra copies of a portion of 12p.[60–62] The role of 12p in the initiation and progression of TGCT is not entirely understood, but studies have shown that 12p amplification is found in "invasive" TGCT, whereas it is generally absent in GCNIS.[63–65] FISH techniques are a reliable way to detect i(12p) and other forms of amplification[66–68] to

support the diagnosis of TGCT. In contrast, most prepubertal germ cell tumors lack i(12p) and rather display loss of 1p and/or 6q[69–71]; prepubertal YST may show aneuploidy, but teratoma is predominantly diploid.[72–75]

Prepubertal type teratomas, and dermoid and epidermoid cysts are not associated with abnormal karyotype, or abnormalities in 12p. Rather, they have a virtually unremarkable molecular and cytogenetic profile, with only occasional copy number aberrations identified[41] and may represent prepubertal teratomas that have persisted into adult life. Postpubertal teratoma is characterized by complex cytogenetic abnormalities, including i12p, and is usually hyperdiploid, similar to other TGCTs. When present as a component of a mixed TGCT, teratoma shows the same cytogenetic abnormalities as the other components.[76]

## Other Molecular Alterations in Testicular Germ Cell Tumor

A number of molecular alterations have been described in TGCT, and a comprehensive review is beyond the scope of this article. Nevertheless, the most common alteration will be discussed in brief, and additional references are available for more in-depth reading.[77–84]

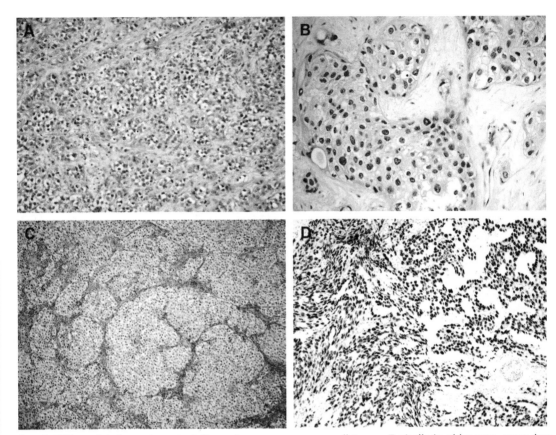

*Fig. 16.* Differential diagnosis: metastatic carcinoma versus germ cell tumor. Typically in older men, secondary involvement of the testis by a malignancy must be considered in some cases. Tumors from the gastrointestinal tract (*A;* esophageal carcinoma) and genitourinary tract (*B;* urothelial carcinoma) may mimic primary testicular germ cell tumors. (*C*) In contrast, fibrous septa with abundant lymphocytes are more commonly seen in seminoma. (*D*) SALL4 is a sensitive and specific marker for germ cell tumors; however, as a very small number of carcinomas may be positive for SALL4, a slightly larger confirmatory immunohistochemical panel is sometimes warranted ([*A, B, C*] hematoxylin-eosin, original magnification [*A*] ×200; [*B*] ×400; [*C*] ×100; [*D*] immunohistochemical stain, original magnification ×200).

## KIT

*C-KIT* mutations are the most common single-nucleotide variation in TGCT, with 10% of all TGCTs and 20% of seminomas harboring a *C-KIT* mutation.[85–88]

## Microsatellite instability

Microsatellite instability (MSI) is associated with chemorefractory TGCT[89–91]; however, in the setting of chemoresistance, MSI TGCT showed a trend for longer progression-free survival in one study,[91] whereas other studies have shown TGCT with MSI to have a higher rate of cancer-specific death.[92,93] In TGCT, loss of mismatch repair (MMR) protein expression is most frequently due to somatic hypermethylation of the *MLH1* promoter,[94,95] rather than germline mutation in MMR genes.

## BRAF

*BRAF* mutations are not infrequent in chemoresistant TGCT,[89] and are associated with MSI tumors,[91] (see previous paragraph). Targeted therapy, including inhibition of BRAF, may be possible, but to date, no evidence of clinical efficacy has been reported.

## Epidermal growth factor receptor

One study has shown evidence for epidermal growth factor receptor (*EGFR*) amplification or polysomy as a possible genetic aberration associated with chemoresistance in EC[96]; however, the effectiveness of anti-EGFR therapy in this setting is unknown. Furthermore, other studies have shown *EGFR* amplification as a frequent event in many types of TGCT.[97]

*Fig. 17.* Karyotype and i12p by FISH on a mixed TGCT. (*A*) A karyotype from a mixed germ cell tumor shows marked aneuploidy, but also the characteristic i12p (*red arrow*). (*B*) The i12p (*orange circle*) may also be identified via FISH analysis.

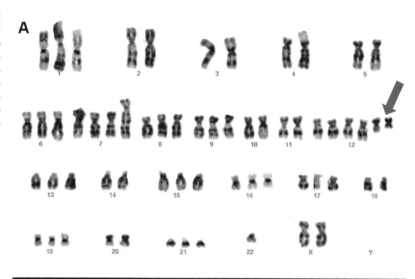

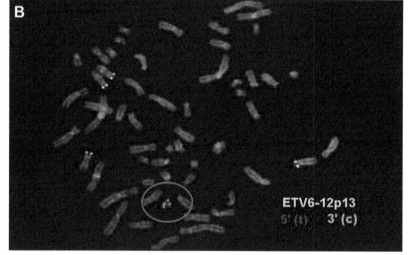

## TP53

*TP53* mutations are not common in TGCT[88]; however, overexpression of wild-type p53 may be seen via immunohistochemistry.[98,99]

## KRAS, NRAS, HRAS

A small subset of TGCTs have mutations in this *RAS* oncogene family, predominantly in seminoma,[88,100,101] but these mutations are of unclear clinical and pathobiologic significance.

## EPIGENETIC ALTERATIONS INCLUDING GENOMIC METHYLATION

Genomic DNA methylation studies have shown a contrast in methylation patterns both between TGCT tissue and normal tissue, as well as in seminoma (generally decreased/hypomethylated) versus nonseminomatous TGCT (generally methylated).[94,102–104]

## TESTICULAR GERM CELL TUMORS IN THE POSTCHEMOTHERAPY SETTING

## MORPHOLOGIC PATTERNS OF TESTICULAR GERM CELL TUMOR MORE COMMON IN THE POSTCHEMOTHERAPY SETTING

Recurrence of TGCT may occur at any stage after treatment. Late recurrences of TGCT are defined as those patients who, following initial treatment, were disease free for at least 2 years before tumor recurrence.[105,106] After treatment, for stage 2 or greater disease, residual masses may be identified in the retroperitoneum or elsewhere that may be surgically excised if persistent. Cases that show pure necrosis or teratoma only following treatment generally have a good prognosis. Residual malignant germ cell elements may be treated with second-line agents but the outlook is far bleaker. Late recurrent TGCT seems to show a different pattern of morphologies and clinical outcomes. Although most of these tumors have a component of teratoma, the most clinically relevant diagnosis is the presence of nonteratomatous elements, namely YST, EC, and somatic-type malignancies. YST is more common in this group,[89,107] and when present, often shows glandular, hepatoid, or parietal-type patterns.[105] Pure teratoma in late recurrence is typically composed of bland cystic elements, and is associated with a much improved prognosis compared with other nonteratomatous late recurrences.[105]

## SOMATIC-TYPE MALIGNANCIES ARISING IN TESTICULAR GERM CELL TUMOR

### Clinical Features

Somatic-type malignancies arising in TGCTs indicate a poor prognosis, as they are typically chemotherapy and radiotherapy resistant.[53,108–111] In general, they are defined as distinct nodules or expansion (at least one 4x field) of tumors lacking features of conventional TGCT, and rather show evidence of sarcomatous or carcinomatous differentiation.[112–114] However, the diagnosis may be extremely challenging in some cases due to morphologic overlap with components of TGCT (ie, stoma associated with

teratoma or EC), and expert advice should be sought for these complex tumors.

### Molecular Features of Somatic-type Malignancies in Testicular Germ Cell Tumor

Somatic-type malignancies arising in TGCT also show i12p by FISH analysis,[110,115,116] supporting the germ cell origin of these tumors. Thus, FISH for 12p is likely to be helpful in questionable cases, especially in the metastatic setting or when the tumor is of unknown primary origin.

### Microscopic Features and Immunohistochemical Profile of Sarcoma Arising in Testicular Germ Cell Tumor

Sarcomatous neoplasms are the most common type of somatic-type malignancy arising in TGCTs, are seen in approximately 10% of late-recurrence TGCTs,[105] and display a wide range of morphologies including rhabdomyosarcoma, angiosarcoma, leiomyosarcoma, liposarcoma, and sarcoma not otherwise specified. Recently, a large subset of sarcomatous tumors showing no specific line of differentiation by morphologic standards were determined to be sarcomatoid YST (Fig. 18A), based on morphologic similarity to myxoid and parietal YST in combination with immunohistochemical evidence (positivity for GPC3, AE1/AE3, and in 60% of cases, SALL4).[53]

### Differential Diagnosis of Sarcomatous Testicular Germ Cell Tumor

The possibility of a truly somatic (ie, primary) sarcoma could be considered, particularly if radiation

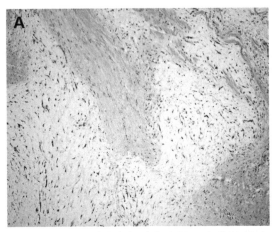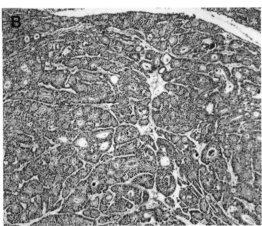

**Fig. 18.** Sarcomatoid and glandular YST. Typically occurring 1 or more years after the initial diagnosis of germ cell tumor, in the postchemotherapy setting, somatic-type malignancies may arise: sarcomas including sarcomatoid YST (A) and carcinomas (not shown), the latter of which may be confused with glandular YST (B). The clinical significance of sarcomatoid and glandular YSTs in treated GCTs is less worrisome when compared with somatic-type malignancies (sarcoma and carcinoma), which are known to have a worse prognosis (hematoxylin-eosin, original magnification ×200).

therapy has been previously administered or the mass is predominantly present in the spermatic cord. A directed immunohistochemical panel may be helpful including more conventional sarcoma biomarkers, but it is also important to remember that somatic-type malignancies in TGCT are not always SALL4 positive, so this is not a discriminatory marker in all cases. Interrogation for extra copies of 12p by FISH is likely to be the most helpful adjunctive study when present.

## Microscopic Features and Immunohistochemical Profile of Carcinomas Arising in Testicular Germ Cell Tumor

Carcinoma arising in TGCT most frequently shows no specific line of differentiation; however, mucinous or enteric differentiation is seen in greater than 25%,[108] whereas other specific types of carcinoma are rare. The pattern of growth is often infiltrative rather than expansile or nodular, and necrotic luminal debris is common. Immunohistochemically, EMA and CK7 are positive along with frequent CDX2 positivity. GPC3 and AFP are negative in carcinomas arising in TGCT.

## Differential Diagnosis of Carcinoma in Testicular Germ Cell Tumor

Glandular YST (see **Fig.** 18B) may be mistaken for a somatic-type carcinoma arising in TGCT. Helpful morphologic features include endometrioid appearance (YST) versus a mucinous or enteric differentiation more commonly seen in somatic-type carcinomas. CDX2, however, is not a helpful IHC marker, as many glandular YSTs are also positive for CDX2.[108] Strong EMA and/or CK7 positivity and GPC3 negativity would support a somatic-type carcinoma.

## CYSTIC TROPHOBLASTIC TUMOR

### Clinical Features

Cystic trophoblastic tumor (CTT) (**Fig.** 19) is a morphologic pattern that may be seen in chemotherapy-treated TGCT, most typically in retroperitoneal lymph node dissections.[117,118] Patients have normal or mildly elevated serum Beta-hCG. Cystic trophoblastic tumor has no adverse effect on outcome and shows no progression to choriocarcinoma. No additional chemotherapy is required.

### Microscopic Features

CTT is composed of small cysts lined by a single layer or a thin stratified layer of trophoblast cells, which occasionally give rise to more complex architecture, such as papillary tufting and cribriform growth. CTT cells are large and often have cytologic atypia but also a smudgy hyperchromasia of degenerative type. The cysts are surrounded by a fibrous stroma. Hemorrhage, necrosis, and mitoses are absent or rare. In one study, all CTTs were associated with teratoma, but no other TGCT elements.[117]

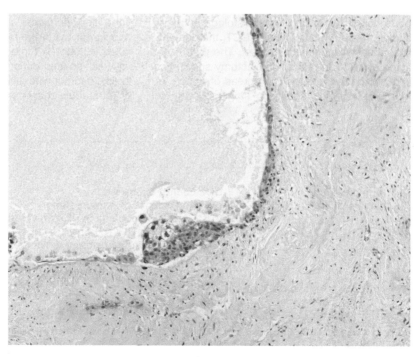

*Fig.* 19. Cystic cytotrophoblastic tumor. This is an uncommon finding, but typically seen in retroperitoneal lymph nodes following chemotherapy and surgical lymphadenectomy. Simple cysts are lined by vacuolated trophoblastic cells with degenerative-type atypia. Solid growth, abundant mitoses, and necrosis are features not typically seen in cystic trophoblastic tumor. If the latter are present, choriocarcinoma and squamous cell carcinomas should be excluded (hematoxylin-eosin, original magnification ×200).

## Differential Diagnosis

The principal differential diagnosis with CTT is choriocarcinoma, which has clinical implications; thus, recognition of CTT is important. Choriocarcinoma is usually more solid, and associated with hemorrhage, necrosis, and frequent mitoses. A distinct biphasic population of syncytiotrophoblast cells and cytotrophoblast cells is present in choriocarcinoma, but absent in CTT. CTT may also mimic squamous cell carcinoma (ie, somatic differentiation) due to the nuclear atypia and eosinophilic nature of the cytoplasm; however, squamous cell carcinoma is typically associated with necrosis and increased mitotic activity.

## Immunohistochemistry and Molecular

Keratin and Beta-hCG are often positive in CTT, similar to other tumors with trophoblastic differentiation; however, in contrast to choriocarcinoma, CTT is typically focally positive for Beta-hCG, whereas choriocarcinoma tends to have a more diffuse staining pattern. Molecular alterations in CTT have not been described.

## THE PATHOLOGY REPORT: STAGING OF TESTICULAR TUMORS AND OTHER PROBLEMATIC ISSUES

## KEY INFORMATION TO INCLUDE IN THE DIAGNOSTIC SURGICAL PATHOLOGY REPORT FOR ORCHIECTOMY

Important information to include in pathology reports include tumor size, tumor histologic subtype, and, in the setting of a mixed TGCT, the percentage of each component present. The pathologic stage of TGCT in radical orchiectomy specimens is based on the location and spread of tumor; tumor size has no impact on staging (Table 3; American Joint Committee on Cancer staging system). Thus, a detailed evaluation of spread beyond the testis including involvement of the tunica vaginalis, rete testis (see later in this article), hilar fat (see later in this article), and spermatic cord should be included in every pathology report. Additionally, lymphovascular invasion (LVI) should be carefully assessed, as this is one of the most important predictors of clinical behavior, particularly for NSGCTs, and guides treatment decisions (see also Bernard and Sweeney, Diagnosis and Treatment of Testicular Cancer: A Clinician's Perspective, Surgical Pathology Clinics, 2015, Volume 8, Issue 4). The presence or absence of GCNIS, or other forms of in situ neoplasia (ie, intratubular seminoma and intratubular EC), should be reported for completeness and to support the diagnosis of malignancy.

## LYMPHOVASCULAR INVASION VERSUS PSEUDO LYMPHOVASCULAR INVASION

The presence of vascular invasion will upstage an otherwise pT1 TGCT to pT2, and influences patient management (see also Bernard and Sweeney, Diagnosis and Treatment of Testicular Cancer: A Clinician's Perspective, Surgical Pathology Clinics, 2015, Volume 8, Issue 4). In TGCTs with LVI (Fig. 20A, B), patients may be offered adjuvant therapy. However, finding tumor cells in lymphovascular spaces is not sufficient for the diagnosis of LVI, as many tumors are friable and may be artifactually pushed into vascular spaces (see Fig. 20C) and similarly into extratesticular tissues and surfaces, particularly in seminoma. Mimics for LVI in the testis that should be recognized include (1) tumor cells displaced into true vascular spaces during processing of the specimen, (2) tumor with retraction artifact from stroma or intratubular tumor mimicking vessels, and (3)

| Table 3  Staging of testicular germ cell tumor | |
|---|---|
| pT (primary tumor characteristics) | pTX: Cannot be assessed  pT0: No evidence of primary tumor  pTis: Germ cell neoplasia in situ (previously intratubular germ cell neoplasia, or "ITGCN") only  pT1: Tumor limited to testis/epididymis without lymphovascular invasion (LVI) and no involvement of tunica vaginalis  pT2: Tumor limited to testis/epididymis with LVI or tumor involving tunica vaginalis  pT3: Spermatic cord invasion (direct)  pT4: Invasion of the scrotum (direct) |

Adapted from Sobin L, Gospodarowicz M, Wittekind C. UICC TNM classification of malignant tumors. 7th edition. New York: Wiley-Liss; 2009.

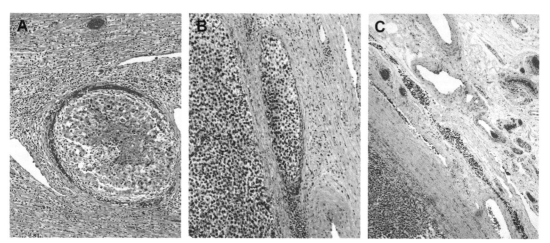

*Fig. 20.* Staging issues: lymphovascular invasion. True lymphovascular invasion is indicated by cohesive tumors cells, partially adherent to the vessel wall, and/or lined by endothelial cells, as demonstrated here with EC (*A*) and seminoma (*B*). Seminoma is frequently pushed into tissue crevices and lymphovascular spaces as discohesive cells (*C*), and this should not be overinterpreted and reported as lymphatic invasion (hematoxylin-eosin, original magnification [*A*] ×400; [*B*] ×200; [*C*] ×100).

nontumor cells, typically histiocytes, mimicking tumor within vessels. In the latter 2 situations, immunohistochemistry may be helpful; CD34, CD31, D2-40, and/or ERG to ensure that the space is truly lymphovascular in nature, and to distinguish between TGCT cells (SALL4 positive) and histiocytes (PU-1, CD163, and/or CD68 positive) to determine the cell type present in the vascular spaces.

Generally, discohesive tumor cells floating in vessels should not be interpreted as LVI. True LVI is best identified at the border of the TGCT in

uninvolved parenchyma, or away from the tumor entirely. Hallmarks of bone fide LVI include a cohesive cluster of cells partly conforming to the vessel shape, attachment of tumor to endothelial lining, and association with thrombosis or fibrin accumulation. In cases of ambiguous LVI, the tumors are best classified as pT1.[119]

## RETE TESTIS INVOLVEMENT AND TUMOR SIZE

Rete testis involvement is not uncommon in TGCT, particularly in the pagetoid form[120,121] (**Fig. 21**A).

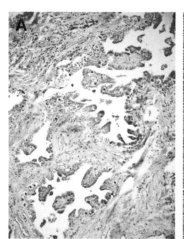
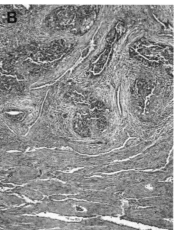
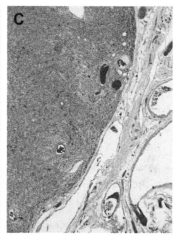

*Fig. 21.* Staging issues: rete testis and hilar soft tissue involvement. The rete testis may be involved by pagetoid (in situ) spread (*A*) or by invasive tumor (*B*) and these findings should be included in the diagnostic pathology report. Although not currently part of any formal staging system, recent studies and the upcoming 2015 World Health Organization (in press) suggest that hilar soft tissue involvement (*C*) be considered pT2 disease, and therefore, the presence or absence of involvement of the soft tissue at the testicular hilum should be documented in the final pathology report (hematoxylin-eosin, original magnification [*A*, *B*] ×200; [*C*] ×100).

Pagetoid invasion probably merely represents spread of GCNIS; however, interstitial invasion (see **Fig. 21**B) may be prognostically significant. Involvement of the rete testis is controversial, as some recent large studies have reported it as a significant prognosticator in multivariate analysis[122–124]; whereas other studies have shown that rete testis involvement is not a significant *independent* prognosticator.[125–127] Nonetheless, most agree for the time being, that the status of the rete testis involvement as pagetoid spread and/or true invasion should be documented for TGCT resections. Additionally, some have shown that rete testis involvement may be a surrogate for tumor size, the latter of which has also been shown to be significantly associated with relapse and progression.[128–130]

## ASSESSING SPERMATIC CORD INVOLVEMENT VERSUS HILAR FAT INVOLVEMENT

Approximately 10% of TGCTs involve the spermatic cord or epididymis, with most cases of extratesticular extension arising via invasion at the hilum (see **Fig. 21**C).[131] However, only direct invasion of the spermatic cord can upstage a tumor to pT3. Involvement of the epididymis is insufficient for this criterion, and although there is no clear definition of what precisely constitutes "spermatic cord invasion,"[132] most require invasion to a level of the spermatic cord containing vas deferens.[133] The significance of hilar fat invasion in isolation is debated, but most consider this to represent pT2 disease.[124,134,135]

## REGRESSION

Occasionally, patients may present with metastatic GCT with no apparent testicular mass or microscopic TGCT identifiable. Although some of these cases are truly extragonadal (typically retroperitoneal or mediastinal) in origin, in a large proportion of these cases, scarring fibrosis is present in the testis, consistent with spontaneous regression of the TGCT. Why the testicular neoplasms regress, and why the sites of metastatic spread do not, is not currently understood. Nevertheless, such a finding is clinically important, as chemotherapy is generally less effective in extragonadal GCTs. Thus, in the presence of a metastatic GCT, the testicular primary may be removed surgically either before or after adjuvant treatment.

The pathologic features of regression include a grossly identifiable area of scarring in most cases (but can be <1 cm[136]) (**Fig. 22**A), associated with microscopic evidence of scarring fibrosis (see **Fig. 22**B), which may have a circumscribed or irregular border. Most cases are associated with atrophy and a lymphoplasmacytic infiltrate (see **Fig. 22**C). Additional helpful clues to support a diagnosis of regressed TGCT include GCNIS, coarse intratubular calcifications, and hemosiderin-laden macrophages.[136]

---

### Differential Diagnosis
#### SEMINOMA VERSUS NON–GERM CELL TUMORS

- Non–germ cell tumors should be considered particularly in older men.
- Absence of ITGCN/GCNIS should raise suspicion for non–germ cell tumor.
- Lymphoma: may also be associated with lymphocytic or granulomatous inflammation.
  - IHC: LCA positive, SALL4 negative.
- Metastatic carcinoma: Often history of other malignancy.
  - IHC: SALL4 and OCT3/4 negative, EMA positive.
- Sex-cord stromal tumors: SALL4 and OCT3/4 negative; SF-1, WT1, and inhibin positive.
- Spermatocytic tumor (previously "spermatocytic seminoma") has 3 different tumor cell morphologies and lacks associated GCNIS (previously "ITGCN") and i12p.
  - IHC: SALL4 positive, OCT3/4 negative; CKIT may be positive.
- Isochromosome 12p present in most germ cell tumors; can be a helpful ancillary test in the differential diagnosis with non–germ cell (negative) tumors and somatic differentiation in metastatic disease (positive)

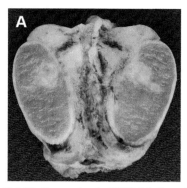
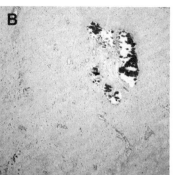
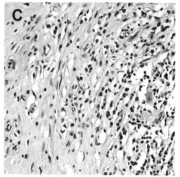

*Fig. 22.* Regression in TGCT. (*A*) Gross features of a regressed germ cell tumor include white to tan scarring; small foci of necrosis and/or calcification may also be present. Histologically, coarse calcifications in a fibrous scar (*B*) and associated lymphoplasmacytic inflammatory infiltrates (*C*) are typical.

## Pitfalls

! Improper fixation hinders morphologic evaluation and may also result in suboptimal IHC

! Not recognizing a nonseminomatous component in a germ cell tumor

! If any unusual growth pattern or cytologic features are present, limited IHC panels should be performed based on morphologic differential diagnosis

! Seminoma versus yolk-sac tumor: OCT3/4, CKIT, GPC3, GATA3

! Seminoma versus embryonal carcinoma: CD30, CKIT, SOX2, SOX17, D2-40

! Cystic trophoblastic tumor is seen in the post-treatment setting and has no clinical significance; this should not be mistaken for choriocarcinoma or squamous cell carcinoma

## ACKNOWLEDGMENTS

The authors thank Dr Thomas Ulbright for allowing us to use microscopic images taken from his vast teaching collection.

## REFERENCES

1. Stang A, Jansen L, Trabert B, et al. Survival after a diagnosis of testicular germ cell cancers in Germany and the United States, 2002–2006: a high resolution study by histology and age. Cancer Epidemiol 2013;37(4):492–7.

2. Sant M, Allemani C, Santaquilani M, et al. EURO-CARE-4. Survival of cancer patients diagnosed in 1995–1999. Results and commentary. Eur J Cancer 2009;45(6):931–91.

3. Stang A, Trabert B, Wentzensen N, et al. Gonadal and extragonadal germ cell tumours in the United States, 1973–2007. Int J Androl 2012;35(4):616–25.

4. Woodward PJ, Heidenreich A, Looijenga LH, et al. Germ cell tumours. In: Eble JN, Sauter G, Epstein JI, et al, editors. Pathology and genetics of tumours of the urinary system and male genital organs. Lyon (France): IARC Press; 2004. p. 221–49.

5. Howlader N, Krapcho M, Garshell J, et al, editors. SEER cancer statistics review, 1975–2011. 2013. Available at: http://seer.cancer.gov/csr/1975_2011/. Accessed December 1, 2014.

6. Nigam M, Aschebrook-Kilfoy B, Shikanov S, et al. Increasing incidence of testicular cancer in the United States and Europe between 1992 and 2009. World J Urol 2015;33(5):623–31.

7. Ulbright TM, Tickoo SK, Berney DM, et al, Members of the IIiDUPG. Best practices recommendations in the application of immunohistochemistry in testicular tumors: report from the International Society of Urological Pathology consensus conference. Am J Surg Pathol 2014;38(8):e50–9.

8. Henley JD, Young RH, Wade CL, et al. Seminomas with exclusive intertubular growth: a report of 12 clinically and grossly inconspicuous tumors. Am J Surg Pathol 2004;28(9):1163–8.

9. Ulbright TM. Germ cell tumors of the gonads: a selective review emphasizing problems in differential diagnosis, newly appreciated, and controversial issues. Mod Pathol 2005;18(Suppl 2):S61–79.

10. Mostofi FK, Davis J Jr, Rehm S. Tumours of the testis. IARC Sci Publ 1994;(111):407–29.

11. Rodriguez PN, Hafez GR, Messing EM. Nonseminomatous germ cell tumor of the testicle: does extensive staging of the primary tumor predict the likelihood of metastatic disease? J Urol 1986; 136(3):604–8.

12. Jacobsen GK, Barlebo H, Olsen J, et al. Testicular germ cell tumours in Denmark 1976–1980.

Pathology of 1058 consecutive cases. Acta Radiol Oncol 1984;23(4):239–47.

13. Berney DM, Warren AY, Verma M, et al. Malignant germ cell tumours in the elderly: a histopathological review of 50 cases in men aged 60 years or over. Mod Pathol 2008;21(1):54–9.

14. Ulbright TM, Young RH. Seminoma with conspicuous signet ring cells: a rare, previously uncharacterized morphologic variant. Am J Surg Pathol 2008;32(8):1175–81.

15. Carriere P, Baade P, Fritschi L. Population based incidence and age distribution of spermatocytic seminoma. J Urol 2007;178(1):125–8.

16. Scully RE. Spermatocytic seminoma of the testis. A report of 3 cases and review of the literature. Cancer 1961;14:788–94.

17. True LD, Otis CN, Delprado W, et al. Spermatocytic seminoma of testis with sarcomatous transformation. A report of five cases. Am J Surg Pathol 1988;12(2):75–82.

18. Ulbright TM. The most common, clinically significant misdiagnoses in testicular tumor pathology, and how to avoid them. Adv Anat Pathol 2008;15(1):18–27.

19. Bishop EF, Badve S, Morimiya A, et al. Apoptosis in spermatocytic and usual seminomas: a light microscopic and immunohistochemical study. Mod Pathol 2007;20(10):1036–44.

20. Jones TD, Ulbright TM, Eble JN, et al. OCT4 staining in testicular tumors: a sensitive and specific marker for seminoma and embryonal carcinoma. Am J Surg Pathol 2004;28(7):935–40.

21. Howitt BE, Brooks JD, Jones S, et al. Identification and characterization of 2 testicular germ cell markers, Glut3 and CyclinA2. Appl Immunohistochem Mol Morphol 2013;21(5):401–7.

22. Cao D, Humphrey PA, Allan RW. SALL4 is a novel sensitive and specific marker for metastatic germ cell tumors, with particular utility in detection of metastatic yolk sac tumors. Cancer 2009;115(12):2640–51.

23. Cao D, Li J, Guo CC, et al. SALL4 is a novel diagnostic marker for testicular germ cell tumors. Am J Surg Pathol 2009;33(7):1065–77.

24. Haroon S, Tariq MU, Fatima S, et al. Spermatocytic seminoma: a 21 years' retrospective study in a tertiary care hospital in Pakistan. Int J Clin Exp Pathol 2013;6(11):2350–6.

25. Kraggerud SM, Berner A, Bryne M, et al. Spermatocytic seminoma as compared to classical seminoma: an immunohistochemical and DNA flow cytometric study. APMIS 1999;107(3):297–302.

26. Kao CS, Badve SS, Ulbright TM. The utility of immunostaining for NUT, GAGE7 and NY-ESO-1 in the diagnosis of spermatocytic seminoma. Histopathology 2014;65(1):35–44.

27. Cummings OW, Ulbright TM, Eble JN, et al. Spermatocytic seminoma: an immunohistochemical study. Hum Pathol 1994;25(1):54–9.

28. Looijenga LH, Hersmus R, Gillis AJ, et al. Genomic and expression profiling of human spermatocytic seminomas: primary spermatocyte as tumorigenic precursor and DMRT1 as candidate chromosome 9 gene. Cancer Res 2006;66(1):290–302.

29. Mostofi FK, Sesterhenn IA, Davis CJ Jr. Developments in histopathology of testicular germ cell tumors. Semin Urol 1988;6(3):171–88.

30. Perrotti M, Ankem M, Bancilla A, et al. Prospective metastatic risk assignment in clinical stage I nonseminomatous germ cell testis cancer: a single institution pilot study. Urol Oncol 2004;22(3):174–7.

31. Bahrami A, Ro JY, Ayala AG. An overview of testicular germ cell tumors. Arch Pathol Lab Med 2007; 131(8):1267–80.

32. Kao CS, Ulbright TM, Young RH, et al. Testicular embryonal carcinoma: a morphologic study of 180 cases highlighting unusual and unemphasized aspects. Am J Surg Pathol 2014;38(5):689–97.

33. Walsh TJ, Grady RW, Porter MP, et al. Incidence of testicular germ cell cancers in U.S. children: SEER program experience 1973 to 2000. Urology 2006; 68(2):402–5 [discussion: 405].

34. Trobs RB, Krauss M, Geyer C, et al. Surgery in infants and children with testicular and paratesticular tumours: a single centre experience over a 25-year-period. Klin Padiatr 2007;219(3):146–51.

35. Norgaard-Pedersen B, Albrechtsen R, Teilum G. Serum alpha-foetoprotein as a marker for endodermal sinus tumour (yolk sac tumour) or a vitelline component of "teratocarcinoma." Acta Pathol Microbiol Scand A 1975;83(6):573–89.

36. Talerman A, Haije WG, Baggerman L. Serum alpha-fetoprotein (AFP) in patients with germ cell tumors of the gonads and extragonadal sites: correlation between endodermal sinus (yolk sac) tumor and raised serum AFP. Cancer 1980;46(2):380–5.

37. Norgaard-Pedersen B, Schultz H, Arends J, et al. Biochemical markers for testicular germ-cell tumors in relation to histology and stage: some experiences from the Danish testicular cancer (DATECA) study from 1976 through 1981. Ann N Y Acad Sci 1983;417:390–9.

38. Jacobsen GK. Alpha-fetoprotein (AFP) and human chorionic gonadotropin (HCG) in testicular germ cell tumours. A comparison of histologic and serologic occurrence of tumour markers. Acta Pathol Microbiol Immunol Scand A 1983;91(3):183–90.

39. Kao CS, Idrees MT, Young RH, et al. Solid pattern yolk sac tumor: a morphologic and immunohistochemical study of 52 cases. Am J Surg Pathol 2012;36(3):360–7.

40. Leibovitch I, Foster RS, Ulbright TM, et al. Adult primary pure teratoma of the testis. The Indiana experience. Cancer 1995;75(9):2244–50.

41. Zhang C, Berney DM, Hirsch MS, et al. Evidence supporting the existence of benign teratomas of

the postpubertal testis: a clinical, histopathologic, and molecular genetic analysis of 25 cases. Am J Surg Pathol 2013;37(6):827–35.

42. Oosterhuis JW, Stoop JA, Rijlaarsdam MA, et al. Pediatric germ cell tumors presenting beyond childhood? Andrology 2014;3(1):70–7.

43. Ehrlich Y, Beck SD, Ulbright TM, et al. Outcome analysis of patients with transformed teratoma to primitive neuroectodermal tumor. Ann Oncol 2010;21(9):1846–50.

44. Michael H, Hull MT, Ulbright TM, et al. Primitive neuroectodermal tumors arising in testicular germ cell neoplasms. Am J Surg Pathol 1997;21(8):896–904.

45. Ulbright TM, Hattab EM, Zhang S, et al. Primitive neuroectodermal tumors in patients with testicular germ cell tumors usually resemble pediatric-type central nervous system embryonal neoplasms and lack chromosome 22 rearrangements. Mod Pathol 2010;23(7):972–80.

46. Alvarado-Cabrero I, Hernandez-Toriz N, Paner GP. Clinicopathologic analysis of choriocarcinoma as a pure or predominant component of germ cell tumor of the testis. Am J Surg Pathol 2014;38(1):111–8.

47. Miettinen M, McCue PA, Sarlomo-Rikala M, et al. GATA3: a multispecific but potentially useful marker in surgical pathology: a systematic analysis of 2500 epithelial and nonepithelial tumors. Am J Surg Pathol 2014;38(1):13–22.

48. Mirkovic J, Elias K, Drapkin R, et al. GATA3 expression in gestational trophoblastic tissues and tumours. Histopathology 2015. [Epub ahead of print].

49. Idrees M, Saxena R, Cheng L, et al. Podoplanin, a novel marker for seminoma: a comparison study evaluating immunohistochemical expression of podoplanin and OCT3/4. Ann Diagn Pathol 2010; 14(5):331–6.

50. Nonaka D. Differential expression of SOX2 and SOX17 in testicular germ cell tumors. Am J Clin Pathol 2009;131(5):731–6.

51. Ulbright TM, Young RH. Seminoma with tubular, microcystic, and related patterns: a study of 28 cases of unusual morphologic variants that often cause confusion with yolk sac tumor. Am J Surg Pathol 2005;29(4):500–5.

52. Compton LA, Buchanan M, Hirsch MS. GATA3 is a sensitive and relatively specific biomarker for testicular choriocarcinoma. Mod Pathol 2014; 27(S2):222A.

53. Howitt BE, Magers JM, Rice KR, et al. Many post-chemotherapy sarcomatous tumors in patients with testicular germ cell tumors are sarcomatoid yolk sac tumors: a study of 33 cases. Am J Surg Pathol 2015;39(2):251–9.

54. Cheng L, Zhang S, MacLennan GT, et al. Interphase fluorescence in situ hybridization analysis of chromosome 12p abnormalities is useful for distinguishing epidermoid cysts of the testis from pure

mature teratoma. Clin Cancer Res 2006;12(19): 5668–72.

55. Al-Abbadi MA, Hattab EM, Tarawneh M, et al. Primary testicular and paratesticular lymphoma: a retrospective clinicopathologic study of 34 cases with emphasis on differential diagnosis. Arch Pathol Lab Med 2007;131(7):1040–6.

56. Ferry JA, Young RH, Scully RE. Testicular and epididymal plasmacytoma: a report of 7 cases, including three that were the initial manifestation of plasma cell myeloma. Am J Surg Pathol 1997; 21(5):590–8.

57. Henley JD, Young RH, Ulbright TM. Malignant Sertoli cell tumors of the testis: a study of 13 examples of a neoplasm frequently misinterpreted as seminoma. Am J Surg Pathol 2002;26(5):541–50.

58. Billings SD, Roth LM, Ulbright TM. Microcystic Leydig cell tumors mimicking yolk sac tumor: a report of four cases. Am J Surg Pathol 1999;23(5):546–51.

59. Ulbright TM, Young RH. Metastatic carcinoma to the testis: a clinicopathologic analysis of 26 nonincidental cases with emphasis on deceptive features. Am J Surg Pathol 2008;32(11):1683–93.

60. Atkin NB, Baker MC. Specific chromosome change, i(12p), in testicular tumours? Lancet 1982;2(8311):1349.

61. Rodriguez E, Houldsworth J, Reuter VE, et al. Molecular cytogenetic analysis of i(12p)-negative human male germ cell tumors. Genes Chromosomes Cancer 1993;8(4):230–6.

62. Suijkerbuijk RF, Sinke RJ, Meloni AM, et al. Overrepresentation of chromosome 12p sequences and karyotypic evolution in i(12p)-negative testicular germ-cell tumors revealed by fluorescence in situ hybridization. Cancer Genet Cytogenet 1993; 70(2):85–93.

63. Oosterhuis JW, Looijenga LH. Current views on the pathogenesis of testicular germ cell tumours and perspectives for future research: highlights of the 5th Copenhagen Workshop on Carcinoma in situ and Cancer of the Testis. APMIS 2003;111(1): 280–9.

64. Skotheim RI, Lothe RA. The testicular germ cell tumour genome. APMIS 2003;111(1):136–50 [discussion: 150–31].

65. Summersgill B, Osin P, Lu YJ, et al. Chromosomal imbalances associated with carcinoma in situ and associated testicular germ cell tumours of adolescents and adults. Br J Cancer 2001;85(2):213–20.

66. Blough RI, Heerema NA, Ulbright TM, et al. Interphase chromosome painting of paraffin-embedded tissue in the differential diagnosis of possible germ cell tumors. Mod Pathol 1998; 11(7):634–41.

67. Blough RI, Smolarek TA, Ulbright TM, et al. Bicolor fluorescence in situ hybridization on nuclei from formalin-fixed, paraffin-embedded testicular germ

cell tumors: comparison with standard metaphase analysis. Cancer Genet Cytogenet 1997;94(2):79–84.

68. Kernek KM, Brunelli M, Ulbright TM, et al. Fluorescence in situ hybridization analysis of chromosome 12p in paraffin-embedded tissue is useful for establishing germ cell origin of metastatic tumors. Mod Pathol 2004;17(11):1309–13.

69. Schneider DT, Schuster AE, Fritsch MK, et al. Genetic analysis of childhood germ cell tumors with comparative genomic hybridization. Klin Padiatr 2001;213(4):204–11.

70. Perlman EJ, Cushing B, Hawkins E, et al. Cytogenetic analysis of childhood endodermal sinus tumors: a Pediatric Oncology Group study. Pediatr Pathol 1994;14(4):695–708.

71. Hu J, Schuster AE, Fritsch MK, et al. Deletion mapping of 6q21–26 and frequency of 1p36 deletion in childhood endodermal sinus tumors by microsatellite analysis. Oncogene 2001;20(55):8042–4.

72. Silver SA, Wiley JM, Perlman EJ. DNA ploidy analysis of pediatric germ cell tumors. Mod Pathol 1994;7(9):951–6.

73. Oosterhuis JW, Castedo SM, de Jong B, et al. Ploidy of primary germ cell tumors of the testis. Pathogenetic and clinical relevance. Lab Invest 1989;60(1):14–21.

74. Mostert M, Rosenberg C, Stoop H, et al. Comparative genomic and in situ hybridization of germ cell tumors of the infantile testis. Lab Invest 2000;80(7):1055–64.

75. Stock C, Ambros IM, Lion T, et al. Detection of numerical and structural chromosome abnormalities in pediatric germ cell tumors by means of interphase cytogenetics. Genes Chromosomes Cancer 1994;11(1):40–50.

76. Kernek KM, Ulbright TM, Zhang S, et al. Identical allelic losses in mature teratoma and other histologic components of malignant mixed germ cell tumors of the testis. Am J Pathol 2003;163(6):2477–84.

77. Sandberg AA, Meloni AM, Suijkerbuijk RF. Reviews of chromosome studies in urological tumors. III. Cytogenetics and genes in testicular tumors. J Urol 1996;155(5):1531–56.

78. Reuter VE. Origins and molecular biology of testicular germ cell tumors. Mod Pathol 2005;18(Suppl 2):S51–60.

79. Netto GJ. Clinical applications of recent molecular advances in urologic malignancies: no longer chasing a "mirage"? Adv Anat Pathol 2013;20(3):175–203.

80. LeBron C, Pal P, Brait M, et al. Genome-wide analysis of genetic alterations in testicular primary seminoma using high resolution single nucleotide polymorphism arrays. Genomics 2011;97(6):341–9.

81. McIntyre A, Summersgill B, Lu YJ, et al. Genomic copy number and expression patterns in testicular

germ cell tumours. Br J Cancer 2007;97(12):1707–12.

82. McIntyre A, Gilbert D, Goddard N, et al. Genes, chromosomes and the development of testicular germ cell tumors of adolescents and adults. Genes Chromosomes Cancer 2008;47(7):547–57.

83. Looijenga LH, Gillis AJ, Stoop H, et al. Dissecting the molecular pathways of (testicular) germ cell tumour pathogenesis; from initiation to treatment-resistance. Int J Androl 2011;34(4 Pt 2):e234–51.

84. Sheikine Y, Genega E, Melamed J, et al. Molecular genetics of testicular germ cell tumors. Am J Cancer Res 2012;2(2):153–67.

85. Kemmer K, Corless CL, Fletcher JA, et al. KIT mutations are common in testicular seminomas. Am J Pathol 2004;164(1):305–13.

86. McIntyre A, Summersgill B, Grygalewicz B, et al. Amplification and overexpression of the KIT gene is associated with progression in the seminoma subtype of testicular germ cell tumors of adolescents and adults. Cancer Res 2005;65(18):8085–9.

87. Coffey J, Linger R, Pugh J, et al. Somatic KIT mutations occur predominantly in seminoma germ cell tumors and are not predictive of bilateral disease: report of 220 tumors and review of literature. Genes Chromosomes Cancer 2008;47(1):34–42.

88. Bamford S. The COSMIC (Catalogue of Somatic Mutations in Cancer) database and website. Br J Cancer 2004;91:355–8.

89. Mayer F, Wermann H, Albers P, et al. Histopathological and molecular features of late relapses in non-seminomas. BJU Int 2011;107(6):936–43.

90. Mayer F, Gillis AJ, Dinjens W, et al. Microsatellite instability of germ cell tumors is associated with resistance to systemic treatment. Cancer Res 2002;62(10):2758–60.

91. Honecker F, Wermann H, Mayer F, et al. Microsatellite instability, mismatch repair deficiency, and BRAF mutation in treatment-resistant germ cell tumors. J Clin Oncol 2009;27(13):2129–36.

92. Velasco A, Corvalan A, Wistuba II, et al. Mismatch repair expression in testicular cancer predicts recurrence and survival. Int J Cancer 2008;122(8):1774–7.

93. Velasco A, Riquelme E, Schultz M, et al. Microsatellite instability and loss of heterozygosity have distinct prognostic value for testicular germ cell tumor recurrence. Cancer Biol Ther 2004;3(11):1152–8 [discussion: 1159–61].

94. Brait M, Maldonado L, Begum S, et al. DNA methylation profiles delineate epigenetic heterogeneity in seminoma and non-seminoma. Br J Cancer 2012;106(2):414–23.

95. Olasz J, Mandoky L, Geczi L, et al. Influence of hMLH1 methylation, mismatch repair deficiency and microsatellite instability on chemoresistance

of testicular germ-cell tumors. Anticancer Res 2005;25(6B):4319–24.

96. Wang X, Zhang S, Maclennan GT, et al. Epidermal growth factor receptor protein expression and gene amplification in the chemorefractory metastatic embryonal carcinoma. Mod Pathol 2009;22(1):7–12.

97. Miyai K, Yamamoto S, Asano T, et al. Protein over-expression and gene amplification of epidermal growth factor receptor in adult testicular germ cell tumors: potential role in tumor progression. Cancer Sci 2010;101(9):1970–6.

98. Heidenreich A, Schenkman NS, Sesterhenn IA, et al. Immunohistochemical and mutational analysis of the p53 tumour suppressor gene and the bcl-2 oncogene in primary testicular germ cell tumours. APMIS 1998;106(1):90–9 [discussion: 99–100].

99. Guillou L, Estreicher A, Chaubert P, et al. Germ cell tumors of the testis overexpress wild-type p53. Am J Pathol 1996;149(4):1221–8.

100. Moul JW, Theune SM, Chang EH. Detection of RAS mutations in archival testicular germ cell tumors by polymerase chain reaction and oligonucleotide hybridization. Genes Chromosomes Cancer 1992; 5(2):109–18.

101. Roelofs H, Mostert MC, Pompe K, et al. Restricted 12p amplification and RAS mutation in human germ cell tumors of the adult testis. Am J Pathol 2000;157(4):1155–66.

102. Furukawa S, Haruta M, Arai Y, et al. Yolk sac tumor but not seminoma or teratoma is associated with abnormal epigenetic reprogramming pathway and shows frequent hypermethylation of various tumor suppressor genes. Cancer Sci 2009;100(4): 698–708.

103. Netto GJ, Nakai Y, Nakayama M, et al. Global DNA hypomethylation in intratubular germ cell neoplasia and seminoma, but not in nonseminomatous male germ cell tumors. Mod Pathol 2008;21(11):1337–44.

104. Lind GE, Skotheim RI, Fraga MF, et al. Novel epigenetically deregulated genes in testicular cancer include homeobox genes and SCGB3A1 (HIN-1). J Pathol 2006;210(4):441–9.

105. Michael H, Lucia J, Foster RS, et al. The pathology of late recurrence of testicular germ cell tumors. Am J Surg Pathol 2000;24(2):257–73.

106. Fedyanin M, Tryakin A, Kanagavel D, et al. Late relapses (>2 years) in patients with stage I testicular germ cell tumors: predictive factors and survival. Urol Oncol 2013;31(4):499–504.

107. George DW, Foster RS, Hromas RA, et al. Update on late relapse of germ cell tumor: a clinical and molecular analysis. J Clin Oncol 2003;21(1): 113–22.

108. Magers MJ, Kao CS, Cole CD, et al. "Somatic-type" malignancies arising from testicular germ cell tumors: a clinicopathologic study of 124 cases with emphasis on glandular tumors supporting frequent yolk sac tumor origin. Am J Surg Pathol 2014; 38(10):1396–409.

109. Tarrant WP, Czerniak BA, Guo CC. Relationship between primary and metastatic testicular germ cell tumors: a clinicopathologic analysis of 100 cases. Hum Pathol 2013;44(10):2220–6.

110. Motzer RJ, Amsterdam A, Prieto V, et al. Teratoma with malignant transformation: diverse malignant histologies arising in men with germ cell tumors. J Urol 1998;159(1):133–8.

111. Rice KR, Magers MJ, Beck SD, et al. Management of germ cell tumors with somatic type malignancy: pathological features, prognostic factors and survival outcomes. J Urol 2014;192(5):1403–9.

112. Ulbright TM, Loehrer PJ, Roth LM, et al. The development of non-germ cell malignancies within germ cell tumors. A clinicopathologic study of 11 cases. Cancer 1984;54(9):1824–33.

113. Guo CC, Punar M, Contreras AL, et al. Testicular germ cell tumors with sarcomatous components: an analysis of 33 cases. Am J Surg Pathol 2009; 33(8):1173–8.

114. Malagon HD, Valdez AM, Moran CA, et al. Germ cell tumors with sarcomatous components: a clinicopathologic and immunohistochemical study of 46 cases. Am J Surg Pathol 2007;31(9): 1356–62.

115. Kum JB, Ulbright TM, Williamson SR, et al. Molecular genetic evidence supporting the origin of somatic-type malignancy and teratoma from the same progenitor cell. Am J Surg Pathol 2012; 36(12):1849–56.

116. Idrees MT, Kuhar M, Ulbright TM, et al. Clonal evidence for the progression of a testicular germ cell tumor to angiosarcoma. Hum Pathol 2010;41(1): 139–44.

117. Ulbright TM, Henley JD, Cummings OW, et al. Cystic trophoblastic tumor: a nonaggressive lesion in postchemotherapy resections of patients with testicular germ cell tumors. Am J Surg Pathol 2004;28(9):1212–6.

118. Little JS Jr, Foster RS, Ulbright TM, et al. Unusual neoplasms detected in testis cancer patients undergoing post-chemotherapy retroperitoneal lymphadenectomy. J Urol 1994;152(4):1144–9.

119. Ye H, Ulbright TM. Difficult differential diagnoses in testicular pathology. Arch Pathol Lab Med 2012; 136(4):435–46.

120. Perry A, Wiley EL, Albores-Saavedra J. Pagetoid spread of intratubular germ cell neoplasia into rete testis: a morphologic and histochemical study of 100 orchiectomy specimens with invasive germ cell tumors. Hum Pathol 1994;25(3):235–9.

121. Lee AH, Theaker JM. Pagetoid spread into the rete testis by testicular tumours. Histopathology 1994; 24(4):385–9.

122. Valdevenito JP, Gallegos I, Fernandez C, et al. Correlation between primary tumor pathologic features and presence of clinical metastasis at diagnosis of testicular seminoma. Urology 2007; 70(4):777–80.

123. Yetisyigit T, Babacan N, Urun Y, et al. Predictors of outcome in patients with advanced nonseminomatous germ cell testicular tumors. Asian Pac J Cancer Prev 2014;15(2):831–5.

124. Yilmaz A, Cheng T, Zhang J, et al. Testicular hilum and vascular invasion predict advanced clinical stage in nonseminomatous germ cell tumors. Mod Pathol 2013;26(4):579–86.

125. Hoskin P, Dilly S, Easton D, et al. Prognostic factors in stage I non-seminomatous germ-cell testicular tumors managed by orchiectomy and surveillance: implications for adjuvant chemotherapy. J Clin Oncol 1986;4(7):1031–6.

126. Vogt AP, Chen Z, Osunkoya AO. Rete testis invasion by malignant germ cell tumor and/or intratubular germ cell neoplasia: what is the significance of this finding? Hum Pathol 2010;41(9): 1339–44.

127. Soper MS, Hastings JR, Cosmatos HA, et al. Observation versus adjuvant radiation or chemotherapy in the management of stage I seminoma: clinical outcomes and prognostic factors for relapse in a large US cohort. Am J Clin Oncol 2014;37(4):356–9.

128. Warde P, Specht L, Horwich A, et al. Prognostic factors for relapse in stage I seminoma managed by surveillance: a pooled analysis. J Clin Oncol 2002;20(22):4448–52.

129. Schultz HP, Arends J, Barlebo H, et al. Testicular carcinoma in Denmark 1976–1980. Stage and selected clinical parameters at presentation. Acta Radiol Oncol 1984;23(4):249–53.

130. Aparicio J, Maroto P, Garcia del Muro X, et al. Prognostic factors for relapse in stage I seminoma: a new nomogram derived from three consecutive, risk-adapted studies from the Spanish Germ Cell Cancer Group (SGCCG). Ann Oncol 2014;25(11):2173–8.

131. Dry SM, Renshaw AA. Extratesticular extension of germ cell tumors preferentially occurs at the hilum. Am J Clin Pathol 1999;111(4):534–8.

132. Sobin L, Gospodarowicz M, Wittekind C. UICC TNM classification of malignant tumors. 7th edition. New York: Wiley-Liss; 2009.

133. Osunkoya AO, Grignon DJ. Practical issues and pitfalls in staging tumors of the genitourinary tract. Semin Diagn Pathol 2012;29(3):154–66.

134. Cortazar JM, Howitt BE, O'Donnell E, et al. Hilar soft tissue involvement by testicular germ cell tumors is associated with advanced stage indicators. Mod Pathol 2014;27(S2):223A.

135. Yilmaz A, Trpkov K. Hilar invasion in testicular germ cell tumors: a potential understaging pitfall. Mod Pathol 2015;28(S2):269A.

136. Balzer BL, Ulbright TM. Spontaneous regression of testicular germ cell tumors: an analysis of 42 cases. Am J Surg Pathol 2006;30(7):858–65.

# Diagnosis and Treatment of Testicular Cancer
## A Clinician's Perspective

Brandon Bernard, MD, Christopher J. Sweeney, MBBS*

**KEYWORDS**

- Testicular cancer • Germ cell tumor • Seminoma • Nonseminoma • Active surveillance
- Cancer of unknown primary

---

**Key points**

- Testicular germ cell tumors (GCTs) include seminoma and nonseminoma; both are highly curable even if metastatic.

- Different adjuvant therapy options exist for clinical stage I (CSI) disease although outcomes are similar to a strategy of surveillance and treatment only for those who relapse.

- LVI is associated with higher relapse rates in CSI nonseminoma but almost 100% can be salvaged with chemotherapy.

- Chance of teratoma in retroperitoneal postchemotherapy residual masses is higher if present in orchiectomy specimen and with increasing size of the mass.

- Histologic concordance rates between the retroperitoneum and lung masses are high; this can influence approach to further treatment.

- Isochromosome of the short arm of chromosome 12 (i12p) and OCT4 can be useful special tests to identify GCT in cancer of unknown primary (CUP).

---

## ABSTRACT

Testicular germ cell tumors (GCTs) include seminoma and nonseminoma. Chance of cure is excellent for clinical stage I disease regardless of whether adjuvant treatment or a surveillance strategy with treatment only for those who relapse is used. Risk of recurrence is greater in nonseminoma with evidence of lymphovascular invasion, but most can be salvaged with chemotherapy and survival rates remain high. This article outlines key pathologic and clinical considerations in clinical stage I seminoma, nonseminoma, advanced disease, and assessment of cancer of unknown primary as a potential GCT.

## OVERVIEW

A majority of testicular cancers are classified as GCTs (see also Howitt and Berney, Tumors of the Testis: Morphologic Features and Molecular Alterations, Surgical Pathology Clinics, 2015, Volume 8, Issue 4). Of these, 2 types exist: seminoma and nonseminoma. Risk factors for the development of GCT include gonadal dysgenesis, cryptorchidism, and positive family history.[1–4] In addition, HIV-positive men have an increased risk of developing seminoma.[5] Moreover, infertility has been linked to an increased risk of developing GCT.[6] Lastly, the finding of testicular microlithiasis on ultrasound is associated with a higher likelihood of diagnosis of GCT.[7]

---

Disclosures: B. Bernard has nothing to disclose. C.J. Sweeney has nothing to disclose related to subject matter of this article.
Dana-Farber Cancer Institute, Lank Center for Genitourinary Oncology, 450 Brookline Avenue, D1230, Boston, MA 02215, USA
* Corresponding author.
E-mail address: christopher_sweeney@dfci.harvard.edu

Surgical Pathology 8 (2015) 717–723
http://dx.doi.org/10.1016/j.path.2015.07.006
1875-9181/15/$ – see front matter © 2015 Elsevier Inc. All rights reserved.

Prognosis and treatment options vary with more advanced American Joint Committee on Cancer clinical TNM stage and International Germ Cell Cancer Collaborative Group classification. CSI is tumor confined to the testis with no radiographic evidence of retroperitoneal or distant metastases and normal tumor markers (β-subunit of human chorionic gonadotropin, alpha fetoprotein [AFP], and lactate dehydrogenase) postorchiectomy.

## CLINICAL STAGE I SEMINOMA

### OVERVIEW

Pure seminoma is a pathologic diagnosis with therapeutic implications.[8] Chance of cure is high even in advanced disease. Seminoma differs from nonseminoma in that men tend to present at an older age, with a median age at diagnosis of approximately 40 years.

---

### Key Features
#### SEMINOMA

1. Pure seminoma accounts for approximately one-half of all GCTs.

2. The median age of diagnosis is approximately 40 years.

3. Light microscopy is often sufficient to distinguish between nonseminoma and seminoma.

4. Sharp cytoplasmic borders, prominent nucleoli, and clear cytoplasm make up the fried egg characteristic appearance.

5. Lymphocytes interspersed with tumor cells is a frequent finding.

6. After orchiectomy, active surveillance is the preferred treatment strategy for CSI given that most relapses are salvaged and survival is near 100%.

7. Most relapses occur within 3 years of orchiectomy.

---

### GROSS FEATURES

Seminomas are bulky, soft, homogeneous masses. A Danish series of 1058 patients with GCT reported a diagnosis of seminoma in 52.4%.[9] It has been reported that risk of metastasis correlates with greater primary tumor size; however, 78% of cases in this series presented with CSI.

## MICROSCOPIC FEATURES

Seminoma is defined by the absence of nonseminomatous components. Histologically, it shows clonal proliferation of cancerous germ cells with sharp cytoplasmic borders, prominent nucleoli, and clear cytoplasm (fried egg appearance) (see also Howitt and Berney, Tumors of the Testis: Morphologic Features and Molecular Alterations, Surgical Pathology Clinics, 2015, Volume 8, Issue 4). Furthermore, groups of lymphocytes are often observed interspersed with tumor cells. Light microscopy is the mainstay of distinguishing from nonseminoma and other testicular cancers.[8] The immunostains, OCT3/4, CKIT, and CD30, are useful, however, if ambiguity exists.

## DIFFERENTIAL DIAGNOSIS

The differential diagnosis for a testicular mass includes torsion, epididymitis, hydrocele, varicocele, hernia, hematoma, spermatocele, and malignancy. Regarding seminoma, other possibilities include a nonseminomatous GCT (in particular, pure embryonal cell carcinoma [EC]) and lymphoma.

---

### Differential Diagnosis
#### SEMINOMA

- Nonseminoma: distinguishing from EC can be problematic if cellular atypia exists; however, EC tends to have less defined cell borders and greater pleomorphism; EC stains positive for CD30 and SOX2 and this can help distinguish it from seminoma, which is in contrast positive for CKIT and D2-40.

- Testicular lymphoma tends to present in older men, invades into the interstitium, and stains positive for markers of lymphoid cell lineage (ie, leukocyte common antigen).

- Sex cord–stromal tumors tend to present in middle age and do not produce tumor markers but may be associated with hormonal abnormalities with consequent symptoms and signs, such as gynecomastia; specifically, antibodies can be used to distinguish from semionoma.

- Mesothelial cell proliferations, such as adenomatoid tumor or, rarely, mesothelioma—the latter can present as a recurrent hydrocele, can be diagnosed from cytology of the aspirate, and can be distinguished with imunostains.

---

## PROGNOSIS

Treatment options for CSI seminoma include active surveillance, adjuvant carboplatin chemotherapy, and radiotherapy. A relapse rate of approximately 17% and a near-100% cause-specific survival has been shown with active surveillance.[10] A retrospective study of active surveillance showed relapse in 13% of patients at a median of 14 months from orchiectomy, with 92% of relapses occurring within 3 years.[11] Alternatively, 1 cycle of adjuvant carboplatin was found noninferior to radiotherapy regarding 5-year relapse-free rate (94.7% vs 96.0%, respectively).[12] In a prospective population-based study, 14.3% of patients relapsed after surveillance, 3.9% after 1 cycle of adjuvant carboplatin, and 0.8% after adjuvant radiotherapy.[13] More recently, surveillance for CSI without risk factors (ie, tumor size <4 cm and no invasion of the rete testis) was associated with a relapse rate of less than 3%.[14]

---

## CLINICAL STAGE I NONSEMINOMA

### OVERVIEW

Nonseminomatous GCT is either of pure or of mixed histology, including carrying amounts of EC, yolk sac tumor (YST), choriocarcinoma, and teratoma (see also Howitt and Berney, Tumors of the Testis: Morphologic Features and Molecular Alterations, Surgical Pathology Clinics, 2015, Volume 8, Issue 4); seminomatous components can also be present. Median age of diagnosis is approximately 30 years. Unlike seminoma, nonseminoma can be associated with an elevated AFP.

---

### Key Features
#### NONSEMINOMA

1. Nonseminoma makes up the other half of testicular GCT.

2. Median age of diagnosis is younger than seminoma, at approximately 30 years.

3. Nonseminoma can produce AFP whereas such a finding is rare in seminoma.

4. Nonseminoma can be of pure or mixed histology comprised of EC, YST, choriocarcinoma, and teratoma.

---

5. Distinguishing subtypes of nonseminoma is primarily via morphologic analysis.

6. Teratoma with transformation to non-GCT (sarcoma or carcinoma) portends a worse prognosis.

7. Lymphovascular invasion (LVI) is the greatest and most validated indicator of risk of relapse; despite this, survival of CSI disease is close to 100%.

---

## GROSS FEATURES

EC is usually smaller than seminoma with poor demarcation; YST may have a shiny surface; choriocarcinoma tends to look like a hemorrhagic nodule; and teratoma can be cystic. In the Danish series, 47% percent of GCTs were nonseminomatous and approximately one-third were pure and two-thirds were of mixed histology; 54% of cases presented as CSI, with pure EC subtypes associated with the highest rate of advanced disease.[9]

## MICROSCOPIC FEATURES

Assessment of nonseminoma can be made secondary to classic morphologic features in most cases (see also Howitt and Berney, Tumors of the Testis: Morphologic Features and Molecular Alterations, Surgical Pathology Clinics, 2015, Volume 8, Issue 4). ECs are epithelial in appearance, with clusters and sheets of cells that exhibit cytologic atypia and stain positive for OCT3/4, SOX2, NANOG, and SALL4, although the latter 2 markers can also be seen in other subtypes of GCT. YSTs are often display lower nuclear grade and are the most varied in appearance. SALL4, AFP, and GATA3 are positive in YST, whereas OCT3/4, NANOG, and SOX2 are negative. Choriocarcinomas notably display hemorrhage and necrosis and are important to making a correct diagnosis; they are composed of both syncytiotrophoblast and cytotrophoblast. Mature teratomas show a heterogeneous amalgamation of differentiated cells or organ-like structures within a fibrous stroma. Comment should be made regarding teratoma with somatic (sarcomatous and/or carcinomatous) differentiation, because such elements are associated with a worse prognosis.

## DIFFERENTIAL DIAGNOSIS

Other potential etiologies for testicular mass, both benign and malignant, are as outlined for seminoma (discussed previously).

## PROGNOSIS

The greatest predictor of recurrence for nonsemi-nomatous GCT is LVI in tumor. Regardless, treatment options are active surveillance, adjuvant platinum-based chemotherapy (eg, bleomycin, etoposide, and cisplatin [BEP]), or primary retro-peritoneal lymph node dissection (RPLND). Surveillance has been associated with relapse rates of 19% to 28% and cause-specific survival up to 100%[10,11]; 44% of patients with LVI relapsed in 1 study; however, less than 1% of patients died of their disease.[11] Such excellent outcomes lend support for a non–risk-adapted approach.[15,16] Alternatively, some investigators endorse a risk-adapted approach with adjuvant platinum-based chemotherapy in an effort to reduce relapse.[17,18] Specifically, relapse rates in patients who received adjuvant BEP × 1 have been reported as 3.2% versus 1.6% for tumors with LVI versus without LVI, respectively, with 5-year cause-specific survival of 100%.[14] Regarding RPLND, a phase III trial in unselected patients showed BEP × 1 modestly superior to surgery at reducing the risk of relapse.[19] Although outcomes are excellent regardless of modality, efforts should be made to reduce diagnostic delay given an association with advanced stage and worse survival.[20] As such, thorough and frequent communication between the clinician and the pathologist is critical in ensuring prompt diagnosis and appropriate therapy.

### Pitfall
### NONSEMINOMA

! Diagnostic delay is associated with increased stage and worse survival.

## RESIDUAL MASS IN ADVANCED DISEASE

### OVERVIEW

The treatment of advanced GCT is orchiectomy plus primary platinum-based chemotherapy. Further management is dictated by the presence or absence of a residual mass on imaging, with recommendation to resect all nonseminoma post-chemotherapy masses greater than 1 cm. Further therapy may be guided by the pathologic evaluation of the resected mass with the absence or presence of viable nonteratomatous tumor critical for treatment decisions.

### Key Features
### RESIDUAL MASS

1. Treatment of metastatic disease is orchiectomy plus 3 to 4 cycles of platinum-based chemotherapy.

2. Nonseminoma residual masses greater than 1 cm postchemotherapy warrant surgical resection.

3. Approximately 5% of resected masses contain viable tumor postchemotherapy.

4. Chance of teratoma in postchemotherapy RPLND masses increases with larger size of the retroperitoneal mass and presence of teratoma in the primary orchiectomy specimen.

5. Concordance rates of pathology between retroperitoneum and lung masses are approximately 70% to 75%.

6. Teratoma in the retroperitoneum mandates consideration of resection of residual lung masses.

7. Complete resection with minimal (<10%) residual viable malignancy is associated with improved survival on resection of the residual GCT.

## MICROSCOPIC FEATURES

Necrosis/fibrosis is found in 40% to 50% of retroperitoneal masses, teratoma in 30% to 40%, and viable nonteratomatous GCT in 5%. The likelihood of finding active disease tends to be higher in those post–multiple lines of chemotherapy.

## DIFFERENTIAL DIAGNOSIS

The differential diagnosis of a postchemotherapy residual mass in advanced nonseminomatous GCT includes fibrosis/necrosis, teratoma, and viable GCT. The likelihood of finding teratoma in an RPLND specimen is higher if teratoma was found in the orchiectomy: 1 study showed 85.6% of primary tumors with teratoma had teratoma at RPLND, whereas 48.0% of primary tumors without had teratoma in the RPLND.[21] Moreover, the chance of teratoma in the retroperitoneum when present in the primary is related to the size of the residual retroperitoneal mass, with 78% of residual masses less than 2.5 cm having teratoma on RPLND compared with 95% of masses greater than 10.0 cm. Within the lung, 1 study found necrosis in 54%, teratoma in 33%, and viable GCT in 13%.[22] Concordance rates of residual lung and retroperitoneal mass pathology showed 77.5% of lung masses show necrosis if present on RPLND, 70% show teratoma if found on RPLND, and 69% show viable GCT if identified on RPLND.[23] Thus, RPLND histology is a strong predictor of histology within the lung and may help guide clinical management regarding residual lung masses.[22]

### Differential Diagnosis
#### RESIDUAL MASS

- Necrosis/fibrosis (40%–50%)

- Teratoma (30%–40%)

- Viable nonteratomatous GCT (5%–10%)

## PROGNOSIS

Clinical stage IIA has a 5-year disease-free survival of approximately 75% after surgical resection without adjuvant chemotherapy, and the presence of extranodal extension does not portend a worse outcome.[24] In stage III disease, the concordance rate of retroperitoneal and lung mass pathology has therapeutic implications. If teratoma is found at RPLND, then lung lesions should be resected given the high chance of teratoma and risk of transformation to more aggressive disease. If no teratoma is found at RPLND and lung lesions are less than 1 cm with normal serum tumor markers, observation is recommended. Lung lesions containing malignant teratoma are associated with a worse survival compared with necrosis/fibrosis and mature teratoma.[25] If cancer is identified, completeness of resection and proportion of malignant cells less than 10% have been associated with improved outcome.[26,27] When tumor markers are persistently elevated after primary chemotherapy, some RPLND specimens may contain necrosis or teratoma (with a consequent favorable prognosis), and cure is still possible even if viable GCT is found with surgery alone.[28,29]

## MIDLINE CANCER OF UNKNOWN PRIMARY

### OVERVIEW

Accurate pathologic assessment of biopsied tissue in CUPs is invaluable and carries consequences regarding prognosis and treatment, especially when considering a highly curable malignancy, such as a GCT. When possible, excisional biopsy is preferred over fine-needle aspiration, because the former has the potential to provide better tissue sampling for diagnosis and ancillary studies if needed.

### Key Features
#### MIDLINE CANCER OF UNKNOWN PRIMARY

1. GCT should always be a consideration in a young man with a midline tumor (anterior mediastinal or retroperitoneal) of unknown etiology.

2. Definitive diagnosis is paramount given the high likelihood of cure with GCT; thorough and frequent communication between the clinical and pathologist is key.

3. Excisional biopsy is recommended over fine-needle aspirate to aid in accurate diagnosis.

4. (i12p) has high prevalence in GCT and can be of diagnostic utility in work-up of CUPs.

5. Immunostains can be helpful in making an accurate distinction of CUP and GCT.

### MICROSCOPIC FEATURES

An i(12p) is a marker of GCT[30] (see also Howitt and Berney, Tumors of the Testis: Morphologic Features and Molecular Alterations, Surgical Pathology Clinics, 2015, Volume 8, Issue 4). Karyotype analysis was shown abnormal in 59% of GCT samples in 1 study, of which 79% displayed i(12p).[31] Comparative genomic hybridization techniques have been shown effective in assessing for i(12p) in paraffin-embedded tissue.[32] SALL4 is broad-spectrum GCT biomarker, and the presence of SALL4 in a CUP supports the diagnosis of a GCT; however, small subsets of non-GCTs may be focally positive for SALL4 and, therefore, should be interpreted as part of a panel of biomarkers and in accordance with the morphologic features. Additionally, the nuclear transcription factor OCT4 has been shown highly sensitive and specific for GCTs with seminomatous and embryonal components via immunohistochemistry.[33]

### DIFFERENTIAL DIAGNOSIS

A midline CUP in a young man may represent thymoma, GCT, lymphoma, thyroid carcinoma, sarcoma, or NUT midline carcinoma.[34] Immunostains are useful in distinguishing these diagnoses, and a prior testicular GCT should always be excluded before diagnosing a midline/mediastinal GCT.

> ⚠️ **Differential Diagnosis**
> MIDLINE CANCER OF UNKNOWN PRIMARY
>
> - Primary malignant GCT (testicular primary must be excluded)
> - Thymoma (if mediastinal)
> - Lymphoma
> - Thyroid carcinoma
> - Sarcoma
> - Midline NUT carcinoma

## PROGNOSIS

Prognosis of a GCT diagnosed from a CUP is the same as for other GCTs. I(12p) copy number has not been shown to have an impact on response to chemotherapy or survival.[31]

## SUMMARY

> **Important Pathologic Findings Required for Appropriate Treatment of Patients with Malignant Germ Cell Tumors**
>
> - The presence or absence of LVI (exclude processing artifacts).
> - Include pathologic findings that accurately stage the patient.
> - Expedite pathologic review for recurrent disease.
> - Report on the presence and percent of residual, viable nonteratomatous GCT after orchiectomy and platinum-based chemotherapy.
> - Report on the presence or absence of teratoma in surgically excised retroperitoneal masses/lymph nodes.
> - Report the presence of somatic differentiation (sarcoma and/or carcinomas).
> - Include GCT in the differential diagnosis of retroperitoneal and mediastinal tumors of unknown origin.

## REFERENCES

1. Gourlay WA, Johnson HW, Pantzar JT, et al. Gonadal tumors in disorders of sexual differentiation. Urology 1994;43(4):537–40.
2. Batata MA, Chu FC, Hilaris BS, et al. Testicular cancer in cryptorchids. Cancer 1982;49(5):1023–30.
3. Forman D, Oliver RT, Brett AR, et al. Familial testicular cancer: a report of the UK family register, estimation of risk and an HLA class 1 sib-pair analysis. Br J Cancer 1992;65(2):255–62.
4. Hemminki K, Chen B. Familial risks in testicular cancer as aetiological clues. Int J Androl 2006; 29(1):205–10.
5. Powles T, Bower M, Daugaard G, et al. Multicenter study of human immunodeficiency virus-related germ cell tumors. J Clin Oncol 2003;21(10):1922–7.
6. Walsh TJ, Croughan MS, Schembri M, et al. Increased risk of testicular germ cell cancer among infertile men. Arch Intern Med 2009;169(4):351–6.
7. Tan IB, Ang KK, Ching BC, et al. Testicular microlithiasis predicts concurrent testicular germ cell tumors and intratubular germ cell neoplasia of unclassified type in adults: a meta-analysis and systematic review. Cancer 2010;116(19):4520–32.
8. Ulbright TM. The most common, clinically significant misdiagnoses in testicular tumor pathology, and how to avoid them. Adv Anat Pathol 2008;15(1): 18–27.
9. Krag Jacobsen G, Barlebo H, Olsen J, et al. Testicular germ cell tumours in Denmark 1976–1980. Pathology of 1058 consecutive cases. Acta Radiol Oncol 1984;23(4):239–47.
10. Groll RJ, Warde P, Jewett MA. A comprehensive systematic review of testicular germ cell tumor surveillance. Crit Rev Oncol Hematol 2007;64(3): 182–97.
11. Kollmannsberger C, Tandstad T, Bedard PL, et al. Patterns of relapse in patients with clinical stage I testicular cancer managed with active surveillance. J Clin Oncol 2015;33(1):51–7.
12. Oliver RT, Mead GM, Rustin GJ, et al. Randomized trial of carboplatin versus radiotherapy for stage I seminoma: mature results on relapse and contralateral testis cancer rates in MRC TE19/EORTC 30982 study (ISRCTN27163214). J Clin Oncol 2011;29(8): 957–62.
13. Tandstad T, Smaaland R, Solberg A, et al. Management of seminomatous testicular cancer: a binational prospective population-based study from the Swedish norwegian testicular cancer study group. J Clin Oncol 2011;29(8):719–25.
14. Cohn-Cedermark G, Stahl O, Tandstad T, et al. Surveillance vs. adjuvant therapy of clinical stage I testicular tumors - a review and the SWENOTECA experience. Andrology 2015;3(1):102–10.
15. Kollmannsberger C, Moore C, Chi KN, et al. Non-risk-adapted surveillance for patients with stage I nonseminomatous testicular germ-cell tumors: diminishing treatment-related morbidity while maintaining efficacy. Ann Oncol 2010;21(6): 1296–301.
16. Sturgeon JF, Moore MJ, Kakiashvili DM, et al. Non-risk-adapted surveillance in clinical stage I

nonseminomatous germ cell tumors: the Princess Margaret Hospital's experience. Eur Urol 2011; 59(4):556–62.

17. Pectasides D, Pectasides E, Constantinidou A, et al. Current management of stage I testicular non-seminomatous germ cell tumours. Crit Rev Oncol Hematol 2009;70:114–23.

18. Tandstad T, Stahl O, Hakansson U, et al. One course of adjuvant BEP in clinical stage I non-seminoma mature and expanded results from the SWENOTECA group. Ann Oncol 2014;25(11): 2167–72.

19. Albers P, Siener R, Krege S, et al. Randomized phase III trial comparing retroperitoneal lymph node dissection with one course of bleomycin and etoposide plus cisplatin chemotherapy in the adjuvant treatment of clinical stage I Nonseminomatous testicular germ cell tumors: AUO trial AH 01/94 by the German Testicular Cancer Study Group. J Clin Oncol 2008;26(18):2966–72.

20. Huyghe E, Muller A, Mieusset R, et al. Impact of diagnostic delay in testis cancer: results of a large population-based study. Eur Urol 2007;52(6): 1710–6.

21. Beck SD, Foster RS, Bihrle R, et al. Teratoma in the orchiectomy specimen and volume of metastasis are predictors of retroperitoneal teratoma in post-chemotherapy nonseminomatous testis cancer. J Urol 2002;168(4 Pt 1):1402–4.

22. Steyerberg EW, Keizer HJ, Messemer JE, et al. Residual pulmonary masses after chemotherapy for metastatic nonseminomatous germ cell tumor. Prediction of histology. ReHiT Study Group. Cancer 1997;79(2):345–55.

23. Tognoni PG, Foster RS, McGraw P, et al. Combined post-chemotherapy retroperitoneal lymph node dissection and resection of chest tumor under the same anesthetic is appropriate based on morbidity and tumor pathology. J Urol 1998;159(6):1833–5.

24. Beck SD, Cheng L, Bihrle R, et al. Does the presence of extranodal extension in pathological stage B1 nonseminomatous germ cell tumor necessitate adjuvant chemotherapy? J Urol 2007;177(3):944–6.

25. Cagini L, Nicholson AG, Horwich A, et al. Thoracic metastasectomy for germ cell tumours: long term survival and prognostic factors. Ann Oncol 1998; 9(11):1185–91.

26. Fizazi K, Tjulandin S, Salvioni R, et al. Viable malignant cells after primary chemotherapy for disseminated nonseminomatous germ cell tumors: prognostic factors and role of postsurgery chemotherapy–results from an international study group. J Clin Oncol 2001;19(2):2647–57.

27. Fizazi K, Oldenburg J, Dunant A, et al. Assessing prognosis and optimizing treatment in patients with postchemotherapy viable nonseminomatous germ-cell tumors (NSGCT): results of the sCR2 international study. Ann Oncol 2008;19(2):259–64.

28. Coogan CL, Foster RS, Rowland RG, et al. Postchemotherapy retroperitoneal lymph node dissection is effective therapy in selected patients with elevated tumor markers after primary chemotherapy alone. Urology 1997;50(6):957–62.

29. Beck SD, Foster RS, Bihrle R, et al. Outcome analysis for patients with elevated serum tumor markers at postchemotherapy retroperitoneal lymph node dissection. J Clin Oncol 2005;23(25): 6149–56.

30. Atkin NB, Baker MC. Specific chromosome change, i(12p), in testicular tumours? Lancet 1982;2(8311): 1349.

31. Bosl GJ, Ilson DH, Rodriguez E, et al. Clinical relevance of the i(12p) marker chromosome in germ cell tumors. J Natl Cancer Inst 1994;86(5): 349–55.

32. Summersgill B, Goker H, Osin P, et al. Establishing germ cell origin of undifferentiated tumors by identifying gain of 12p material using comparative genomic hybridization analysis of paraffin-embedded samples. Diagn Mol Pathol 1998;7(5): 260–6.

33. Cheng L. Establishing a germ cell origin for metastatic tumors using OCT4 immunohistochemistry. Cancer 2004;101(9):2006–10.

34. French CA. NUT midline carcinoma. Cancer Genet Cytogenet 2010;203(1):16–20.

# Adrenal Tumors in Adults

Andre Pinto, MD, Justine A. Barletta, MD*

## KEYWORDS

• Adrenal • Adrenal adenoma • Adrenocortical carcinoma • Pheochromocytoma

## ABSTRACT

Although most adrenal tumors are not diagnostic dilemmas, there are cases that are challenging. This may be due to the tissue provided, for example fragmented tissue received in the setting of morcellation, or it may be due to inherently challenging histology, such as in cases with equivocal features of malignancy. Additionally, much has been learned about the molecular alterations of adrenal tumors, especially pheochromocytomas. Many of these alterations represent germline mutations with significant clinical implications for patients and their families. The aim of this review is to provide an overview of the most common adrenal tumors in adults so that pathologists can tackle these interesting tumors.

## OVERVIEW

This article will present an overview of the most common adrenal tumors in adults. It will start with a discussion of adrenal incidentalomas, including what they represent and when they are removed. Next adrenal cortical adenomas, the most common adrenal neoplasm, and a tumor that is generally diagnostically straight-forward will be covered. From there adrenocortical carcinomas will be reviewed, concentrating on gross and microscopic findings and histologic features of malignancy. The article will finish with pheochromocytomas, addressing not only what they look like, but also discussing important hereditary associations.

## ADRENAL INCIDENTALOMA

Adrenal incidentalomas are defined as adrenal masses larger than 1 cm that are inadvertently discovered in the course of diagnostic evaluation or treatment of another medical condition.[1] This excludes masses found in the setting of imaging performed to detect metastatic disease in a patient with a known malignancy since 75% of such masses are metastases.[2] Adrenal incidentalomas are estimated to be present in 1.5% to 9.0% of people and are found in up to 5.0% of patients undergoing computed tomography of the abdomen.[3] In general, the lesions are small (<3–4 cm), men and women are equally affected, and they are most commonly detected in patients in their sixth decade of life.[4] A list of underlying lesions responsible for incidentalomas is presented in Table 1.[1] There are 2 main factors to consider when deciding whether an incidentaloma should be surgically removed. The first is the functional status of the tumor, and the second is the risk of malignancy. Roughly 10% of incidentalomas are functional and fewer than 5% are malignant (see Table 1).[1] A 2002 National Institutes of Health state-of-the-science statement regarding the management of patients with incidentalomas elaborated the following abbreviated conclusions.[2] Patients with biochemical evidence of a pheochromocytoma should be surgically treated. Additionally, surgery should be considered for patients with clinically apparent functional cortical tumors. Data were deemed insufficient to advocate for surgery or nonsurgical management of tumors with subclinical hyperfunctioning adrenal cortical adenomas. Because of the higher risk of malignancy with increased tumor size (adrenal cortical carcinomas account for <2% of tumors that are ≤4 cm, 6% of tumors that are 4.1–6 cm, and 25% of those >6 cm), it was advised that tumors larger than 6 cm should be surgically removed, those smaller than 4 cm could be followed, and those 4 to 6 cm require additional clinical data to determine whether surgery is appropriate.

The authors have no conflicts of interest to disclose.
Department of Pathology, Brigham and Women's Hospital, Harvard Medical School, 75 Francis Street, Boston, MA 02115, USA
* Corresponding author.
E-mail address: jbarletta@partners.org

Surgical Pathology 8 (2015) 725–749
http://dx.doi.org/10.1016/j.path.2015.07.005
1875-9181/15/$ – see front matter © 2015 Elsevier Inc. All rights reserved.

Table 1
Etiology of incidentalomas

| Cause | Prevalence, %, Approximate |
|-------|----------------------------|
| Adrenal cortical adenoma | 80 |
| Functional | 10 |
| Adrenal cortical carcinoma | 2 |
| Pheochromocytoma | 3 |
| Metastases | 1 |
| Other causes[a] | 15% |

[a] Includes adrenal cortical nodules, adrenal cysts, myelolipomas, hematomas/hemorrhage, infection.
Data from Cawood TJ, Hunt PJ, O'Shea D, et al. Recommended evaluation of adrenal incidentalomas is costly, has high false-positive rates and confers a risk of fatal cancer that is similar to the risk of the adrenal lesion becoming malignant; time for a rethink? Euro J Endocrinol 2009;161(4):513–27.

## ADRENAL CORTICAL ADENOMA

When evaluating an adrenal cortical adenoma, it is helpful to know the functional status of the tumor. Tumors that produce aldosterone are almost always benign; whereas, production of sex steroids is an ominous sign because there are only rare reports of benign adenomas with sex steroid production. Production of glucocorticoids is seen with adenomas and carcinomas, although because of the much higher frequency of adrenal adenomas compared with adrenal cortical carcinoma, the vast majority of tumors that produce cortisol will be adenomas. Most adenomas are small (<5 cm) and solitary. Grossly, most adenomas are yellow, solid, homogeneous, and well circumscribed (Fig. 1A). Some tumors may appear heterogeneous depending on variable cytoplasmic lipid content of tumor cells: a brighter yellow color is seen with higher cytoplasmic lipid and a more tan color with lipid depletion. Secondary changes, such as cystic degeneration and hemorrhage, also can occur (see Fig. 1B). Grossly, aldosterone-producing tumors may be slightly brighter yellow ("canary yellow") compared with cortisol-producing tumors. Rarely, cortisol-producing adenomas can be dark or even black in color (see Fig. 1C). Ultimately, functional status cannot be determined with certainty by gross evaluation.

Histologically, most adenomas are well circumscribed with a pushing border; however, in some cases a thin fibrous capsule is present (Fig. 2A). Most adenomas are similar in appearance to the zona fasciculata (see Fig. 2B). The architecture is generally nested or alveolar and less frequently corded or trabecular. The cells are slightly larger than those of fasciculata, but have the same vacuolated clear cytoplasm, small nuclei, and variably distinct nucleoli. The vacuolated cytoplasm is secondary to the high lipid content, which can be demonstrated by an oil-red-O stain. Some tumors have a more heterogeneous microscopic appearance (see Fig. 2C). Adenomas associated with aldosterone production are predominantly composed of cells similar to fasciculata; however, some tumors may have populations of cells that appear like fasciculata, glomerulosa, and reticularis admixed. Tumors resected in the setting of spironolactone treatment for an aldosterone-producing adenoma may demonstrate "spironolactone bodies," which are cytoplasmic laminated inclusions composed of aldosterone seen in compact cells with eosinophilic cytoplasm (glomerulosa-like cells of the adenoma) (see Fig. 2D). Adenomas associated with cortisol production are often also composed of cells similar to fasciculata, but again there may be some heterogeneity with lipid-depleted cells admixed. Lipofuscin pigment is often present in these lipid-depleted cells (see Fig. 2E), and abundant lipofuscin explains the black adenomas described previously. Functional status cannot be determined with certainty with histologic evaluation. However, tumors associated with cortisol production more frequently have intracytoplasmic lipofuscin and myelolipomatous metaplasia, whereas spironolactone bodies are virtually diagnostic of spironolactone treatment, and thus an aldosterone-producing adenoma. Additionally, non-neoplastic cortical atrophy can often be discerned with cortisol-producing adenomas. In contrast, the cortex adjacent to aldosterone-producing adenomas may be normal or even show hyperplasia of the glomerulosa layer ("paradoxic hyperplasia") with the normally patchy glomerulosa layer forming a thick band beneath the adrenal capsule. Scattered cells or small clusters with marked nuclear atypia (Fuhrman nuclear grade 3 or 4) can be seen in benign adenomas regardless of functional status (see Fig. 2F). This atypia alone does not warrant a diagnosis of malignancy. In contrast, mitoses are very rarely seen in adenomas (<1 mitosis/50 high-power fields [HPFs] is typical), and atypical mitoses are virtually confined to carcinomas.

Adrenal cortical adenomas are not typically a diagnostic dilemma; however, occasionally, distinguishing an adenoma from a non-neoplastic adrenal cortical nodule or even normal cortex can be a challenge. Non-neoplastic adrenal cortical nodules are frequently seen in the setting of old age, hypertension, and diabetes. These nodules are

*Fig. 1.* Gross photographs of adrenal cortical adenomas showing (*A*) the typical well-circumscribed, solid, yellow appearance; (*B*) a tumor with cystic degeneration; and (*C*) a cortisol-producing adenoma with abundant lipofuscin imparting a brown color grossly.

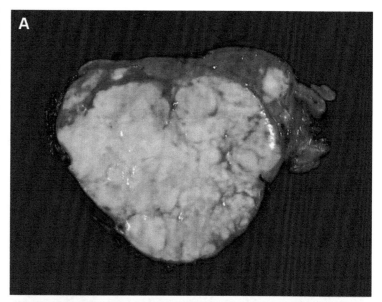

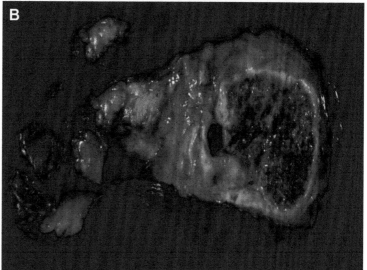

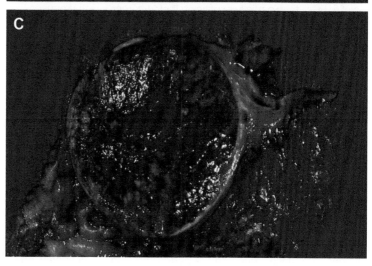

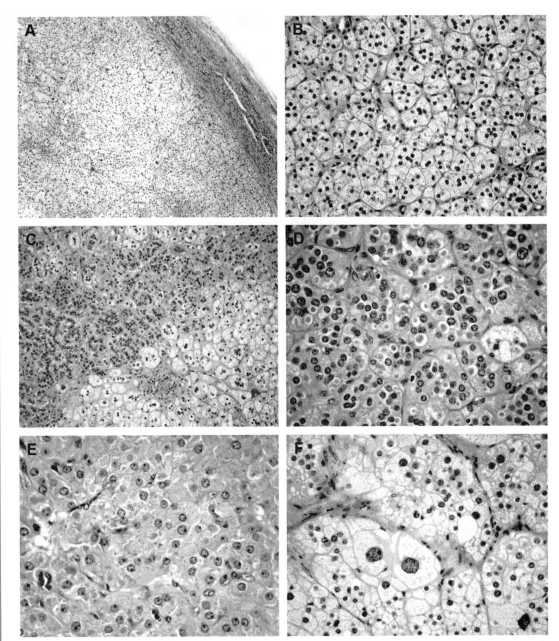

*Fig. 2.* Histology of adrenal cortical adenomas showing (*A*) a tumor at low power that has a thin fibrous capsule, (*B*) the typical morphology with tumor cells appearing similar to those of zona fasciculata, (*C*) a tumor that is more heterogeneous histologically with cells resembling fasciculata admixed with others more similar in appearance to glomerulosa, (*D*) an aldosterone-producing adenoma that was treated with spironolactone showing numerous spironolactone bodies, (*E*) a cortisol-producing adenoma with abundant lipofuscin pigment, and (*F*) an adenoma with scattered cells demonstrating a high Fuhrman nuclear grade.

thought to be compensating for adjacent adrenal atrophy arising as a result of vascular insufficiency of adrenal arterioles. Non-neoplastic nodules also can be seen in patients with aldosterone-producing adenomas, and these nodules are thought to arise due to hypertension. In most cases, non-neoplastic adrenal cortical nodules are multifocal and bilateral; however, dominant nodules can occur and so occasionally clinical/radiologic correlation may be required to differentiate a nonfunctional adenoma from a dominant non-neoplastic adrenal cortical nodule.

Occasionally it can be difficult to distinguish a benign adenoma from normal adrenal cortex due to the tissue provided (i.e, limited tissue in the setting of the rare adrenal core biopsy or fragmented tissue in the setting of morcellation). If a biopsy is entirely composed of cells that are similar in appearance to fasciculata cells, this could favor adenoma; however, it should be noted that the cells of an adenoma are somewhat larger when compared with the normal fasciculata cells. As noted previously, some adenomas are composed of cells with a more heterogeneous appearance. In core biopsies of such cases, knowing that adenomas can appear cytologically heterogeneous is helpful. Finally, correlating the histologic features with clinical and radiologic findings is important.

## ADRENOCORTICAL CARCINOMA

### OVERVIEW

In contrast to adrenal cortical adenomas, adrenocortical carcinomas (ACCs) are extremely rare, with an estimated annual incidence of 0.5 to 2.0 cases per million.[5] The average age at presentation is slightly under 50 years (though ACC demonstrates a bimodal distribution with a first peak in early childhood and a second higher peak in adults), and a female predominance is reported in most studies.[6–9] Approximately half of ACCs are functional.[6,8] Cortisol production is most common, either alone or in combination with a sex steroid; less commonly, sex steroids are produced in isolation, and, although rare, aldosterone-producing ACCs do occur.[6,8] In an analysis of Surveillance, Epidemiology, and End Results data, approximately 40% of patients had localized disease, whereas more than half had locally invasive disease, lymph node involvement, or distant metastases.[9] The overall 5-year survival for patients with ACC is 35% to 40%,[6,8,9] with patients with localized disease demonstrating a significantly better outcome than those with distant metastatic disease at presentation (5-year survival 62% compared with 7%, respectively).[9] Most patients develop distant metastatic disease during follow-up, with lung, liver, and bone being the most frequent metastatic sites.[6]

### GROSS FEATURES

ACCs are usually large, heavy tumors. The average size is 10 to 12 cm, and the average weight is approximately 300 g.[6,7,9] Although a large size and weight are worrisome features for an adrenal cortical tumor, tumors smaller than 5 cm and less than 100 g can pursue an aggressive

clinical course.[9,10] The tumors are yellow/tan to red/brown depending on the associated steroid production (cortisol-producing tumors are generally yellow/tan whereas sex-steroid–producing ACCs are red/brown). Fibrous septa, necrosis, and hemorrhage are frequent findings, and rare cases of ACC are cystic.[11] Many ACCs are clearly malignant on gross examination alone, based on a combination of tumor size, presence of necrosis, invasion into adjacent tissues, or gross involvement of associated lymph nodes (Fig. 3).

## MICROSCOPIC FEATURES AND CRITERIA FOR MALIGNANCY

Histologically, ACCs can range from fairly uniform to highly heterogeneous. Many ACCs are predominantly composed of small cuboidal cells with eosinophilic cytoplasm with scattered markedly enlarged cells with bizarre nuclei (Fig. 4A, B). Necrosis and increased mitotic activity, including atypical mitoses, is common (see Fig. 4C, D). Tumors can be very hepatoid in appearance (a fact to keep in mind when evaluating core biopsy specimens of a "liver mass") or can show a rhabdoid cytomorphology (which is significant when considering whether a biopsy might represent a high-grade renal cell carcinoma with a rhabdoid component vs an ACC; the former is PAX8 positive and the latter is PAX8 negative; see later in this article for more detail). In some tumors clear cells predominate. In cases with this morphology, metastatic disease and pleomorphic liposarcoma should be considered in the differential diagnosis (approximately a quarter of pleomorphic liposarcomas have an epithelioid morphology resulting in a striking overlap with ACC). Although most tumors are histologically malignant throughout, some tumors have areas that may not be diagnostic of malignancy (Fig. 5). This is an important fact to keep in mind when evaluating core biopsy specimens of adrenal masses. Thus, although some core biopsy specimens may be diagnostic of malignancy, others are not. In core biopsies lacking histologic features of malignancy, it is prudent to indicate that although no features of malignancy are seen in this small core biopsy specimen, clinical and radiologic correlation is required.

The most widely used criteria for malignancy were proposed by Weiss[12] 3 decades ago based on the investigator's assessment of 43 adrenocortical tumors. The 9 histologic features of the Weiss criteria are as follows: mitotic activity (>5 per 50 HPFs), presence of atypical mitoses, necrosis, high nuclear grade, venous invasion,

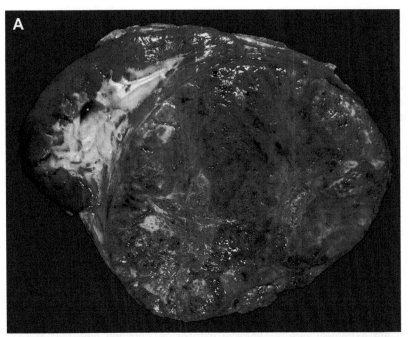

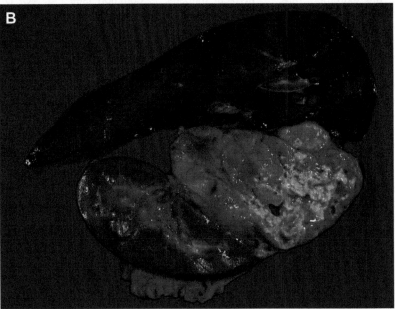

*Fig. 3.* Gross photographs of adrenocortical carcinoma showing (*A*) a large tumor with hemorrhage and necrosis that grossly distorted the kidney, and (*B*) a tumor with central necrosis that grossly invaded the inferior vena cava and liver.

sinusoidal invasion, capsular invasion, diffuse growth accounting for more than one-third of the tumor, and clear cells comprising ≤25% of the tumor (**Table 2**). Mitotic activity should be assessed by evaluating the most proliferative area of 5 tumor slides (with 10 HPFs assessed on each slide); however, if fewer than 5 tumor slides are available, then more fields should be counted per slide so that a total of 50 fields is achieved. Atypical mitoses are defined as those with an abnormal

chromosomal distribution or an excessive number of mitotic spindles resulting in a multipolar appearance. Necrosis requires the involvement of a confluent area of cells (ie, apoptotic cells alone do not suffice). High nuclear grade is based on Fuhrman criteria, with Fuhrman grade 3 or 4 warranting a designation as high grade. In heterogeneous tumors, nuclear grade is based on the highest degree of atypia within the tumor, even if that atypia is focal. Venous invasion implies

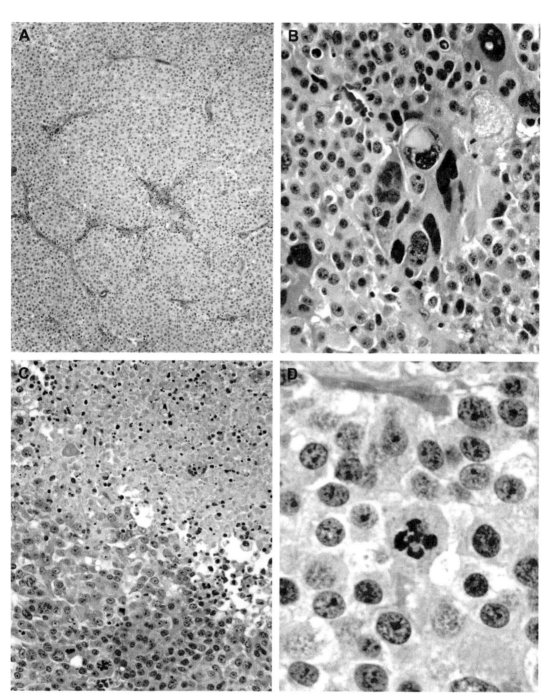

*Fig. 4.* Histology of adrenocortical carcinoma showing (*A*) a tumor at low power that has a diffuse architecture and is composed entirely of cells with eosinophilic cytoplasm, (*B*) high Fuhrman nuclear grade that is present in most tumors, (*C*) necrosis, and (*D*) atypical mitoses.

invasion of an endothelial-lined structure with a wall containing smooth muscle, whereas sinusoidal invasion reflects invasion of vessels that lack smooth muscle. In both cases, the tumor should appear as plugs of cells or polypoid projections of tumor. Because free-floating tumor in vessels can be artifactual, this finding should be excluded when considering venous and sinusoidal invasion. Capsular invasion is defined as tumor invading into or entirely through the adrenal capsule with an associated stromal reaction. Diffuse architecture requires a sheeted-appearance, with all other

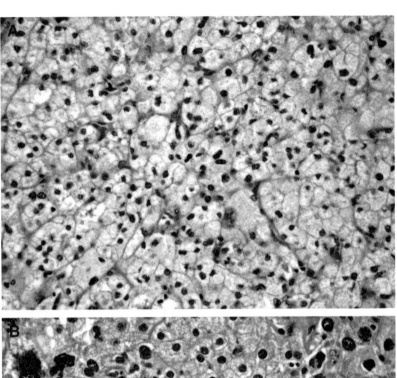

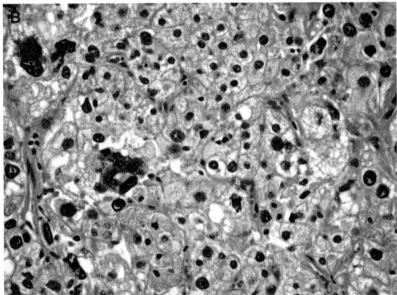

*Fig. 5.* Some adrenocortical carcinomas have areas that may not be diagnostic of malignancy as seen in (*A*), whereas other areas of the tumor (*B*) showed high Fuhrman nuclear grade, marked mitotic activity, and atypical mitoses.

growth patterns (ie, nested, trabecular, corded) considered nondiffuse. And last, clear cells imply cells similar in appearance to the cells of zona fasciculata.

Each histologic feature receives 1 point when present (no weighting of features) resulting in a total score of 0 to 9. Although the score for malignancy was initially set at 4 or more, in a study Weiss published 5 years later, the threshold was lowered from 4 to 3 based on a patient with a tumor with a score of 3 who developed local recurrence and subsequently died due to disease.[10] In this later study by Weiss, 76% of ACCs showed a mitotic count of more than 5 per 50 HPFs, 70% had

atypical mitoses, 90% had necrosis, 88% demonstrated a high Fuhrman nuclear grade, 50% had venous invasion, 57% had sinusoidal invasion, 57% had capsular penetration, 71% had a diffuse architecture comprising more than a third of the tumor, and 90% were composed of 25% or fewer cells with clear cytoplasm.[10] All tumors with fewer than 3 criteria pursued a benign clinical course, whereas 91% of patients with a tumor score of 3 or more developed recurrent or metastatic disease. The strongest predictor of clinical outcome was mitotic count. The investigators reported that patients with tumors with a mitotic count of more than 20 mitoses per 50 HPFs had a median survival

*Table 2*
**Weiss criteria for the assessment of malignant potential of adrenocortical tumors**

| Histologic Feature | Prevalence, % |
| --- | --- |
| >5 mitoses per 50 HPFs | 76 |
| Atypical mitoses | 70 |
| Necrosis | 90 |
| High nuclear grade | 88 |
| Venous invasion | 50 |
| Sinusoidal invasion | 57 |
| Capsular invasion | 57 |
| Diffuse growth >1/3rd of tumor | 71 |
| Clear cells ≤25% of the tumor | 90 |

3 or more criteria are required for a diagnosis of adrenocortical carcinoma.

*Adapted from* Weiss LM, Medeiros LJ, Vickery AL Jr. Pathologic features of prognostic significance in adrenocortical carcinoma. Am J Surg Pathol 1989;13(3):202–6.

of 14 months, whereas those with tumors with 20 or fewer mitoses per 50 HPFs had a median survival of 58 months (*P* = .02). Based on this finding, they proposed that tumors with more than 20 mitoses per 50 HPFs should be considered high grade, whereas those with 20 or fewer mitoses per 50 HPFs should be considered low grade. Subsequently, others have advocated for this grading system based on the fact that mitotic count is not only predictive of survival (with a doubling of the mitotic rate resulting in a 4.7-fold increase in relative risk of dying of ACC in the subsequent 5-year period), but also correlates with gene expression profiling.[13] Although many pathologists do not grade ACCs, all reports should indicate mitotic count per 50 HPFs because it clearly is of prognostic significance, and in some settings, may guide treatment (see also Elfiky, Adrenal Cortical Carcinoma: A Clinician's Perspective, Surgical Pathology Clinics, 2015, Volume 8, Issue 4).

Other systems have been proposed to distinguish benign from malignant adrenal cortical tumors. The system proposed by Hough and colleagues[14] weighs pathologic findings, including tumor mass, diffuse growth, vascular invasion, tumor necrosis, fibrous bands, capsular invasion, mitotic index, and nuclear pleomorphism, and in addition takes into account clinical data, including urinary ketosteroids, response to adrenocorticotropic hormone, presence (or absence) of Cushing syndrome or virilization, and weight loss. Because many of these clinical parameters are often not available to a pathologist, this system is not readily applied in most cases. In the system proposed by van Slooten and colleagues,[15] histologic findings

are weighted. Regressive changes (necrosis, hemorrhage, fibrosis, or calcification) receive 5.7 points, loss of normal structure 1.6 points, nuclear atypia 2.1 points, nuclear hyperchromasia 2.6 points, abnormal nucleoli 4.1 points, mitotic count of 2 per 10 HPFs 9 points, and capsular or vascular invasion 3.3 points. A score of more than 8 is associated with malignancy. Again, this system is not as easily used as the Weiss criteria. In 2002, Aubert and colleagues[16] proposed a modification of the Weiss system by eliminating criteria more prone to low interobserver reproducibility. Instead of the 9 histologic features assessed in the original Weiss system, 5 criteria were kept. Diffuse architecture, sinusoidal invasion, nuclear grade, and venous invasion were all eliminated because they had kappa values of less than 0.60. The following features were kept because all demonstrated substantial interobserver reproducibility (kappa value >0.60): mitotic count greater than 5 per 50 HPFs, 25% or fewer clear cells, abnormal mitoses, necrosis, and capsular invasion. A mitotic count of more than 5 per 50 HPFs and 25% or fewer clear cells both receive 2 points, whereas abnormal mitoses, necrosis, and capsular invasion all receive 1 point. A tumor can achieve a score of 0 to 7, and similar to the Weiss system, a score of 3 or more is considered indicative of malignancy. The validity of this modified Weiss system has subsequently been confirmed.[17] In 2009, an Italian group, again citing issues of reproducibility for some parameters of the Weiss system, proposed the "reticulin algorithm."[18] This algorithm defines malignancy through an altered reticulin framework associated with 1 of 3 additional parameters: necrosis, high mitotic rate (>5 per 50 HPFs), and venous invasion. An altered reticulin network is defined as either a quantitative loss of the reticulin network that is seen in normal or adenomatous cortex or a qualitative change. Tumors with a quantitative change demonstrate areas of tumor lacking the reticulin network altogether (**Fig. 6**), whereas cases with a qualitative change have an intact network composed of irregularly thickened or frayed fibers. A subsequent study demonstrated substantial interobserver reproducibility in assessing whether the reticulin network is normal or altered.[19] Although the modified Weiss system and reticulin algorithm both seem valid and potentially reproducible, the original Weiss criteria are still used by most pathologists to assess the malignant potential of adrenocortical tumors.

## VARIANT ADRENOCORTICAL TUMORS

There are 2 rare adrenocortical "variants" that deserve special mention because assessment of

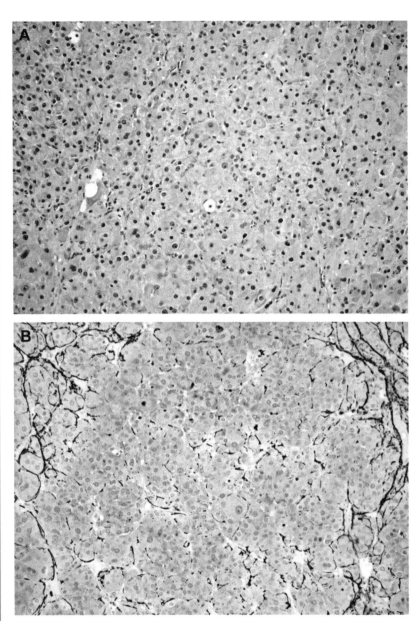

Fig. 6. An adrenocortical carcinoma. (A) Hematoxylin and eosin (H&E) showing a tumor with a vaguely hepatoid appearance. (B) A paired reticulin stain showing a quantitative loss in the normal reticulin network.

their malignant potential is especially challenging. Oncocytic adrenocortical tumors are rare with only 147 cases described in the literature as of 2012.[20] These tumors are usually incidentally discovered (20%–50% are functional, most commonly producing cortisol, although sex steroid and aldosterone production have also been reported), present at a mean age of 47 years (range 27–72), and demonstrate a female predominance (2.5:1.0).[20,21] Oncocytic adrenocortical tumors are typically larger than their non-oncocytic counterparts with a mean size of 8 cm (range 2–20 cm).[20] They are grossly well circumscribed and have a brown/mahogany cut surface. They

are composed entirely or nearly entirely of oncocytic cells with abundant granular eosinophilic cytoplasm secondary to an accumulation of mitochondria within the cytoplasm. As Lin and colleagues[22] discussed in their description of 7 oncocytic adrenocortical neoplasms, these tumors by definition have 25% or fewer clear cells, and nearly always have a diffuse growth pattern, as well as high-grade nuclear atypia with frequent eosinophilic nuclear pseudo-inclusions (Fig. 7A, B), regardless of whether they are benign or malignant. As a result, most oncocytic adrenocortical tumors inherently have a Weiss score of 3. Due to this observation, in 2004 Bisceglia and

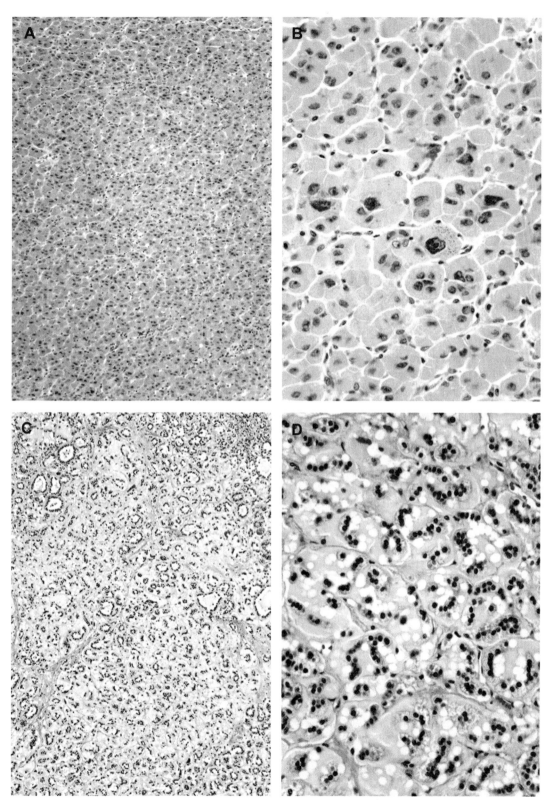

*Fig. 7.* Variant adrenocortical tumors. An oncocytic adrenocortical tumor: (*A*) at low power the tumor has a diffuse architecture, and (*B*) at high power the cells have abundant granular eosinophilic cytoplasm and nuclei with a focally high Fuhrman nuclear grade. A myxoid adrenocortical tumor: (*C*) at low power the tumor cells appear to be floating within a myxoid stroma, and (*D*) at high power the cells have a corded architecture, are small, uniform and bland.

colleagues[23] recommended altered criteria to assess malignancy in pure (defined as tumors with >90% oncocytic cells) oncocytic adrenocortical neoplasms. The major criteria of this system (often referred to as the Lin-Weiss-Bisceglia system) include a mitotic count of greater than 5 per 50 HPFs, atypical mitoses, and venous invasion, whereas minor criteria include a size larger than 10 cm or a weight of more than 200 g, necrosis, capsular invasion, or sinusoidal invasion (Box 1). If any major criteria are present, the tumor should be considered malignant, if any minor criteria are present, the tumor should be considered of uncertain malignant potential, and if no criteria are present, then the tumor can be considered benign. These criteria are not to be used for adrenocortical tumors with fewer than 90% oncocytic cells. In cases with a lesser oncocytic component, use of Weiss criteria has been advocated. However, given the rarity of such cases, a note indicating some degree of uncertainty of malignant potential is probably warranted. Interestingly, the reticulin algorithm (described previously) has been shown to be helpful in both pure oncocytic adrenocortical tumors and those with a lesser oncocytic component.[19] The prognosis of oncocytic ACCs appears to be somewhat better than that of non-oncocytic ACCs, and most, although not all, borderline tumors have pursued a benign clinical course.[19,21]

Even more uncommon than oncocytic tumors are myxoid adrenocortical tumors. These tumors are often functional (most commonly producing cortisol, although sex steroid and aldosterone production have also been reported), present at a mean age of roughly 50, and demonstrate a female predominance.[24] The mean tumor size is approximately 12 cm (range 2–20 cm), and on cut section, tumors with an abundant myxoid component appear translucent gray or white.[24] Histologically, the myxoid component can comprise 5% to 95% of the tumor. Tumors that are largely myxoid are characterized by a uniform population of small regular cells (often with cells reminiscent to those of zona glomerulosa) with a corded, nested, pseudoglandular, or microcystic architecture (see Fig. 7C, D). ACCs may also show focal myxoid change. In these cases, the cells resemble conventional ACC. Myxoid tumors are evaluated by Weiss criteria. Although benign myxoid adrenocortical tumors with reasonable follow-up time have been reported, the amount of follow-up data are limited and there is one case in the literature that pursued a malignant course despite a Weiss score of 1.[24,25] Therefore, for cases with myxoid features that do not meet Weiss criteria for malignancy, it might be best to consider these tumors of uncertain malignant potential.

## IMMUNOHISTOCHEMISTRY

The immunohistochemical profile of ACCs is summarized in Table 3. ACCs are positive for inhibin, synaptophysin, A103 (Melan-A), calretinin, and SF-1 (steroidogenic factor 1); negative to weakly positive for keratins (Cam5.2 shows the most expression); negative for PAX8; and virtually always negative for chromogranin.[26] Markers like inhibin and Melan-A are highly specific for ACC. Pheochromocytomas and virtually all carcinomas that might metastasize to the adrenal are negative for these 2 markers. However, the sensitivity of inhibin and Melan-A is 70% to 90%, with inhibin being more sensitive than Melan-A.[26,27] As a result, SF-1 has become a very useful stain, as nuclear SF-1 expression is both very specific and very sensitive for ACC, with a sensitivity of 95% (Fig. 8).[27,28] This transcription factor is expressed in steroidogenic organs like the adrenal glands, testes, and ovaries, and plays a key role in the development of steroidogenic tissue and the regulation of steroid biosynthesis.[27] Additionally, there is some evidence that tumors with a high level of SF-1 expression may be more clinically aggressive than tumors with low-level SF-1 expression.[27] Chromogranin is often used when trying to differentiate an ACC from a pheochromocytoma because pheochromocytomas are positive for both synaptophysin and chromogranin. The vast majority of ACCs are negative for chromogranin; however, rare cases of ACC may show some degree of chromogranin expression.[26]

*Table 3*
Immunohistochemical profile of pheochromocytomas and adrenocortical carcinomas

| | Pheochromocytoma | Adrenocortical Carcinoma |
|---|---|---|
| Chromogranin | Positive | Negative[a] |
| Synaptophysin | Positive | Positive |
| MelanA103/Mart-1 | Negative[a] | Positive |
| Calretinin | Negative[a] | Positive |
| Inhibin | Negative[a] | Positive |
| PAX8 | Negative | Negative |
| Keratins | Negative[a] | Weak/Negative |
| SF-1 | Negative | Positive |
| GATA3 | Positive | Usually negative[b] |

[a] <5% of cases are positive.
[b] ~10% of cases are positive.

Although these rare cases do not decrease the utility of chromogranin, they do indicate that immunohistochemical stains should be part of a broader panel and their results need to be interpreted in the context of the morphology of the tumor.

There are also several immunohistochemical stains that have been reported either to aid in the assessment of malignant potential of adrenocortical tumors or have prognostic value in the setting of ACC. The Ki-67 proliferative index has been consistently shown to be higher in ACC than in adenomas. However, while the vast majority of adenomas have a Ki-67 proliferative index of less than 5%,[29,30] not all ACCs will demonstrate a proliferative index of greater than 5%. This means that although a proliferative index above 5% warrants concern, tumors with a proliferative index less than 5% cannot be assumed to be benign. As a consequence, many pathologists do not routinely report a Ki-67 proliferative index. But this may soon change, because a recent study by Beuschlein and colleagues[7] has provided compelling evidence that Ki-67 is a strong predictor of outcome that could guide therapy in localized ACCs (see also Elfiky, Adrenal Cortical Carcinoma: A Clinician's Perspective, Surgical Pathology Clinics, 2015, Volume 8, Issue 4). They found that Ki-67 indices of less than 10%, 10% to 19%, and 20% or more provided highly significant differences for both recurrence-free survival (RFS) and overall survival (OS), translating into a median RFS and a median OS of 53.2 and 180.5 months for patients with tumors with a Ki-67 proliferative index of less than 10%, 31.6 and 113.5 months for patients with tumors with a Ki-67 proliferative index of 10% to 19%, and 9.4 and 42.0 months for patients with tumors with a Ki-67 proliferative index

of 20% or more. Moreover, they demonstrated that the prognostic value of the Ki-67 proliferative index was maintained in multivariate analysis, and they confirmed the prognostic significance of the Ki-67 proliferative index in a second validation cohort. Additional markers that are preferentially expressed in ACCs compared with adenomas include insulin-like growth factor-2 (IGF2), matrix metalloprotease type 2 (MMP2), p53, and aberrant cytoplasmic/nuclear localization of B-catenin.[29,31,32] Erickson and colleagues[31] reported that IGF2 is expressed at a higher frequency and at a higher level in ACCs compared with carcinomas, but their results also indicated that IGF2 expression does not definitively reflect malignancy. Volante and colleagues[32] reported that approximately 75% of ACCs showed focal to diffuse MMP2 expression compared with only 2% of adenomas; thus, MMP2 expression could be used to support a malignant diagnosis, but could not be used to exclude it. Similarly, although p53 overexpression is virtually confined to carcinomas, it is seen in a relatively small percentage of ACCs.[33] Finally, although diffuse aberrant cytoplasmic/nuclear B-catenin expression has been seen more in the setting of ACCs compared with adrenocortical adenomas, a subset of adenomas harbor B-catenin mutations, and therefore aberrant B-catenin expression is not definitive for malignancy.[34]

## PHEOCHROMOCYTOMA

### OVERVIEW

Pheochromocytomas arise from catecholamine-producing chromaffin cells of the adrenal medulla. They are rare tumors with an average age at diagnosis of 40 to 45 years and a roughly equal

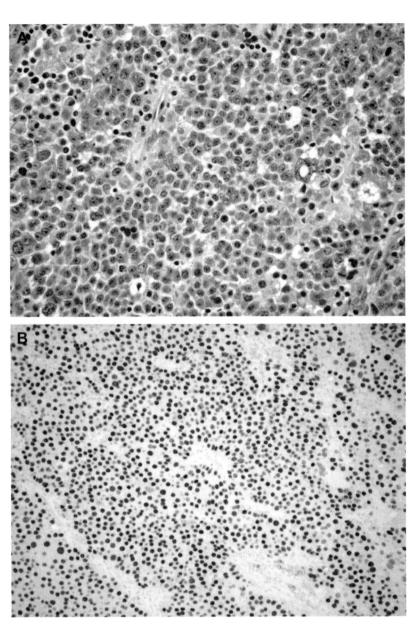

*Fig. 8.* An ACC. (*A*) H&E showing a tumor composed of cells with scant amphophilic cytoplasm, and (*B*) a paired SF-1 immunohistochemical stain, a highly sensitive and specific stain for ACC.

sex distribution.[35] The signs and symptoms of pheochromocytoma are secondary to catecholamine excess and include hypertension (either sustained or paroxysmal), tachycardia, headaches, palpitations, diaphoresis, chest pain, anxiety, and weight loss. Although most patients are hypertensive, roughly 10% are not. It is commonly thought that 10% of pheochromocytomas are malignant; however, that percentage is closer to 5% with the 10% reflecting inclusion of extra-adrenal sympathetic paragangliomas (see also Arias-Stella and Williamson, Updates in Benign Lesions of the Genitourinary Tract, Surgical Pathology Clinics, 2015, Volume 8, Issue 4), which have a higher

rate of malignancy.[35] For patients with malignant pheochromocytomas, the 5-year survival is approximately 50%.[36]

## GROSS FEATURES

Pheochromocytomas are encapsulated or well-circumscribed tumors with a pink/tan cut surface (**Fig. 9**A). Hemorrhage is frequent, and larger tumors may also demonstrate cystic change (see **Fig. 9**B, C). It may be evident that the tumor is arising from the medulla; however, this can be difficult to appreciate when the tumor is large. Sporadic pheochromocytomas are almost always

*Fig. 9.* Gross photographs of a pheo-chromocytoma showing (*A*) the typical well-circumscribed, solid, tan/pink appearance, (*B*) a tumor with areas of hemorrhage, and (*C*) a tumor with cystic degeneration.

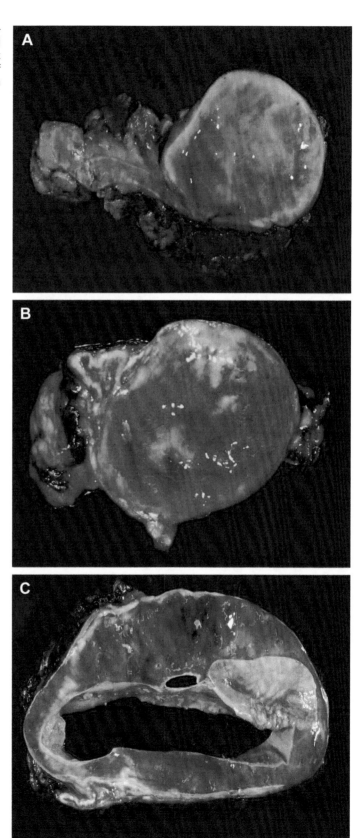

solitary masses, whereas familial cases are more frequently bilateral and, in the setting of multiple endocrine neoplasia 2 (MEN) 2, may arise in a background of diffuse or nodular medullary hyperplasia.

## MICROSCOPIC FEATURES

Pheochromocytomas are microscopically well demarcated from the adjacent adrenal tissue with some tumors demonstrating a thin fibrous capsule. Characteristically these tumors have "zellballen" (cell balls) morphology; that is, an alveolar architecture with nests of neuroendocrine cells surrounded by delicate blood vessels and sustentacular cells (Fig. 10A). The zellballen architecture in some tumors is difficult to appreciate with the architecture appearing more diffuse or solid (see Fig. 10B). The cytology of the tumor cells typically resembles non-neoplastic chromaffin cells: they are intermediate to large in size with abundant amphophilic to basophilic, granular cytoplasm (see Fig. 10). However, in some cases the cells may be smaller and may have clear cytoplasm (Fig. 11A), mimicking an adrenal cortical adenoma or a renal cell carcinoma. Other tumors may have a moderate amount of eosinophilic cytoplasm (see

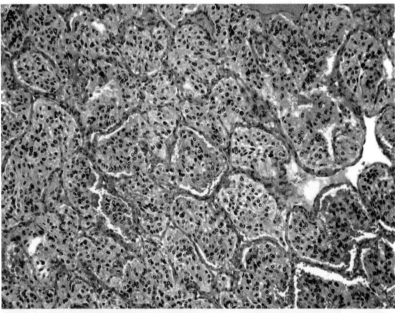

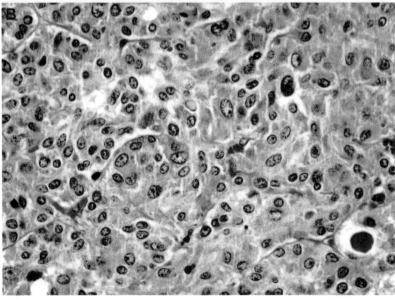

*Fig. 10.* Histology of pheochromocytomas showing (*A*) the zellballen growth pattern, and (*B*) the typical cytomorphology, with tumor cells with abundant granular amphophilic cytoplasm.

*Fig. 11.* Some pheochromocytomas (*A*) are composed of smaller cells with clear cytoplasm (that may raise the differential diagnosis of an adrenocortical adenoma or a renal cell carcinoma), whereas others (*B*) are composed of cells with eosinophilic cytoplasm (that may raise the diagnosis of adrenocortical carcinoma).

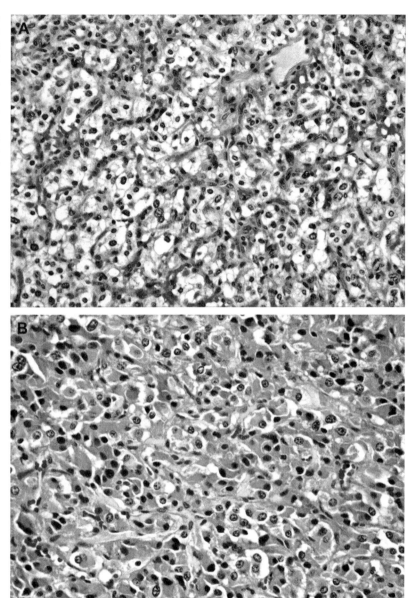

Fig. 11B), resulting in a tumor that resembles ACC. Intracytoplasmic eosinophilic hyaline globules are often present (these Periodic-acid-Schiff–positive globules are likely derived from the membrane components of secretory granules) (**Fig. 12A**). The tumor cell nuclei may be pleomorphic, hyperchromatic, or spindled (see **Fig. 12B**). Sustentacular cells within pheochromocytomas are generally inconspicuous on hematoxylin and eosin, but can be highlighted by S100 immunohistochemical staining (**Fig. 13A, B**). These support cells, although actually non-neoplastic, can even populate metastatic deposits.

## CRITERIA FOR MALIGNANCY

There are no universally accepted histologic findings to classify a pheochromocytoma as benign or malignant. Instead, malignancy is defined simply by the presence of metastatic disease. To exclude multicentric disease, the metastatic site must be one that normally lacks chromaffin tissue (ie, lymph nodes, bone, liver, and lung). Surprisingly, both locally invasive growth and lymphovascular invasion are poor predictors of metastasis, as tumors that are confined to the adrenal may subsequently metastasize, and benign tumors

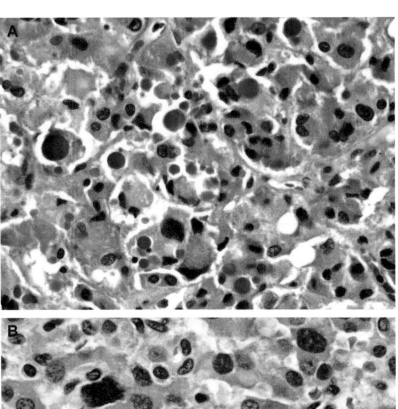

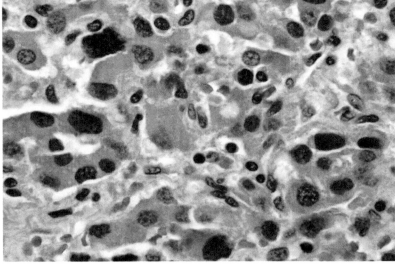

*Fig. 12.* Some pheochromocytomas (*A*) have numerous eosinophilic hyaline globules. (*B*) Nuclear atypia and hyperchromasia is often seen in pheochromocytomas and is not indicative of malignancy.

without known metastatic disease may show lymphovascular invasion. In a 1990 study by Linnoila and colleagues,[37] the investigators evaluated 120 pheochromocytomas and extra-adrenal sympathetic paragangliomas and found that more than 70% could be classified as benign or malignant on the basis of extra-adrenal location (with a significantly higher percentage of extra-adrenal sympathetic paragangliomas being malignant than pheochromocytomas, 52% compared with 6%, respectively), coarse nodularity of the primary tumor, confluent necrosis, and absence of hyaline globules. Most (71%) malignant tumors had 2 to 3 of these characteristics, whereas 89% of benign

tumors had only 1 or none of these features. In 2002, Thompson[36] proposed the "pheochromocytoma of the adrenal gland scaled score" (PASS) to separate benign from malignant tumors. He evaluated 100 pheochromocytomas from the files of the Armed Forces Institute of Pathology, 50 of which were malignant based on his histologic criteria and 50 of which were benign. Neither size nor weight distinguished benign from malignant cases, and no one histologic parameter predicted malignancy. However, malignant pheochromocytomas more frequently demonstrated vascular invasion (1 point), capsular invasion (1 point), invasion into periadrenal adipose tissue (2 points),

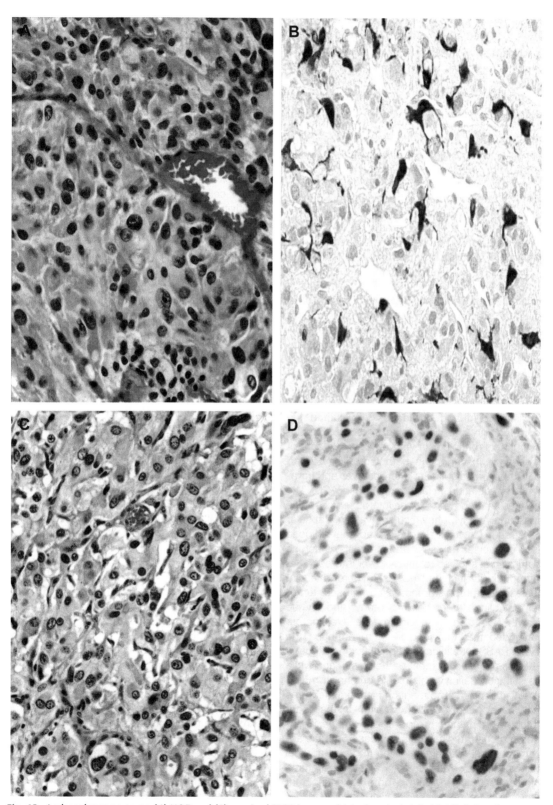

*Fig. 13.* A pheochromocytoma (*A*) H&E and (*B*) a paired S100 immunohistochemical stain highlighting the sustentacular cells within the tumor. A pheochromocytoma (*C*) H&E and (*D*) a paired GATA3 immunohistochemical stain that is often positive in pheochromocytomas and paragangliomas.

focal or confluent necrosis (2 points), large nests (defined as 3–4 times the size of a zellballen nest) or confluent growth (2 points), high cellularity (2 points), a mitotic count greater than 3 per 10 HPFs (2 points), atypical mitoses (2 points), tumor cell spindling (2 points), cellular monotony (2 points), profound nuclear pleomorphism (1 point), and hyperchromasia (1 point). Tumors with a PASS score of 4 or more were deemed to have potential for biologically aggressive behavior, with 33 of 50 tumors in this category demonstrating a malignant clinical course. Tumors with a score of less than 4 all demonstrated a benign clinical course over a 10-year follow-up period. Appropriately, the investigator indicated that a score of 4 or more could not be equated with malignancy, given that 34% of such tumors in his cohort were not clinically malignant; however, he indicated that these tumors are more at risk for pursuing a malignant clinical course and so deserve closer clinical follow-up. Thompson[36] also found that malignant tumors had a decrease in the number of sustentacular cells as assessed by S100 immunohistochemical staining. This finding is consistent with other reports, and likely reflects the histologic observation that malignant tumors tend to have a more diffuse architecture. After the PASS was published, Wu and colleagues[38] evaluated the reproducibility of PASS among a group of 5 multi-institutional pathologists with at least 10 years of experience in endocrine pathology. They found that there was significant interobserver and intraobserver variation in assignment of PASS. The features that showed higher interobserver reproducibility were lymphovascular invasion, capsular penetration, invasion into extra-adrenal adipose tissue, atypical mitoses, and necrosis, whereas features that showed relatively lower interobserver reproducibility included nuclear hyperchromasia, nuclear pleomorphism, increased mitoses, tumor cell spindling, tumor cell monotony, and diffuse growth. Based on these findings, the investigators concluded that they could not recommend the use of PASS for clinical prognostication. Although PASS is not used by most pathologists, and while we still lack definitive histologic criteria of malignancy, it is prudent to mention histologic features that have been associated with a malignant outcome in a pathology report. For example, if a tumor demonstrates necrosis, increased mitotic activity, atypical mitoses, invasion into peri-adrenal adipose tissue, or vascular invasion, these features should be reported, with a note indicating that although there are no definite histologic criteria for malignancy in pheochromocytomas, the tumor demonstrates concerning histologic findings and close clinical follow-up is advised.

## IMMUNOHISTOCHEMISTRY

The immunohistochemical profile of pheochromocytomas is summarized in Table 3. Pheochromocytomas exhibit immunopositivity for synaptophysin and chromogranin A. Keratins are almost always negative (which is useful when distinguishing a pheochromocytoma/paraganglioma from a neuroendocrine carcinoma), although cases of pheochromocytoma with keratin positivity have been reported.[36] The sustentacular cells are positive for S-100 protein, and rarely the chromaffin cells may exhibit some degree of S100 positivity. Pheochromocytomas are negative for SF1, inhibin, calretinin, and Melan-A. Recently the transcription factor GATA3 has been shown to be positive in pheochromocytomas and paragangliomas (see Fig. 13C, D). Miettinen and colleagues[39] reported GATA3 positivity in 82% of paragangliomas and 92% of pheochromocytomas. Along with keratins, it appears that GATA3 can be helpful in differentiating pheochromocytoma/paraganglioma from other neuroendocrine tumors, such as small cell carcinoma, Merkel cell carcinoma, pulmonary carcinoid, and small intestine and pancreatic neuroendocrine tumors, as all these tumors lacked GATA3 expression in the cohort of Miettinen and colleagues.[39] It should be noted that GATA3 was positive in 11% of ACCs evaluated in this study; thus, it is not a good stain to use to differentiate pheochromocytoma from an ACC.

### Hereditary Syndromes

For years it was thought that 10% of pheochromocytomas were hereditary; however, we now know that the percentage is roughly doubled if considering pheochromocytomas alone and more than tripled if pheochromocytomas and paragangliomas are grouped together.[35,40] Pheochromocytomas were known to be associated with MEN2A and 2B (with an underlying activating mutation in the RET proto-oncogene that results in activation of the encoded tyrosine kinase receptor), VHL disease (with an underlying inactivating mutation in the tumor suppressor gene VHL), and NF1 (with an underlying mutation in the NF1 tumor suppressor gene) (Table 4). The risk of developing a pheochromocytoma in these syndromes is 50% for MEN2A and 2B, 10% to 26% for VHL disease, and 0.1% to 6% for NF1.[41] Although MEN2 syndromes demonstrate the highest penetrance for the development of a pheochromocytoma, given that VHL disease is more common, VHL accounts for a higher percentage of hereditary pheochromocytomas. Although patients with VHL and NF1 develop pheochromocytomas more frequently

**Table 4**
Main hereditary syndromes with pheochromocytomas and/or paragangliomas

| Syndrome | Mutation | Proportion of All PCCs/PGLs, % | Penetrance of PCC/PGL, % | Frequency of Malignancy, % |
|---|---|---|---|---|
| MEN2 | RET | 5 | 50 | 3 |
| VHL | VHL | 9.0 | 10–26 | 3 |
| NF1 | NF1 | 3 | 0.1–6 | 9 |
| HPGL/PCC | SDHD | 7 | 86 | 3.5 |
| HPGL/PCC | SDHC | 0.5 | Unknown | 0 |
| HPGL/PCC | SDHB | 5.5 | 77 | 31 |
| Sporadic | None | 70 | Not applicable | 9 |

*Abbreviations:* HPGL/PCC, Hereditary paraganglioma/pheochromocytoma syndrome; MEN2, multiple endocrine neoplasia 2; SDH, succinate dehydrogenase.
*Data from* Welander J, Soderkvist P, Gimm O. Genetics and clinical characteristics of hereditary pheochromocytomas and paragangliomas. Endocr Relat Cancer 2011;18(6):R253–76.

than paragangliomas, paragangliomas are also associated with these syndromes. In contrast, patients with MEN2 virtually never develop paragangliomas. Very rarely, pheochromocytomas can be seen in the setting of Carney triad, Carney-Stratakis syndrome, and multiple endocrine neoplasia type 1 (MEN 1).[41]

In a landmark study by Neumann and colleagues,[42] the investigators found that not 10%, but 24% of patients who presented with nonsyndromic pheochromocytomas (or paragangliomas) without a family history had germline mutations. This was in part due to more frequent germline mutations in RET and VHL than previously recognized, but also because succinate dehydrogenase (SDH) mutations were now assessed. SDH is an enzyme complex localized to the inner mitochondrial membrane that plays a role in cellular metabolism, participating in both the Krebs cycle and the electron transport chain.[43] It is a heterotetrameric complex composed of 4 protein subunits (SDHA, SDHB, SDHC, and SDHD). The SDH genes act as tumor suppressor genes: tumors demonstrate loss of heterozygosity in combination with germline inactivating mutations. In pheochromocytomas the rate of SDH deficiency is 4% to 5% (the rate is significantly higher in paragangliomas, up to approximately 50% in some studies), with a roughly equal number of SDHB and SDHD mutations.[35,44,45] SDHC mutations do not significantly contribute to the development of pheochromocytomas, and only rare pheochromocytomas harbor an SDHA mutation.[46,47] SDHAF2, a gene encoding a protein that is involved in stabilization of the SDH complex, germline mutations have been reported in head and neck paragangliomas, but not in pheochromocytomas.[48,49]

Recently, 2 additional genes have been linked to the development of hereditary pheochromocytomas. TMEM127 encodes a transmembrane protein that functions as a tumor suppressor. Yao and colleagues[50] evaluated a cohort of 990 patients with pheochromocytomas or paragangliomas that were negative for RET, VHL, and SDH mutations and found germline TMEM127 mutations in 2% of cases. Only a quarter of these patients had a clear family history, suggesting a fairly low penetrance. Additionally, MAX, the MYC-associated factor X gene, mutations have been found to be responsible for approximately 1% of pheochromocytomas/paragangliomas in patients without evidence of other known mutations.[51] MAX acts as a tumor suppressor gene, shows a paternal mode of inheritance, and is frequently associated with bilateral pheochromocytomas.[51,52] Finally, it is worth noting that many sporadic tumors harbor somatic mutations of the genes responsible for the development of the familial syndromes discussed previously. Approximately 10% of pheochromocytomas/paragangliomas harbor somatic VHL mutations, 10% harbor NF1 mutations, 5% have RET mutations, and 2.5% have MAX mutations.[51,53,54]

Although clinical history can significantly aid in identifying patients with pheochromocytomas that are most likely to have an underlying hereditary syndrome, clinical history may be deceiving. As the study by Neumann and colleagues[42] demonstrated, 24% of patients with an underlying germline mutation lack a positive family history. This can be because of gaps in a patient's knowledge of his or her relatives' medical history, due to a new germline mutation in the patient that was not present in the parents, due to incomplete penetrance of syndromes, or confounding

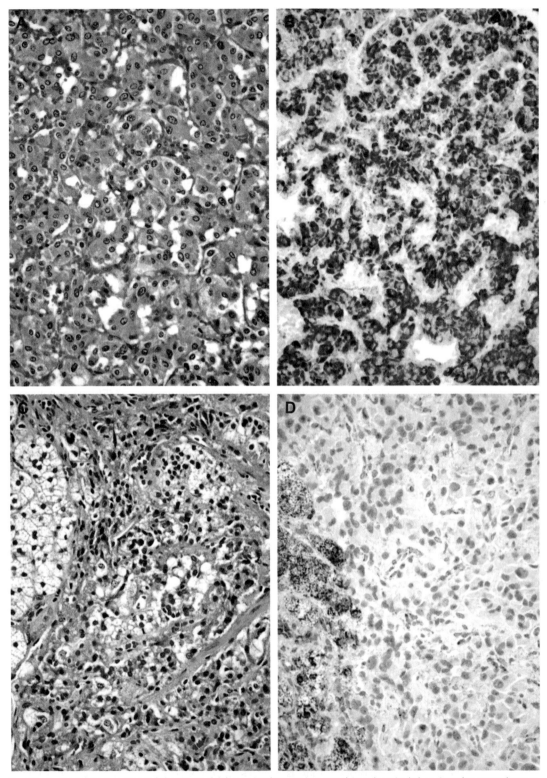

*Fig. 14.* A pheochromocytoma (*A*) H&E and (*B*) a paired SDHB immunohistochemical showing the granular cytoplasmic staining seen in tumors that lack an underlying SDH mutation. A pheochromocytoma (*C*) H&E and (*D*) a paired SDHB immunohistochemical showing loss of SDHB expression within the tumor (indicating an underlying SDH mutation) with intact staining seen in the adjacent adrenal cortical tissue, blood vessels, and sustentacular cells within the tumor.

effects of a paternal mode of inheritance. Besides family history, other factors such as age, multifocality, and adrenal versus an extra-adrenal location can be used to stratify risk of an underlying hereditary syndrome. Neumann and colleagues[42] found that younger age, multifocal tumors, and extra-adrenal location were significantly associated with the presence of a mutation. However, among the patients who were positive for mutations, only 32% had multifocal tumors, and 35% presented after the age of 30 years, with 8% presenting after the age of 40. In a large Italian cohort, of the 278 patients who presented with unilateral pheochromocytomas, 21% were associated with germline mutations (9% VHL, 6% RET, 3% NF1, 2% SDHB, and 1% SDHD mutation).[35]

Identifying patients with hereditary syndromes has significant clinical implications. For one, identification of a syndrome prompts evaluation/screening for other tumors associated with each syndrome, such as medullary thyroid carcinoma in the setting of MEN 2A or 2B, or renal cell carcinoma and hemangioblastoma in the setting of VHL disease. Additionally, identification of a hereditary syndrome can prompt genetic counseling and evaluation of family members at risk of disease. Finally, the underlying mutation may have prognostic significance (see Table 4). The rate of malignancy in pheochromocytomas in patients with germline RET or VHL germline mutations is significantly lower than that of sporadic pheochromocytomas. The reported rate of malignancy for tumors with SDHB mutations ranges from 21% to 71%, which is significantly higher than that for tumors with SDHD mutations (approximately 3%) and SDHC mutations (virtually always benign).[35,41,42] Moreover, even among patients with malignant pheochromocytomas and paragangliomas, the presence of SDHB mutations confers a worse prognosis, with a significant and independent association with mortality (relative risk 2.7).[55] The fact that SDHB mutations are prognostically significant is especially important, given that there are no reliable histologic features that predict malignancy for paragangliomas and pheochromocytomas. Additionally, it appears that MAX mutations also may be associated with a higher risk of malignancy.[52]

Can tumors associated with a genetic syndrome be recognized in pathology? The answer is sometimes. As mentioned previously, pheochromocytomas in patients with MEN2A and 2B often arise in a background of diffuse or nodular medullary hyperplasia. There is also some indication that pheochromocytomas occurring in the context of VHL have certain histologic features, such as a thick fibrous capsule, myxoid or hyalinized stroma, more clear cells, and a lack of hyaline globules.[56] However, VHL-associated tumors are not histologically distinct enough to allow for definitive identification based on histologic characteristics alone; thus, genetic testing is ultimately required to assess for a VHL mutation. Pheochromocytomas and paragangliomas arising in the setting of an SDH mutation may show worrisome features, such as increased mitotic activity; however, overall these tumors lack unique histologic features. Immunohistochemistry, on the other hand, is excellent at identifying tumors with an underlying SDH mutation. A mutation in any one of the SDH genes (SDHA, B, C, or D) not only results in a lack of SDH enzyme activity, it also causes destabilization of the SDH protein complex. Destabilization of the complex, as a result of a mutation in any of the 4 SDH genes, can be identified by immunohistochemical analysis for SDHB. Although SDHB is ubiquitously expressed (including in normal tissues of patients harboring a germline mutation in an SDH subunit gene), SDH-deficient tumors nearly always lack SDHB expression by immunohistochemistry (loss of SDHB staining is both very sensitive and specific for the detection of an underlying SDH germline mutation) (Fig. 14).[57] For the rare pheochromocytomas with germline SDHA mutations, immunohistochemical staining for SDHA can be used specifically to detect the SDHA mutation. Tumors with SDHB, SDHC, or SDHD germline mutations will show loss of staining for SDHB but intact staining for SDHA (why the SDHA protein is not degraded in the presence of SDHB, SDHC, or SDHB mutations is not currently known). In contrast, tumors with SDHA germline mutations will show loss of immunohistochemical staining for both SDHB and SDHA.[46]

## REFERENCES

1. Cawood TJ, Hunt PJ, O'Shea D, et al. Recommended evaluation of adrenal incidentalomas is costly, has high false-positive rates and confers a risk of fatal cancer that is similar to the risk of the adrenal lesion becoming malignant; time for a rethink? Eur J Endocrinol 2009;161(4):513–27.
2. NIH state-of-the-science statement on management of the clinically inapparent adrenal mass ("incidentaloma"). NIH Consensus State Sci Statements 2002; 19(2):1–25.
3. Gopan T, Remer E, Hamrahian AH. Evaluating and managing adrenal incidentalomas. Cleve Clin J Med 2006;73(6):561–8.
4. Reginelli A, Di Grezia G, Izzo A, et al. Imaging of adrenal incidentaloma: our experience. Int J Surg 2014;12(Suppl 1):S126–31.

5.  Dackiw AP, Lee JE, Gagel RF, et al. Adrenal cortical carcinoma. World J Surg 2001;25(7):914–26.
6.  Ayala-Ramirez M, Jasim S, Feng L, et al. Adrenocortical carcinoma: clinical outcomes and prognosis of 330 patients at a tertiary care center. Eur J Endocrinol 2013;169(6):891–9.
7.  Beuschlein F, Weigel J, Saeger W, et al. Major prognostic role of Ki67 in localized adrenocortical carcinoma after complete resection. J Clin Endocrinol Metab 2015;100(3):841–9.
8.  Crucitti F, Bellantone R, Ferrante A, et al. The Italian Registry for Adrenal Cortical Carcinoma: analysis of a multiinstitutional series of 129 patients. The ACC Italian Registry Study Group. Surgery 1996;119(2):161–70.
9.  Paton BL, Novitsky YW, Zerey M, et al. Outcomes of adrenal cortical carcinoma in the United States. Surgery 2006;140(6):914–20 [discussion: 919–20].
10. Weiss LM, Medeiros LJ, Vickery AL Jr. Pathologic features of prognostic significance in adrenocortical carcinoma. Am J Surg Pathol 1989;13(3):202–6.
11. Erickson LA, Lloyd RV, Hartman R, et al. Cystic adrenal neoplasms. Cancer 2004;101(7):1537–44.
12. Weiss LM. Comparative histologic study of 43 metastasizing and nonmetastasizing adrenocortical tumors. Am J Surg Pathol 1984;8(3):163–9.
13. Giordano TJ. The argument for mitotic rate-based grading for the prognostication of adrenocortical carcinoma. Am J Surg Pathol 2011;35(4):471–3.
14. Hough AJ, Hollifield JW, Page DL, et al. Prognostic factors in adrenal cortical tumors. A mathematical analysis of clinical and morphologic data. Am J Clin Pathol 1979;72(3):390–9.
15. van Slooten H, Schaberg A, Smeenk D, et al. Morphologic characteristics of benign and malignant adrenocortical tumors. Cancer 1985;55(4):766–73.
16. Aubert S, Wacrenier A, Leroy X, et al. Weiss system revisited: a clinicopathologic and immunohistochemical study of 49 adrenocortical tumors. Am J Surg Pathol 2002;26(12):1612–9.
17. van't Sant HP, Bouvy ND, Kazemier G, et al. The prognostic value of two different histopathological scoring systems for adrenocortical carcinomas. Histopathology 2007;51(2):239–45.
18. Volante M, Bollito E, Sperone P, et al. Clinicopathological study of a series of 92 adrenocortical carcinomas: from a proposal of simplified diagnostic algorithm to prognostic stratification. Histopathology 2009;55(5):535–43.
19. Duregon E, Fassina A, Volante M, et al. The reticulin algorithm for adrenocortical tumor diagnosis: a multicentric validation study on 245 unpublished cases. Am J Surg Pathol 2013;37(9):1433–40.
20. Mearini L, Del Sordo R, Costantini E, et al. Adrenal oncocytic neoplasm: a systematic review. Urol Int 2013;91(2):125–33.
21. Wong DD, Spagnolo DV, Bisceglia M, et al. Oncocytic adrenocortical neoplasms–a clinicopathologic study of 13 new cases emphasizing the importance of their recognition. Hum Pathol 2011;42(4):489–99.
22. Lin BT, Bonsib SM, Mierau GW, et al. Oncocytic adrenocortical neoplasms: a report of seven cases and review of the literature. Am J Surg Pathol 1998;22(5):603–14.
23. Bisceglia M, Ludovico O, Di Mattia A, et al. Adrenocortical oncocytic tumors: report of 10 cases and review of the literature. Int J Surg Pathol 2004;12(3):231–43.
24. Papotti M, Volante M, Duregon E, et al. Adrenocortical tumors with myxoid features: a distinct morphologic and phenotypical variant exhibiting malignant behavior. Am J Surg Pathol 2010;34(7):973–83.
25. Brown FM, Gaffey TA, Wold LE, et al. Myxoid neoplasms of the adrenal cortex: a rare histologic variant. Am J Surg Pathol 2000;24(3):396–401.
26. Weissferdt A, Phan A, Suster S, et al. Adrenocortical carcinoma: a comprehensive immunohistochemical study of 40 cases. Appl Immunohistochem Mol Morphol 2014;22(1):24–30.
27. Sbiera S, Schmull S, Assie G, et al. High diagnostic and prognostic value of steroidogenic factor-1 expression in adrenal tumors. J Clin Endocrinol Metab 2010;95(10):E161–71.
28. Duregon E, Volante M, Giorcelli J, et al. Diagnostic and prognostic role of steroidogenic factor 1 in adrenocortical carcinoma: a validation study focusing on clinical and pathologic correlates. Hum Pathol 2013; 44(5):822–8.
29. Schmitt A, Saremaslani P, Schmid S, et al. IGFII and MIB1 immunohistochemistry is helpful for the differentiation of benign from malignant adrenocortical tumours. Histopathology 2006;49(3):298–307.
30. Vargas MP, Vargas HI, Kleiner DE, et al. Adrenocortical neoplasms: role of prognostic markers MIB-1, P53, and RB. Am J Surg Pathol 1997;21(5):556–62.
31. Erickson LA, Jin L, Sebo TJ, et al. Pathologic features and expression of insulin-like growth factor-2 in adrenocortical neoplasms. Endocr Pathol 2001; 12(4):429–35.
32. Volante M, Sperone P, Bollito E, et al. Matrix metalloproteinase type 2 expression in malignant adrenocortical tumors: diagnostic and prognostic significance in a series of 50 adrenocortical carcinomas. Mod Pathol 2006;19(12):1563–9.
33. Reincke M, Karl M, Travis WH, et al. p53 mutations in human adrenocortical neoplasms: immunohistochemical and molecular studies. J Clin Endocrinol Metab 1994;78(3):790–4.
34. Tissier F, Cavard C, Groussin L, et al. Mutations of beta-catenin in adrenocortical tumors: activation of the Wnt signaling pathway is a frequent event in both benign and malignant adrenocortical tumors. Cancer Res 2005;65(17):7622–7.

35. Mannelli M, Castellano M, Schiavi F, et al. Clinically guided genetic screening in a large cohort of Italian patients with pheochromocytomas and/or functional or nonfunctional paragangliomas. J Clin Endocrinol Metab 2009;94(5):1541–7.

36. Thompson LD. Pheochromocytoma of the Adrenal gland Scaled Score (PASS) to separate benign from malignant neoplasms: a clinicopathologic and immunophenotypic study of 100 cases. Am J Surg Pathol 2002;26(5):551–66.

37. Linnoila RI, Keiser HR, Steinberg SM, et al. Histopathology of benign versus malignant sympathoadrenal paragangliomas: clinicopathologic study of 120 cases including unusual histologic features. Hum Pathol 1990;21(11):1168–80.

38. Wu D, Tischler AS, Lloyd RV, et al. Observer variation in the application of the Pheochromocytoma of the Adrenal Gland Scaled Score. Am J Surg Pathol 2009;33(4):599–608.

39. Miettinen M, McCue PA, Sarlomo-Rikala M, et al. GATA3: a multispecific but potentially useful marker in surgical pathology: a systematic analysis of 2500 epithelial and nonepithelial tumors. Am J Surg Pathol 2014;38(1):13–22.

40. Dluhy RG. Pheochromocytoma–death of an axiom. N Engl J Med 2002;346(19):1486–8.

41. Welander J, Soderkvist P, Gimm O. Genetics and clinical characteristics of hereditary pheochromocytomas and paragangliomas. Endocr Relat cancer 2011;18(6):R253–76.

42. Neumann HP, Bausch B, McWhinney SR, et al. Germ-line mutations in nonsyndromic pheochromocytoma. N Engl J Med 2002;346(19):1459–66.

43. Barletta JA, Hornick JL. Succinate dehydrogenase-deficient tumors: diagnostic advances and clinical implications. Adv Anat Pathol 2012;19(4):193–203.

44. Amar L, Bertherat J, Baudin E, et al. Genetic testing in pheochromocytoma or functional paraganglioma. J Clin Oncol 2005;23(34):8812–8.

45. Burnichon N, Rohmer V, Amar L, et al. The succinate dehydrogenase genetic testing in a large prospective series of patients with paragangliomas. J Clin Endocrinol Metab 2009;94(8):2817–27.

46. Korpershoek E, Favier J, Gaal J, et al. SDHA immunohistochemistry detects germline SDHA gene mutations in apparently sporadic paragangliomas and pheochromocytomas. J Clin Endocrinol Metab 2011;96(9):E1472–6.

47. Schiavi F, Boedeker CC, Bausch B, et al. Predictors and prevalence of paraganglioma syndrome associated with mutations of the SDHC gene. JAMA 2005;294(16):2057–63.

48. Bayley JP, Kunst HP, Cascon A, et al. SDHAF2 mutations in familial and sporadic paraganglioma and phaeochromocytoma. Lancet Oncol 2010;11(4):366–72.

49. Hao HX, Khalimonchuk O, Schraders M, et al. SDH5, a gene required for flavination of succinate dehydrogenase, is mutated in paraganglioma. Science 2009;325(5944):1139–42.

50. Yao L, Schiavi F, Cascon A, et al. Spectrum and prevalence of FP/TMEM127 gene mutations in pheochromocytomas and paragangliomas. JAMA 2010;304(23):2611–9.

51. Burnichon N, Cascon A, Schiavi F, et al. MAX mutations cause hereditary and sporadic pheochromocytoma and paraganglioma. Clin Cancer Res 2012;18(10):2828–37.

52. Comino-Mendez I, Gracia-Aznarez FJ, Schiavi F, et al. Exome sequencing identifies MAX mutations as a cause of hereditary pheochromocytoma. Nat Genet 2011;43(7):663–7.

53. Burnichon N, Buffet A, Parfait B, et al. Somatic NF1 inactivation is a frequent event in sporadic pheochromocytoma. Hum Mol Genet 2012;21(26):5397–405.

54. Burnichon N, Vescovo L, Amar L, et al. Integrative genomic analysis reveals somatic mutations in pheochromocytoma and paraganglioma. Hum Mol Genet 2011;20(20):3974–85.

55. Amar L, Baudin E, Burnichon N, et al. Succinate dehydrogenase B gene mutations predict survival in patients with malignant pheochromocytomas or paragangliomas. J Clin Endocrinol Metab 2007;92(10):3822–8.

56. Koch CA, Mauro D, Walther MM, et al. Pheochromocytoma in Von Hippel-Lindau disease: distinct histopathologic phenotype compared to pheochromocytoma in multiple endocrine neoplasia type 2. Endocr Pathol 2002;13(1):17–27.

57. van Nederveen FH, Gaal J, Favier J, et al. An immunohistochemical procedure to detect patients with paraganglioma and phaeochromocytoma with germline SDHB, SDHC, or SDHD gene mutations: a retrospective and prospective analysis. Lancet Oncol 2009;10(8):764–71.

# Adrenocortical Carcinoma
## A Clinician's Perspective

Aymen Elfiky, MD, MA, MPH, MSc

## KEYWORDS

- Adrenocortical carcinoma • Adrenal cortex tumors • Rare malignancies • Mitotane
- Platinum-based chemotherapy

---

### Key points

- Adrenocortical carcinoma (ACC) diagnosis management often requires a multidisciplinary approach.
- Most cases are sporadic, although specific cancer syndromes have been identified with increased incidence of ACC.
- Approximately 60% of ACC tumors are functional and present with signs and symptoms related to production of excess hormones.
- Careful consideration should be given to the clinical context and manifestations of an adrenal tumor before obtaining pathology specimens.
- Although multidisciplinary approaches to ACC may result in long-term disease control and survival, conventional chemotherapy is not curative and newer targeted therapies have not yielded any significant impact on disease trajectory.

---

## ABSTRACT

Within the category of orphan diseases and rare malignancies, adrenocortical carcinoma (ACC) represents an aggressive entity with high mortality and morbidity. While localized tumors which are diagnosed early can be cured with surgical intervention, there are prognostic factors which predict for micrometastases and consequent recurrent and advanced disease. In such cases, mitotane and cytotoxic chemotherapy have been utilized with a modest degree of benefit. The poor prognosis of recurrent and advanced ACC has underscored the interest in nuanced characterization of ACC cases to guide the personalized use of immunotherapeutic and novel targeted therapies.

## OVERVIEW

Adrenocortical carcinoma (ACC) is a rare and aggressive malignancy of the adrenal cortex with an annual US incidence of approximately 1 to 2 new cases per million population.[1,2] Overall, ACC carries a poor prognosis, with the most consistent prognostic factor being the tumor stage at the time of diagnosis.[3] Unfortunately, retrospective studies have reported a 5-year survival rate of 24% for stage III and 0% for stage IV disease.[4]

ACC diagnosis (see also Pinto and Barletta, Adrenal Tumors, Surgical Pathology Clinics, 2015, Volume 8, Issue 4) and management often requires a multidisciplinary approach, frequently involving a medical oncologist, an endocrine surgeon, an endocrinologist, a pathologist (preferably one with endocrine expertise), and other disciplines. Approximately 80% of patients with localized disease will recur after complete resection.[5–7] With regard to recurrent or advanced disease, ACC is modestly responsive to standard cytotoxic chemotherapies, although various combinations have shown palliative benefit. Radiation and ablative techniques have been used with variable benefit depending on the clinical scenario.

---

Disclosures: None.
Dana-Farber Cancer Institute/Brigham and Women's Hospital, Lank Center for Genitourinary Oncology, 450 Brookline Avenue, Boston, MA 02215, USA
E-mail address: Aymen_Elfiky@dfci.harvard.edu

Surgical Pathology 8 (2015) 751–754
http://dx.doi.org/10.1016/j.path.2015.07.002

## PATHOGENESIS

Most cases are sporadic, although specific cancer syndromes have been identified with increased incidence of ACC (Table 1). Sporadic cases have been proposed to develop through a sequence of genetic defects that are progressively acquired, ultimately resulting in malignant transformation.[8–11] TP53 is a frequently mutated gene in ACC and has been implicated in approximately one-third of sporadic ACC cases; loss of heterozygosity (LOH) at the 17p13 locus has been a frequent associated finding. Similarly, overexpression of insulinlike growth factor (IGF)-II, whose gene is located on chromosome 11, has been associated with sporadic ACC cases resulting from LOH at the 11p15 locus.[12,13]

Constitutive activation of beta-catenin in the Wnt signaling pathway as a result of activating somatic mutation of the *CTNNB1* gene has been identified as a frequent alteration in malignant adrenocortical tumors.[14] Wnt/beta-catenin pathway activation has been shown to be an independent predictor of less favorable disease-free and overall survival in patients with resected primary adrenal carcinoma.[15] Using present day exome sequencing techniques and nucleotide polymorphism arrays, a spectrum of mutations can be revealed in any given sporadic case. Although each such finding is not clinically actionable, we do appreciate that such genetic features can help differentiate patients with ACC with poor or good outcomes.

## CLINICAL

Approximately 60% of ACC tumors are functional and present with signs and symptoms related to production of excess hormones. Cushing syndrome is a notable cause of morbidity and is the most frequent presentation in 45% of cases as compared with a mixed Cushing and virilization syndrome characterized by both glucocorticoid and androgen excess in 25%.[16,17] Glucocorticoid excess causes weight gain, fatigue, muscle weakness, and insomnia progressing over the course of months. Feminization and hyperaldosteronism occur in fewer than 10% of cases.[16] Virilization alone manifests in fewer than 10% of cases, but in the context of an adrenal lesions, this finding tends to be most suggestive of ACC.

In contrast, nonfunctioning ACCs include those with normal or subclinical production of hormones. These tumors are usually discovered incidentally when imaging is obtained for other reasons or as a consequence of a local mass effect or metastatic disease progression.

## DIFFERENTIAL CONSIDERATIONS

Careful consideration should be given to the clinical context and manifestations of an adrenal tumor before obtaining pathology specimens. Suspicion of pheochromocytoma, for example, must be approached by biochemical testing as opposed to biopsy. Findings of hyperaldosteronism, hyperandrogenism, or Cushing syndrome provide added insight into the differential of an adrenal tumor. In attempting to rule out an ACC, cytology from a specimen obtained by fine-needle aspiration (FNA) is typically not adequate to distinguish between a benign mass and ACC (see also Pinto and Barletta, Adrenal Tumors, Surgical Pathology Clinics, 2015, Volume 8, Issue 4). Instead, FNA of an adrenal mass is more useful to characterize a metastatic lesion if there is sufficient suspicion that a different primary malignancy has metastasized to the adrenal gland.[18]

Several markers, such as alpha-inhibin, Melan A, and SF-1, can confirm the primary adrenal origin of a tumor (see also Pinto and Barletta, Adrenal Tumors, Surgical Pathology Clinics, 2015, Volume 8, Issue 4), but to distinguish ACC from a benign

---

**Table 1**
Cancer syndromes associated with increased incidence of ACC

| Syndrome | Characteristics |
| --- | --- |
| Li-Fraumeni syndrome | Inactivating mutations of the *TP53* tumor suppressor gene on chromosome 17p with risk of breast cancer, soft tissue and bone sarcoma, brain tumors, and ACC. |
| Beckwith-Wiedemann syndrome | Abnormalities in 11p15 with risk of Wilms tumor, neuroblastoma, hepatoblastoma, and ACC. |
| Multiple endocrine neoplasia type 1 (MEN1) | Inactivating mutations of the *MEN1* gene on chromosome 11q. With risk of parathyroid, pituitary, and pancreatic neuroendocrine tumors, adrenal adenomas, and carcinomas. |

*Abbreviation:* ACC, adrenocortical carcinoma.

adrenal lesion, an experienced pathologist is required to use the microscopic Weiss criteria.[19–22] The 5 criteria used in the updated/modified Weiss system include the following:

- Greater than 6 mitoses/50 high-power fields
- ≤25% clear tumor cells in cytoplasm
- Abnormal mitoses
- Necrosis
- Capsular invasion

Each criterion is scored 0 when absent, or 2 for the first 2 criteria and 1 for the last 3 when present; the threshold for malignancy is a total score ≥3.[21]

Other immunohistochemical criteria can be used to provide added insight into the malignant potential of ACC, although specific cutoff criteria have not been consistently validated. The Ki-67 proliferation index of malignant lesions can vary from 1.5% to 10.0%,[23] but when considered in the context of other factors, such as stage, patient age, and comorbidities, it can be used to tailor treatment decisions. In contrast, ACC often overexpresses *TP53*, IGF-2, and cyclin E[23]; however, such findings do not provide added insight on which to base management decisions. Most recently, PD-L1 expression has been evaluated in malignant ACC samples.[24] Although PD-L1 positivity was noted in both tumor cells and tumor-infiltrating mononuclear cells, there was no significant association with higher stage at diagnosis Union for International Cancer Control (UICC) or European Network for the Study of Adrenal Tumors (ENSAT), higher tumor grade, excessive hormone secretion, or overall survival (OS).[24]

## TREATMENT AND PROGNOSIS

Malignant ACC is a rare and often very aggressive disease, and therefore distinction from benign cortical adrenal tumors and medullary based tumors is critical (see also Pinto and Barletta, Adrenal Tumors, Surgical Pathology Clinics, 2015, Volume 8, Issue 4). Although multidisciplinary approaches to ACC may result in long-term disease control and survival, conventional chemotherapy is not curative and newer targeted therapies have not yielded any significant impact on disease trajectory.

Platinum-based chemotherapies form the cornerstone of first-line ACC therapy, which have response rates ranging from 11% to 48%, affected in part by patient selection.[25,26] Specifically, the combination of etoposide/doxorubicin/cisplatin chemotherapy given in conjunction with mitotane

offers the current standard approach based on a Phase III clinical trial result.[27] Despite no differences in OS being found, this study provides the most robust evidence for the systemic treatment of advanced ACC. Emerging genomic insights as well as immunotherapeutic strategies provide optimism in realizing novel therapeutics and improved patient outcomes.

## REFERENCES

1. Third national cancer survey: incidence data. Natl Cancer Inst Monogr 1975;(41):i–x, 1–454.
2. Kebebew E, Reiff E, Duh QY, et al. Extent of disease at presentation and outcome for adrenocortical carcinoma: have we made progress? World J Surg 2006;30(5):872–8.
3. Bilimoria KY, Shen WT, Elaraj D, et al. Adrenocortical carcinoma in the United States: treatment utilization and prognostic factors. Cancer 2008;113:3130–6.
4. Khorram-Manesh A, Ahlman H, Jansson S, et al. Adrenocortical carcinoma: surgery and mitotane for treatment and steroid profiles for follow-up. World J Surg 1998;22:605–11 [discussion: 611–2].
5. Dackiw AP, Lee JE, Gagel RF, et al. Adrenal cortical carcinoma. World J Surg 2001;25(7):914–26.
6. Koch CA, Pacak K, Chrousos GP. The molecular pathogenesis of hereditary and sporadic adrenocortical and adrenomedullary tumors. J Clin Endocrinol Metab 2002;87:5367.
7. Sidhu S, Sywak M, Robinson B, et al. Adrenocortical cancer: recent clinical and molecular advances. Curr Opin Oncol 2004;16:13.
8. Bernard MH, Sidhu S, Berger N, et al. A case report in favor of a multistep adrenocortical tumorigenesis. J Clin Endocrinol Metab 2003;88:998.
9. Libé R, Bertherat J. Molecular genetics of adrenocortical tumours, from familial to sporadic diseases. Eur J Endocrinol 2005;153:477.
10. Gicquel C, Bertagna X, Gaston V, et al. Molecular markers and long-term recurrences in a large cohort of patients with sporadic adrenocortical tumors. Cancer Res 2001;61:6762.
11. Bourcigaux N, Gaston V, Logié A, et al. High expression of cyclin E and G1 CDK and loss of function of p57KIP2 are involved in proliferation of malignant sporadic adrenocortical tumors. J Clin Endocrinol Metab 2000;85:322.
12. Stojadinovic A, Ghossein RA, Hoos A, et al. Adrenocortical carcinoma: clinical, morphologic, and molecular characterization. J Clin Oncol 2002;20:941.
13. Latronico AC, Pinto EM, Domenice S, et al. An inherited mutation outside the highly conserved DNA-binding domain of the p53 tumor suppressor protein in children and adults with sporadic adrenocortical tumors. J Clin Endocrinol Metab 2001; 86:4970.

14. Mazzuco TL, Durand J, Chapman A, et al. Genetic aspects of adrenocortical tumours and hyperplasias. Clin Endocrinol (Oxf) 2012;77:1.

15. Gaujoux S, Grabar S, Fassnacht M, et al. β-catenin activation is associated with specific clinical and pathologic characteristics and a poor outcome in adrenocortical carcinoma. Clin Cancer Res 2011; 17:328.

16. Ng L, Libertino JM. Adrenocortical carcinoma: diagnosis, evaluation and treatment. J Urol 2003;169:5.

17. Wajchenberg BL, Albergaria Pereira MA, Medonca BB, et al. Adrenocortical carcinoma: clinical and laboratory observations. Cancer 2000; 88:711.

18. Kocijancic K, Kocijancic I, Guna F. Role of sonographically guided fine-needle aspiration biopsy of adrenal masses in patients with lung cancer. J Clin Ultrasound 2004;32:12.

19. Weiss LM, Medeiros LJ, Vickery AL Jr. Pathologic features of prognostic significance in adrenocortical carcinoma. Am J Surg Pathol 1989;13:202.

20. Medeiros LJ, Weiss LM. New developments in the pathologic diagnosis of adrenal cortical neoplasms. A review. Am J Clin Pathol 1992;97:73.

21. Aubert S, Wacrenier A, Leroy X, et al. Weiss system revisited: a clinicopathologic and immunohistochemical study of 49 adrenocortical tumors. Am J Surg Pathol 2002;26:1612.

22. Tissier F. Pathological pattern of adrenal cortical carcinoma. In: Bertagna X, editor. Adrenal cancer. Montrouge, France: John Libbey Eurotext Ltd; 2006. p. 25.

23. Lau SK, Weiss LM. The Weiss system for evaluating adrenocortical neoplasms: 25 years later. Hum Pathol 2009;40:757.

24. Fay AP, Signoretti S, Callea M, et al. Programmed death ligand-1 expression in adrenocortical carcinoma: an exploratory biomarker study. J Immunother Cancer 2015;3:3.

25. Ahlman H, Khorram-Manesh A, Jansson S, et al. Cytotoxic treatment of adrenocortical carcinoma. World J Surg 2001;25(7):927–33.

26. Sperone P, Ferrero A, Daffara F, et al. Gemcitabine plus metronomic 5-fluorouracil or capecitabine as a second-/third-line chemotherapy in advanced adrenocortical carcinoma: a multicenter phase II study. Endocr Relat Cancer 2010;17(2):445–53.

27. Fassnacht M, Terzolo M, Allolio B, et al. Combination chemotherapy in advanced adrenocortical carcinoma. N Engl J Med 2012;366(23):2189–97.

# Updates in Benign Lesions of the Genitourinary Tract

Javier A. Arias-Stella III, MD, Sean R. Williamson, MD*

## KEYWORDS

- Renal tumors • Urinary bladder pathology • Prostate pathology • Testis pathology
- Benign neoplasms

## ABSTRACT

The genitourinary tract is a common site for new cancer diagnosis, particularly for men. Therefore, cancer-containing specimens are very common in surgical pathology practice. However, many benign neoplasms and nonneoplastic, reactive, and inflammatory processes in the genitourinary tract may mimic or cause differential diagnostic challenges with malignancies. Emerging clinicopathologic, immunohistochemical, and molecular characteristics have shed light on the pathogenesis and differential diagnosis of these lesions. This review addresses differential diagnostic challenges related to benign genitourinary tract lesions in the kidney, urinary bladder, prostate, and testis, with emphasis on recent advances in knowledge and areas most common in diagnostic practice.

## KIDNEY

### MIXED EPITHELIAL AND STROMAL TUMOR AND CYSTIC NEPHROMA

#### Introduction

Mixed epithelial and stromal tumors (MESTs) of the kidney and cystic nephroma are benign renal tumors composed of a mixture of cysts and spindle cell stroma, both of which occur predominantly in adult women.[1–7] In light of the female predilection[8] of both tumors, immunohistochemical positivity for estrogen and progesterone receptors (greater in MESTs),[9] foci of overlapping morphology, and areas reminiscent of ovarian-type stroma in both tumors (although greater in MESTs), it has been debated whether these tumors should be considered a spectrum of a single entity or unique neoplasms. As such, the term, *renal epithelial and stromal tumor*, has been proposed by some investigators to encompass both lesions.[7] In most cases, however, classification into 1 of the 2 categories is readily achievable.[8] Although it was previously hypothesized that only the stroma is neoplastic,[10] recent molecular evidence suggests that the epithelium and stroma are both neoplastic in MESTs.[11] In the pediatric age group, tumors previously classified as cystic nephromas are currently thought best regarded as cystic partially differentiated nephroblastomas (Wilms tumors), in which areas of morphologically apparent nephroblastoma may be scant.

#### Gross Features

Grossly, cystic nephroma forms a circumscribed mass, often located centrally within the kidney, composed entirely of cysts with thin fibrous septa separating the cystic cavities. Some investigators have found this septal thickness consistently less than 5 mm, in line with the absence of a solid component in these tumors.[7] In contrast, MEST forms a solid and cystic renal mass, and in some cases, the solid component may be predominant, raising diagnostic suspicion for another subtype of solid mesenchymal neoplasm.[7]

#### Microscopic Features

Microscopically, heterogeneous cyst lining epithelium may show a variety of patterns in both tumors, including flattened, hobnail-like, cuboidal,

Conflicts of Interest and Source of Funding: None declared.

Department of Pathology and Laboratory Medicine, Henry Ford Health System, Detroit, MI, USA

* Corresponding author. Department of Pathology, Henry Ford Hospital, K6, 2799 West Grand Boulevard, Detroit, MI 48202.

E-mail address: sr.williamson@yahoo.com

Surgical Pathology 8 (2015) 755–787

http://dx.doi.org/10.1016/j.path.2015.09.001

columnar, or urothelial-like lining cells.[1,7] The stroma has also been reported to show a spectrum of morphologies, including areas that range from hypocellular and collagenous to more cellular, composed of spindle-shaped cells or smooth muscle-like cells.[1,7] Foci resembling ovarian stroma have been described in both tumors (Fig. 1A). Stromal cellularity, however, is generally low in cystic nephroma, with a greater predominance of hypocellular, collagenous stroma. Entrapped tubules may be seen in some of the septae. In MESTs, the epithelial elements also vary substantially in size, ranging from small

clusters of tubules (see Fig. 1B) to larger cystic spaces. In MEST, stroma sometimes invaginates into epithelial structures, forming large polypoid phyllodes tumor-like papillary structures (Fig. 2A). Immunohistochemically, the stromal cells are often positive for estrogen (see Fig. 2B) and progesterone receptors, and some positivity has been reported for CD10, calretinin, and inhibin, generally greater in MESTs than in cystic nephroma.[1,3,7] Stromal cells are also typically positive for smooth muscle actin,[1,3] and in MESTs there is often substantial stromal positivity for desmin,[1] even sometimes in areas without overt

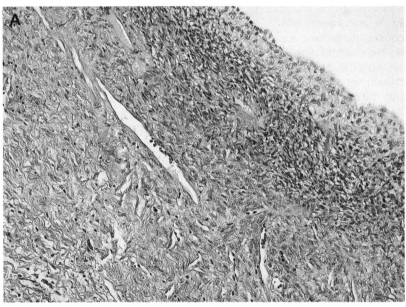

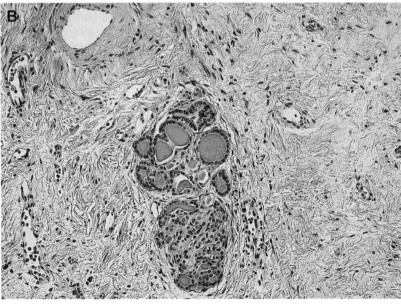

*Fig. 1.* MESTs of the kidney may contain (*A*) large cystic structures with condensation of ovarian-like stroma just under the lining epithelium or (*B*) smaller clusters of renal tubular elements in solid areas of fibrous or cellular stroma (H&E stain, original magnification ×20).

*Fig. 2.* (*A*) MESTs of the kidney sometimes contain invaginations of cellular stroma into epithelial elements, resembling phyllodes tumor of the breast (H&E stain, original magnification ×40). (*B*) Immunohistochemical staining for estrogen receptor is typically positive in the stromal cell nuclei (IHC stain, original magnification ×40).

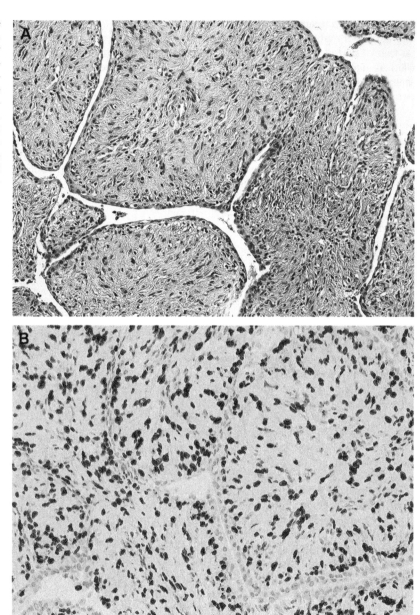

smooth muscle morphology. Labeling for HMB-45 is consistently negative,[1–3] whereas melan-A has been much less extensively studied in these tumors.

## Differential Diagnosis

Regardless of whether these 2 entities are considered a spectrum of a single disease or distinct tumor types, distinguishing them from malignancies is likely of greater clinical significance. Cystic renal cell carcinomas that might be considered in the differential diagnosis include multilocular cystic renal cell carcinoma (or multilocular cystic clear cell renal neoplasm of low malignant potential[8]), clear cell papillary (also known as tubulopapillary) renal cell carcinoma, and tubulocystic renal cell carcinoma (see also Mehra, et al. Emerging Entities in Renal Neoplasia. Surgical Pathology Clinics, 2015, Volume 8, Issue 4). Differential diagnostic considerations among mesenchymal tumors include synovial sarcoma and angiomyolipoma with epithelial cysts (AMLEC). Multilocular cystic renal cell carcinoma has long been regarded as variant of clear cell renal carcinoma,[12] based on overlapping morphology and shared genetic alterations.[13,14] To date, however, no example of metastasis or aggressive behavior has been reported, suggesting that they be reclassified as neoplasms of low malignant potential.[8] Similar to MESTs and cystic nephroma, these tumors are composed of cysts separated by fibrous septa; however, a spindle cell stroma is lacking and a key distinguishing characteristic is the presence of small clusters of neoplastic cells within the fibrous septa, similar to the epithelial cells of low-grade clear cell renal cell carcinoma. These cells may be morphologically challenging to distinguish from lymphocytes or histiocytes in some cases; however, immunohistochemical staining confirms their epithelial nature (keratins, carbonic anhydrase IX, PAX8, and so forth).[15] Labeling for estrogen and progesterone receptors is typically absent.[15] Cystic clear cell papillary (tubulopapillary) renal cell carcinomas demonstrate the characteristic picket fence nuclei with clear cytology that line the cystic spaces and small papillary structures. These tumors are immunoreactive for CK7 and CAIX and are negative for AMACR and CD10. In tubulocystic renal cell carcinoma, the epithelium is more uniform, with moderate amounts of eosinophilic cytoplasm and prominent nucleoli. Stroma is generally dense and fibrotic rather than cellular.[8]

Angiomyolipomas are usually solid, composed of a mixture of abnormal smooth muscle cells, fat, and thick-walled blood vessels; however, infrequent examples have recently been recognized that contain a cystic epithelial component, which can raise a differential diagnostic challenge with MESTs.[16,17] Several other similarities in both tumors include myoid spindle-shaped cells, positivity for hormone receptors, thick-walled blood vessels, rare fat in MESTs, and increased density of cells adjacent to the cysts. Positivity immunoreactivity for melanocytic antigens (HMB-45 and melan-A), however, in angiomyolipoma but not MESTs readily resolves this differential diagnosis.[16,17] Among mesenchymal neoplasms, distinguishing MEST from synovial sarcoma is likely of greatest importance. Synovial sarcoma uncommonly arises as a primary renal neoplasm; however, a cystic epithelial component in synovial sarcoma can mimic other renal tumors clinically and pathologically.[10,18,19] The spindle-shaped cells of synovial sarcoma are more homogeneous with ovoid, hyperchromatic nuclei, and readily identifiable mitotic figures, although marked pleomorphism is usually lacking.[18,19] Despite the presence of epithelial cysts in renal synovial sarcomas, the cyst-forming epithelium is thought to be nonneoplastic, entrapped renal tubular epithelium, because it lacks immunohistochemical positivity for TLE1 and shows positive labeling for PAX8

and PAX2.[10,19] Therefore, primary renal synovial sarcomas seem largely of monophasic rather than biphasic type. Labeling of the spindle-shaped cells for keratins is a helpful clue to the diagnosis of synovial sarcoma, although this may be minor in extent.[18,19] Labeling of the spindle-shaped cells for EMA seems more sensitive for synovial sarcoma, and, in diagnostically challenging cases, confirmation of the presence of *SS18* gene rearrangement (formerly SYT) by molecular techniques can confirm the diagnosis.[18,19]

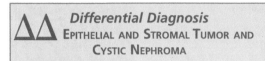

**Differential Diagnosis**
**EPITHELIAL AND STROMAL TUMOR AND CYSTIC NEPHROMA**

- Synovial sarcoma
- AMLEC
- Multilocular cystic renal cell carcinoma (also known as multilocular cystic clear cell renal neoplasm of low malignant potential)
- Cystic clear cell papillary (tubulopapillary) renal cell carcinoma
- Tubulocystic renal cell carcinoma

### Diagnosis

Diagnosis of MEST and cystic nephroma depends on integration of the clinicopathologic features with immunohistochemical or ancillary studies as necessary to exclude other differential diagnostic possibilities (discussed previously).

### Prognosis

MESTs and cystic nephroma are benign tumors; however, rare examples with malignant-appearing overgrowth of the epithelial or stromal component have been reported.[20–23] If a diagnosis of renal synovial sarcoma has been excluded, it remains open to debate whether such tumors truly represent sarcomatous or carcinomatous transformation of MEST or another unknown subtype of primary renal sarcoma that similarly incorporates tubular elements.

## ANGIOMYOLIPOMA

Angiomyolipomas are common mesenchymal neoplasms of the kidney, composed of a mixture of abnormal smooth muscle cells, thick-walled blood vessels, and fat. In a given tumor, 1 or 2 of these components may predominate, making the diagnosis less obvious. Originally regarded as hamartomas, molecular studies have found clonal similarity between the histologic components, supporting their classification as benign neo-plasms.[24] Angiomyolipoma is the prototypical member of the perivascular epithelioid cell family of tumors (PEComas), which together are characterized by cells with abnormal positivity for both smooth muscle and melanocytic antigens. Multiple angiomyolipomas of the kidney are a hallmark of tuberous sclerosis complex, although most tumors likely occur sporadically.[25–27]

## Gross Features

The gross appearance of angiomyolipoma varies depending on the predominant histologic tissue type. Tumors with a predominance of myoid cells may resemble a smooth muscle neoplasm (Fig. 3), whereas tumors with a predominance of fat may be resemble normal fat or a lipomatous tumor. Because radiologic identification of an adipose tissue component can establish the diagnosis without tissue sampling, the tumors more likely encountered as surgical specimens are those that have a paucity of fat, raising clinical suspicion for a renal cell neoplasm, or those that become large, raising concern for rupture or impingement on other vital structures.

## Microscopic Features

Microscopically, although angiomyolipomas contain a smooth muscle component, these cells usually contrast in appearance to normal smooth muscle and are composed of spindle-shaped or epithelioid cells with pale, faint eosinophilic cytoplasm (Fig. 4A), rather than the dense eosinophilic cytoplasm and well-defined fascicles of normal smooth muscle. Blood vessels characteristically have thickened, hyalinized walls (see Fig. 4B),

and epithelioid cells may be preferentially located near blood vessels or radially arranged around them (see Fig. 4C), leading to the "perivascular epithelioid" descriptor for this tumor family.[25–27] Some tumors may be composed almost entirely of fat, although careful examination typically reveals focal myoid cells with pale eosinophilic cytoplasm intervening between the adipocytes. Usual angiomyolipomas do not typically pose a differential diagnostic challenge; however, unusual patterns include epithelioid angiomyolipoma, which is typically composed of epithelioid cells with substantial cytologic atypia, and AMLEC (see Fig. 4D).

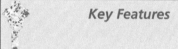

## Key Features

- Myoid spindle-shaped cells with pale eosinophilic cytoplasm
- Thick-walled blood vessels
- Epithelioid smooth muscle cells arranged around blood vessels
- Positive reactivity for HMB-45 and melan-A (may be focal)
- Diffuse reactivity for cathepsin K

## Differential Diagnosis

The differential diagnosis of angiomyolipoma depends on the predominant cell type. Tumors composed predominantly of muscle cells may mimic a smooth muscle neoplasm, such as leiomyoma or leiomyosarcoma, a sarcomatoid carcinoma, or another mesenchymal neoplasm

*Fig. 3.* This smooth muscle–predominant angiomyolipoma grossly demonstrates a white-tan, fibrous cut surface, similar to leiomyoma or leiomyosarcoma.

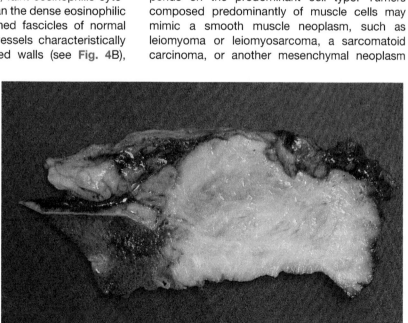

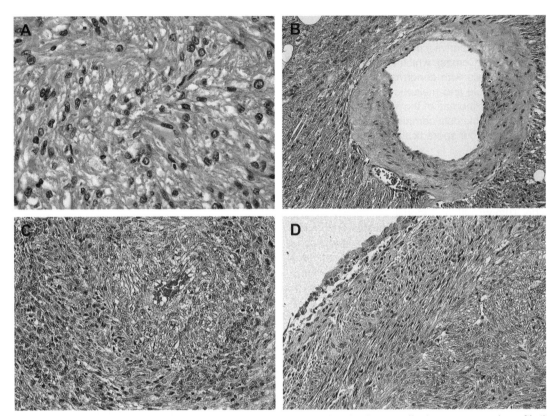

*Fig. 4.* (*A*) Angiomyolipoma contains spindle-shaped smooth muscle cells that usually demonstrate pale or fibrillary cytoplasm, compared with the dense eosinophilic cytoplasm of pure smooth muscle tumors (H&E stain, original magnification ×60). (*B*) Blood vessels in angiomyolipoma often have thickened, hyalinized walls (H&E stain, original magnification ×20), and (*C*) sometimes the cells adjacent to the blood vessels have an epithelioid cell appearance (H&E stain, original magnification ×40). (*D*) A recently recognized, rare variant of angiomyolipoma is AMLEC, with cystic structures composed of renal tubular epithelium entrapped in the tumor (H&E stain, original magnification ×40).

involving the kidney. True renal leiomyomas are rare compared with angiomyolipomas.[28] Distinction between these 2 lesions is often apparent based on the pale cytoplasmic characteristics and lack of well-formed muscular fascicles in the latter. Both of these tumors may show reactivity for smooth muscle markers by immunohistochemistry, such as smooth muscle actin or desmin; however, positivity for melanocytic antigens (HMB-45 or melan-A) confirms the diagnosis of angiomyolipoma. Some renal leiomyomas have been reported to have positivity for HMB-45, in particular those that appear to arise from the renal capsule,[29] although it remains open to debate whether such lesions should truly be regarded as pure/predominant smooth muscle angiomyolipomas. Reactivity for melanocytic markers in angiomyolipoma may be limited to scattered cells and small clusters of cells; however, cathepsin K has recently emerged as a marker of the PEComas and typically shows diffuse strong cytoplasmic positivity in PEComas, including angiomyolipoma. However, positive

staining for cathepsin K is not entirely restricted to PEComas.[30–32] For large, smooth muscle–predominant tumors, leiomyosarcoma might also be a differential diagnostic consideration. Leiomyosarcomas can arise from the kidney or renal pelvic structures, and some demonstrate limited cytologic atypia, making this distinction important; however, unlike angiomyolipoma, necrosis is usually present in a leiomyosarcoma, which aids in the diagnosis.[33] For difficult cases, recognizing the unique cytologic features of the myoid cells in angiomyolipoma, the subtle vascular or adipose components, and positive labeling for melanocytic antigens is important to avoid misclassification of a benign tumor as a sarcoma.

Epithelioid angiomyolipoma, in contrast to usual angiomyolipoma, does not necessarily pursue an entirely benign clinical course, with a subgroup of tumors demonstrating disease progression, including recurrence, metastasis, or death.[8,34–38] Morphologically, epithelioid angiomyolipomas are characterized by a predominance of epithelioid cells with substantive cytologic atypia, and, therefore, differential diagnosis for such tumors is more likely to include carcinoma or sarcoma, rather than usual angiomyolipoma. In such cases, factors associated with disease progression in some of the larger studies have included association with tuberous sclerosis complex, necrosis, large size (>7 cm), extrarenal extension, renal vein involvement, 70% or more atypical epithelioid cells, 2 or more mitotic figures per 10 high-power fields, and atypical mitotic figures.[8,34–38] In contrast, however, foci of epithelioid smooth muscle cells without substantial atypia and occasional multinucleated giant cells may be observed in usual angiomyolipomas. The differential diagnosis of AMLEC is discussed previously with MESTs.

## Diagnosis

Diagnosis of angiomyolipoma of the kidney is usually straightforward; however, morphologic patterns with a predominance of a single-cell type (predominant smooth muscle pattern or predominant epithelioid cells) may introduce diagnostic complexity. In most cases, recognition of the unique morphology of the myoid cells and positive immunohistochemistry for melanocytic markers resolve these problems.

## Prognosis

Usual angiomyolipoma is a benign neoplasm, although large tumors may cause morbidity via tumor rupture or impingement on vital structures. In epithelioid angiomyolipoma, at least a minor subgroup of tumors has been reported to pursue a more aggressive course, including local recurrence, distant metastasis, and death from disease.[8,34–38] Rates of such aggressive behavior have varied slightly between studies, likely due to the rarity of these tumors and differing study inclusion criteria. In general, the authors reserve use of the diagnosis of epithelioid angiomyolipoma (and potential for more aggressive behavior) for tumors with pure or predominant epithelioid morphology and substantial cytologic atypia. In contrast, the authors do not specifically report the presence of a focal, cytologically bland epithelioid component or scattered giant cells in an otherwise usual triphasic angiomyolipoma.

## ONCOCYTOMA

Renal oncocytoma is now widely accepted as a benign renal neoplasm,[39] typically comprising less than 5% to 10% of adult renal epithelial tumors. Despite widespread recognition, however, several challenges with regard to its diagnosis remain incompletely resolved, particularly distinguishing oncocytoma from the eosinophilic variant of chromophobe renal cell carcinoma and in the use of diagnostic immunohistochemical and molecular markers to confirm the diagnosis.[40,41]

### Gross Features

Grossly, oncocytoma characteristically demonstrates a red-brown or mahogany cut surface, often similar in color to the normal renal parenchyma. A central scar or stellate area of fibrosis is a prototypical gross feature, although this finding is not uniformly present and not pathognomonic for oncocytoma. Because detection of renal neoplasms incidentally by imaging studies has increased in recent years, the size range of surgically resected oncocytomas is now wide, ranging from small nodules removed via partial nephrectomy to large masses of greater than 10 cm diameter.

### Microscopic Features

Microscopically, oncocytomas are composed of nests and tubular structures, lined by cells with moderate to voluminous amounts of eosinophilic, granular cytoplasm (**Fig. 5**A), resulting from the dense composition of the cytoplasm by mitochondria.[39] Characteristically, these tubules and nests are often at least partly dispersed in fibrous or edematous stroma[42]; however, other areas may show a more compact arrangement with scant intervening stroma. Nuclei are round and monomorphic with smooth nuclear contours; however, a subset of tumors contains prominent zones of so-called degenerative cytologic atypia, characterized by enlarged, irregular nuclei with smudged nuclear chromatin, binucleation, and intranuclear cytoplasmic inclusions (see **Fig. 5**B).[42,43] These cells are often clustered together in small patches but rarely occur more diffusely.[41,42] Microscopically, the areas corresponding to the gross central scar may contain tubular structures with a jagged, irregular growth pattern and scant to clear cytoplasm.[43] Often, nonneoplastic renal tubules are entrapped within the tumor, usually extending in linear rows into the tumor from the adjacent normal parenchyma. Although oncocytomas are benign, it is relatively well accepted that some cases invade or intermingle with the perinephric fat. A minority of oncocytomas have also been reported to invade large vein branches or the renal vein.[44] Despite these potentially worrisome features, it seems that if other findings remain in line with those of oncocytoma, the benign behavior of such tumors remains unaltered,[44] at least in the limited number of studied examples to date.

Histochemically, the colloidal iron staining technique (Hale or modified Mowry method) generally

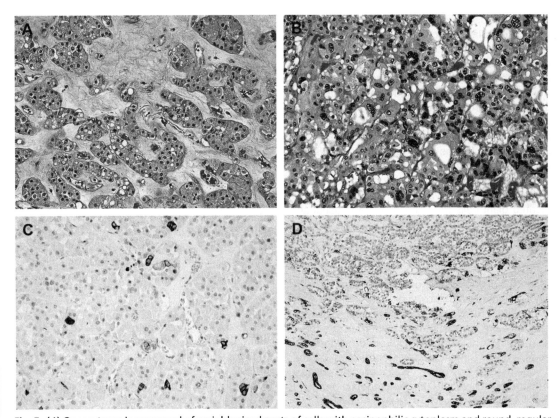

*Fig. 5.* (*A*) Oncocytoma is composed of variably sized nests of cells with eosinophilic cytoplasm and round, regular nuclei, usually dispersed in fibrous or edematous stroma (H&E stain, original magnification ×20). (*B*) Some areas may exhibit increased nuclear pleomorphism with degenerative-appearing, smudged nuclear chromatin, usually distributed in patches throughout the tumor. This finding does not have any known impact on the benign behavior of oncocytoma. Mitotic activity remains inconspicuous even in these areas (H&E stain, original magnification ×40). Immunohistochemistry for CK7 in oncocytoma (*C*) usually reveals positivity in only scattered single cells and small clusters of cells, although in the areas (CK7 IHC stain, original magnification ×20) of (*D*) scar or hyalinized stroma, labeling for CK7 or vimentin may be increased (CK7 IHC stain, original magnification ×10).

demonstrates a negative cytoplasmic staining reaction in oncocytoma, compared with diffuse cytoplasmic labeling in chromophobe renal cell carcinoma[45]; however, technical challenges and uncertainty regarding borderline (apical) staining patterns have impeded the widespread use of this histochemical technique in current practice.[46] Using immunohistochemistry, a large number of potential markers have been studied for differentiating oncocytoma from chromophobe renal cell carcinoma, as reviewed recently by Ng and colleagues.[40] For the most part, however, none of these antibodies has clearly emerged as optimal for resolving this challenge in all cases. Oncocytomas characteristically exhibit staining of scattered cells and small clusters of cells for cytokeratin 7 (CK7) in a small fraction of the overall tumor (see **Fig. 5**C), whereas chromophobe renal cell carcinomas often exhibit more diffuse membranous positivity.[46] A limitation of this antibody is that patchy or perhaps even absent reactivity has

been noted by some investigators in eosinophilic chromophobe renal cell carcinomas, the subgroup that is likely to pose the greatest diagnostic challenge.

---

### Key Features

- Nests and tubular structures dispersed in edematous or fibrous stroma

- Round nuclei with smooth nuclear contours

- Patchy degenerative atypia in some tumors, with enlarged nuclei, smudged chromatin

- Reactivity for CK7 in scattered cells and clusters of cells

- Vimentin, CD10, and colloidal iron (cytoplasmic pattern) typically negative

## Differential Diagnosis

The most common differential diagnostic consideration with renal oncocytoma is the eosinophilic variant of chromophobe renal cell carcinoma,[47] which in general lacks, or only subtly demonstrates, the pale cytoplasm, prominent cell borders, and characteristic nuclear features of usual chromophobe renal cell carcinoma. Diffuse positivity for CK7 or a diffuse cytoplasmic staining reaction with colloidal iron supports a diagnosis of chromophobe renal cell carcinoma, although with both of these staining techniques, the significance of an intermediate staining pattern is a subject of uncertainty. When available, fluorescence in situ hybridization or cytogenetic analyses may provide insight into this diagnostic challenge. In general, oncocytoma shows a normal karyotype; loss of material from chromosome 1, 14, X or Y; or translocation or rearrangement involving 11q13.[48] In contrast, chromophobe renal cell carcinomas typically exhibit multiple losses of chromosomes, most commonly Y, 1, 2, 6, 10, 13, 17, and 21, including the eosinophilic variant.[47,48] Recently, multiple chromosomal gains have also been reported in some chromophobe renal cell carcinomas.[49]

If other subtypes of renal cell carcinoma are differential diagnostic considerations, such as clear cell renal cell carcinoma with a predominance of eosinophilic cells or papillary renal cell carcinoma with an oncocytic pattern, other immunohistochemical antibodies may be helpful in resolving these challenges. KIT (CD117) often demonstrates membranous positivity in oncocytoma and chromophobe renal cell carcinoma, but this pattern is typically lacking in clear cell and papillary renal cell carcinomas.[46,50] Similarly, oncocytoma and chromophobe renal cell carcinoma are negative for vimentin and CD10, in contrast to positivity in clear cell and papillary renal cell carcinomas.[46] The tubular structures entrapped in the central scar or fibrous areas of oncocytoma, however, often show a discordant staining pattern, with positivity for vimentin[51] or CK7 (see **Fig. 5D**). It is unusual to capture only such areas in a needle biopsy specimen; however, another diagnostic pitfall in this situation is that cells in these central fibrous zones of oncocytoma can also take on an appearance of clear cytoplasm (**Fig. 6**),[43] mimicking clear cell renal cell carcinoma, albeit focally. Minor papillary tufts sometimes protrude into the lumina of tubules or cysts in oncocytoma; however, prominent well-formed papillary structures argue against the diagnosis and are in favor of an oncocytic pattern of papillary renal cell carcinoma or an unclassified renal cell carcinoma with oncocytic features.

It is now recognized that succinate dehydrogenase (SDH)-deficient renal cell carcinoma is a unique tumor type that has overlapping morphologic features with oncocytoma.[52–55] Although these tumors are usually composed of monomorphic eosinophilic cells that can mimic the cytologic features of oncocytoma, characteristic clues to the diagnosis include a predominantly solid growth pattern (absence of tubules or nests in fibrous stroma) and prominent cytoplasmic vacuoles or inclusions of eosinophilic material (**Fig. 7**).[52–55] In contrast to oncocytoma, these tumors are typically negative for KIT (although numerous mast cells may be highlighted by the antibody) and usually entirely negative for CK7, in contrast to the scattered cell positivity of oncocytoma.[52]

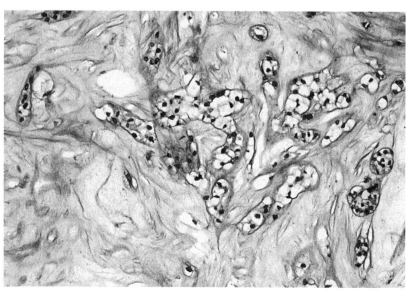

*Fig. 6.* Rarely, areas of central scar within oncocytoma contain cytoplasmic clearing, which could mimic a clear cell renal cell carcinoma in a needle biopsy sample (H&E stain, original magnification ×40).

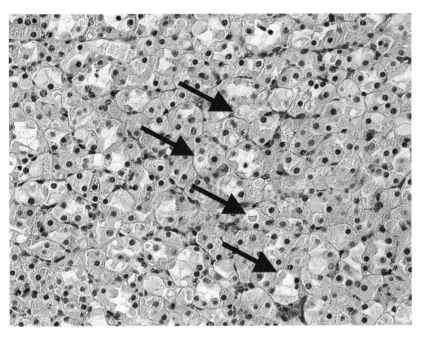

*Fig. 7.* SDH-deficient renal cell carcinoma has been recently recognized as a unique renal cell carcinoma subtype. These tumors often demonstrate unique morphology that mimics oncocytoma, composed of cytologically monomorphic cells with eosinophilic cytoplasm and vacuole-like structures containing flocculent or eosinophilic material (*arrows*). Recognition of this morphology is important, because metastases and death from renal cell carcinoma have been described in a subgroup of patients (H&E stain, original magnification ×40).

Reactivity for epithelial markers in general may be minor.[52] Absence of detectable SDHB protein by immunohistochemistry in these tumors resolves this differential diagnostic challenge and points to the possibility of germline mutation of the SDH subunit genes.[52–55] Recognition and distinction of these tumor types are clinically important, because metastasis and death of disease have been reported in some SDH-deficient renal cell carcinomas,[55,56] even in the absence of pleomorphic cytologic features.[52] Finally, an uncommon mimic of oncocytoma is angiomyolipoma, for which rare cases have been described to have an oncocytoma-like pattern.[57]

### Diagnosis

Despite all efforts to accurately differentiate renal oncocytoma and chromophobe renal cell carcinoma, borderline tumors that do not fit cleanly into either category will doubtlessly remain. In this situation, several approaches for diagnostic terminology may be used, and, therefore, open communication between pathologists and clinicians is necessary to guide proper management. The authors often use descriptive terminology in this context, such as *oncocytic renal neoplasm*, with a description in a note of borderline features of oncocytoma and chromophobe renal cell carcinoma, to convey to clinical colleagues that a follow-up course similar to that of chromophobe renal cell carcinoma may be reasonable, without applying a label of outright malignancy. If some of the cytologic features of chromophobe renal cell carcinoma are present, such as foci of perinuclear cytoplasmic clearing or wrinkling of nuclear contours, the authors often report chromophobe renal cell carcinoma as the favored diagnosis. Some urologic pathologists choose to designate such borderline tumors as unclassified renal cell carcinomas. When using this approach, however, it is important to convey to clinicians the differential diagnosis and the designation of *low-grade* or *uncertain malignant potential*, because the term, *unclassified*, typically conjures a mental image of a poorly differentiated malignancy that evades classification, whereas it is likely that these borderline tumors pursue an indolent course. In regard to a needle biopsy diagnosis of renal oncocytoma, some pathologists generally argue against making an unequivocal diagnosis of oncocytoma (because a hybrid tumor cannot be excluded); however, others are comfortable doing so if appropriate morphologic and immunohistochemical criteria are met.[41]

 **Pitfalls**

! Oncocytoma may invade perinephric fat.

! Rare cases with renal vein invasion still seem to follow a benign course.

! Unexpected positivity for CK7 and vimentin in sclerotic areas differs from the overall staining pattern and may cause confusion.

## Prognosis

Oncocytoma is a benign neoplasm and the favorable outcome seems unaffected by even potentially worrisome pathologic features, such as scattered cytologic atypia, large size[39,42]; microscopic infiltration of perinephric fat[42,43]; or extension into vein branches.[44] Nonetheless, distinction from these malignancies may be facilitated by integration of histologic, immunohistochemical, and molecular features.

## HEMANGIOMA

Hemangiomas and arteriovenous malformations of the kidney are rare, in contrast to renal cell carcinomas; however, several recent studies have called attention to primary renal vascular tumors and shed light on the pathology of renal hemangiomas.[58–64] In particular, there is growing evidence that many primary renal hemangiomas are of the newly recognized anastomosing hemangioma subtype,[58] with morphologic similarity to spleen sinusoids[58,62–64] and potential for confusion with angiosarcoma.[58] An association of renal hemangiomas with end-stage renal disease has also been recently noted.[61,64] Some arteriovenous malformations are thought congenital, whereas others are thought the result of trauma or procedure, such as percutaneous biopsy.[59,63] Although hemangiomas of the urinary bladder are associated with Klippel-Trénaunay-Weber syndrome, there is no known syndromic association for renal hemangiomas.

## Gross Features

Grossly, renal hemangiomas form brown, spongy masses with prominent vascularity that may mimic hemorrhagic renal cell carcinomas.[59,62,63] Those that seem to involve the renal cortex may be challenge to distinguish from renal cell carcinomas; however, some lesions have been described as occurring in the renal hilar area or adjacent to the kidney, which may be a clue to their nonepithelial nature. Intravascular papillary endothelial hyperplasia (Masson tumor) has also been rarely described involving the renal vein.[65,66]

## Microscopic Features

Microscopically, renal arteriovenous malformations are composed of large interconnecting vascular channels with variably thick and thin walls, resembling arterial and venous vascular structures.[59,63] Using elastic stains, some of these vessels may contain a partial elastic lamina.[59] Hemangiomas are typically composed of compact arrangements of capillary vascular channels, often showing at least some anastomosing sinusoidal-like growth patterns, resembling splenic sinusoids, representing the so-called anastomosing hemangioma subtype (Fig. 8A).[62] Larger tumors may contain zones of sclerosis and collagen deposition or tufted vascular proliferation within larger spaces.[62] Non-neoplastic renal tubules are sometimes entrapped.[63] Intratumoral extramedullary hematopoiesis and cytoplasmic globules of hyaline material (see Fig. 8B) are also unique findings that have been described in these anastomosing hemangiomas.[62] In end-stage kidneys, multiple small multifocal tumors have also been described.[61,64] Although in the past renal hemangiomas have been classified under a variety of different subtypes, the authors' recent experience is that many of these tumors likely fit in the novel anastomosing hemangioma category.

## Differential Diagnosis

The foremost and probably most important differential diagnostic consideration for renal hemangioma is renal cell carcinoma. Although most renal cell carcinomas include a morphologically apparent epithelial component, recent examples have been characterized with a predominantly hemangioma-like appearance and inconspicuous epithelium (Fig. 9), leading to potential for misdiagnosis.[67,68] Areas of collagenous fibrosis or other degenerative changes are common in clear cell renal cell carcinoma in general, and representation of such areas in a biopsy sample may reveal collagenous stroma, prominent capillary vascular structures, and a paucity of epithelium.[69] In this situation, immunohistochemical staining can be of great aid and should be strongly considered before rendering a diagnosis of a primary benign vascular tumor of the kidney.[68] A panel of antibodies directed against multiple antigens, such as broad-spectrum keratins, epithelial membrane antigen, carbonic anhydrase IX, and PAX8, may be helpful in this situation, because a given renal cell carcinoma might show negative reactivity for a particular keratin antibody.[68] Such staining often highlights a much greater number of epithelial cells than are morphologically obvious.[15,69] The proclivity of anastomosing hemangioma to mimic angiosarcoma has also been noted in a few reports.[58,62] The absence of cytologic atypia, papillary endothelial tufting or multilayering, spindle-cell growth pattern, and substantial mitotic activity, however, are clues to the diagnosis of these tumors.[58,62]

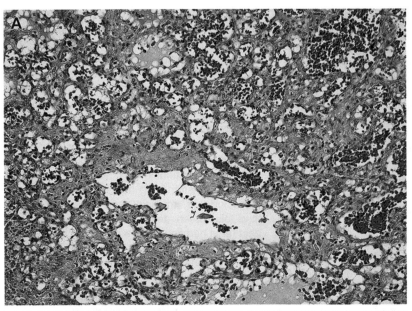

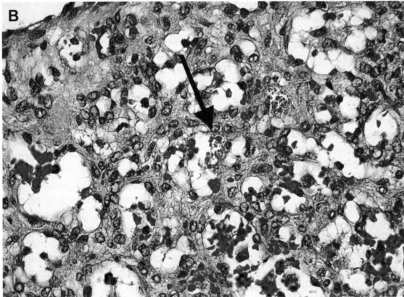

*Fig. 8.* Anastomosing hemangioma of the kidney has been recently recognized as a common form of unique benign vascular tumor, composed of (*A*) interconnecting vascular channels that resemble spleen sinusoids (H&E stain, original magnification ×10). (*B*) Cytoplasmic hyaline globules (*arrow*) within endothelial cells are often present. Immunohistochemistry is typically useful to exclude a highly vascular renal cell carcinoma (H&E stain, original magnification ×40).

Primary renal hemangioblastoma might be another differential diagnostic consideration for renal hemangioma. Although rare, a few recent reports have highlighted the occurrence of hemangioblastomas as primary renal tumors, contrasting to their usual occurrence in the nervous system.[70,71] An unexpected finding in this location is that immunohistochemical staining may reveal positivity for PAX8, suggesting a renal tubular epithelial neoplasm. Vacuolated stromal cells with scant reactivity for keratins, however, and immunohistochemical positivity for alpha-inhibin, neuron-specific enolase, and S-100 are helpful clues to the diagnosis of primary renal hemangioblastoma.[70,71] Angiomyolipoma is an unlikely mimic of renal hemangioma, because a predominance of vascular growth is not typical. Pale-staining, spindle-shaped, or epithelioid myoid cells intervening between vessels likewise argue against a diagnosis of renal hemangioma.

## Pitfalls

! Renal cell carcinoma may have a hemangioma-like pattern with inconspicuous epithelium.

! Multiple immunohistochemical antibodies may be necessary to exclude an epithelial component (keratin, EMA, PAX8, carbonic anhydrase IX, and so forth).

## Diagnosis

Primary renal hemangiomas are uncommon but may show a predilection for end-stage renal disease. A critical challenge in diagnosis is adequately excluding the possibility of a low-grade renal cell carcinoma, in particular clear cell renal cell carcinoma, in which the epithelial component is inconspicuous.[67,68] Application of immunohistochemical staining techniques (discussed previously) can aid greatly in resolving this challenge. Additionally, the presence of a vascular biomarker, such as ERG, argues against a renal epithelial neoplasm and supports the diagnosis of a vascular lesion.

## Prognosis

Renal hemangiomas are benign and thus far it seems that they do not recur after treatment. Some patients have multifocal lesions.

## URINARY BLADDER

## VON BRUNN NESTS, CYSTITIS CYSTICA, AND CYSTITIS GLANDULARIS

von Brunn nests, cystitis cystica, and cystitis glandularis are benign proliferative processes of the urothelium that may clinically or pathologically raise the differential diagnosis of a neoplasm. Histologically, these may be particularly challenging when compared with the variants of bladder cancer that are known to have a deceptively bland cytologic appearance.[72] von Brunn nests are invaginations of the urothelium that extend into the lamina propria, often appearing detached from the surface epithelium as 3-D structures are cut into 2-D tissue sections. Similar structures with a central cystic lumen are referred to as cystitis cystica, and those with apical glandlike orientation of the cytoplasm and/or the presence of goblet-cells are referred to as cystitis glandularis.

### Gross Features

Grossly, these 3 entities, when pronounced, may appear as raised submucosal nodules. Although usually small, cystitis cystica may form larger translucent nodules evident at cystoscopy.[73] Alternatively, these lesions can also be encountered incidentally in surgical pathology specimens without clinical suspicion of a mass or lesion.

### Microscopic Features

von Brunn nests are small nests of urothelial cells without significant cytologic atypia, located in the

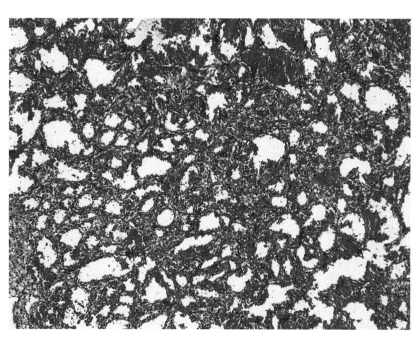

*Fig. 9.* This renal cell carcinoma contains alveolar spaces filled with blood, mimicking hemangioma; however, immunohistochemistry revealed diffuse labeling of the lining of these structures for epithelial markers and labeling of only the surrounding vascular network for endothelial markers (H&E stain, original magnification ×10).

superficial lamina propria, paralleling the urothelial surface (**Fig. 10**). The urothelial cells maintain their normal architectural polarity and the nuclei have open chromatin and occasional inconspicuous nucleoli. When florid von Brunn nest proliferation is present, it maintains this regular shape and orderly spatial arrangement, at a uniform depth from the epithelial surface and without an infiltrative or invasive growth pattern. In the upper urinary tract, von Brunn nests may appear smaller with a more haphazard arrangement; however, this uniform depth without deeper infiltration is maintained (see **Fig. 10**). Cystitis cystica and cystitis glandularis similarly consist of von Brunn nests with central lumina forming small cystic cavities and glands, lined by cuboidal to columnar urothelial or glandlike or goblet cells (**Fig. 11**).

---

### Key Features

- Cytologically bland nests and glandular structures lined by urothelial cells

- Maintains a uniform depth under the surface epithelium without deeper invasion

- Lobular configuration

- Smaller, haphazard nests in upper urinary tract and ureter

---

## Differential Diagnosis

von Brunn nests, cystitis cystica, and cystitis glandularis may raise a differential diagnosis with invasive urothelial carcinoma, particularly in small biopsy specimens, in which the architectural growth pattern is more difficult to assess.[74] Nested variant of urothelial carcinoma in particular is a rare, deceptively benign-appearing variant that closely resembles von Brunn nests,[72] yet which has a high rate of muscle invasion, extravesical disease, and metastasis.[75] Histologically, the invasive nests in nested variant urothelial carcinoma have little or no atypia (**Fig. 12**A); however, foci with enlarged nucleoli and coarse nuclear chromatin are often evident at least focally, especially in the deep aspect of the tumor.[76] Other morphologic clues to the diagnosis of nested urothelial carcinoma are the disordered proliferation of discrete, small variably sized nests or tubules, a jagged and infiltrative tumor stroma interface, and deep extension into the bladder wall often involving the muscularis propria (see **Fig. 12**B).[75] In contrast, benign von Brunn nests extend only to a uniform depth from the surface epithelium. Immunohistochemically, Ki67 (MIB-1), p53, p27, and CK20 have been explored and found to have slight differences in staining patterns between benign von Brunn nests and nested variant urothelial carcinoma, although these differences are likely not specific enough to be useful in routine practice, leaving histologic features as the major

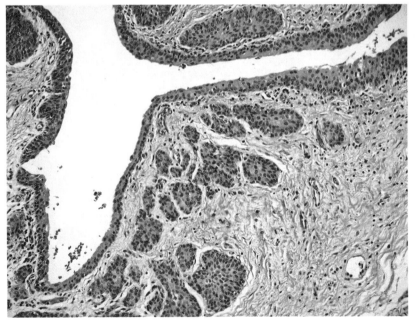

*Fig. 10.* von Brunn nests are small nests of urothelial cells that invaginate from the surface epithelium. In the ureter and upper urinary tract (as depicted in this figure), the nests are often smaller with a haphazard arrangement, which could raise suspicion for a urothelial neoplasm; however, their restriction to a uniform, superficial depth under the surface is a clue to the benign nature (H&E stain, original magnification ×20).

*Fig. 11.* (*A*) Cystitis cystica and cystitis glandularis are nests of urothelial cells similar to von Brunn nests that contain cystic spaces or glandlike lumina (H&E stain, original magnification ×40). (*B*) Cystitis glandularis exhibits apical polarization of the cytoplasm (*black arrow*), whereas cystitis cystica (*red arrow*) contains a cystic space without glandlike polarization of cytoplasm (H&E stain, original magnification ×40).

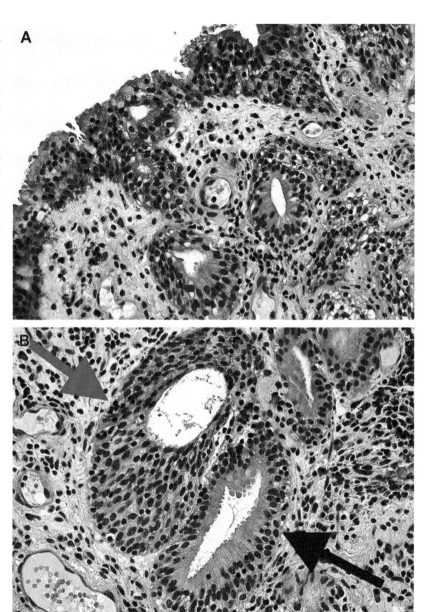

determinant.[74] Similarly, microcystic variant of urothelial carcinoma and urothelial carcinoma with small tubules are rare, infiltrative carcinomas composed of variably sized tubular and cystic structures with bland cytologic features that may be confused with cystitis cystica.[72,77] As with von Brunn nests, a helpful feature favoring a diagnosis of cystitis cystica is the confinement of the cystic epithelial proliferation to a uniform depth, without deeper infiltration.

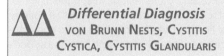

**Differential Diagnosis**
VON BRUNN NESTS, CYSTITIS CYSTICA, CYSTITIS GLANDULARIS

- Nested variant urothelial carcinoma

- Microcystic variant urothelial carcinoma

- Urothelial carcinoma with small tubules

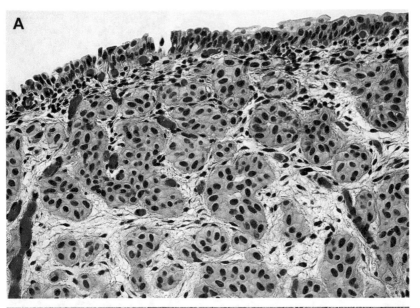

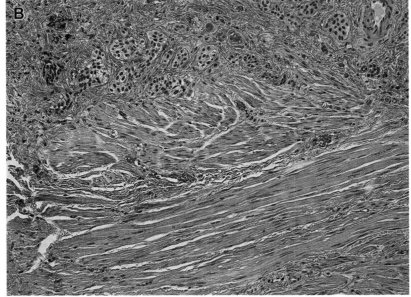

*Fig. 12.* Nested variant urothelial carcinoma exhibits minimal cytologic atypia and may be confused with von Brunn nests. (*A*) In this example of nested variant urothelial carcinoma, the tumor cell nests are more monotonous and somewhat smaller than expected of von Brunn nests (H&E stain, original magnification ×40). (*B*) The infiltrative configuration of the nests and extension to muscularis propria are clues to the diagnosis of carcinoma. Atypia may be better appreciated in the deeper nests in some cases (H&E stain, original magnification ×20).

### Diagnosis

Careful assessment of the histologic features is of great importance for the diagnosis and differentiating these benign lesions from urothelial carcinoma variants with deceptively bland cytologic features. For all of these lesions, distinguishing features include a noninfiltrative pattern with a uniform lobular or linear arrangement of the nests and glandular structures at a uniform depth from the surface epithelium and absence of cytologic atypia.

### Prognosis

von Brunn nests, cystitis cystica, and cystitis glandularis are benign, reactive conditions, which currently are not regarded as conferring any risk for progression to urothelial neoplasia.[73] A possible exception is intestinal metaplasia (cystitis glandularis, intestinal type), which contains intestinal type epithelium with goblet cells and has been hypothesized to represent a precursor to adenocarcinoma,[78] although this remains debated.

## NEPHROGENIC ADENOMA

Nephrogenic adenoma is a benign proliferative lesion composed of small tubules, papillary structures, and cysts that morphologically resemble renal tubules. Although originally these lesions were regarded as a metaplastic change of the urothelium in response to irritation, such as previous surgery, calculi, trauma, or inflammation,[79–81] it has been more recently recognized that nephrogenic adenoma arises from implantation of shed renal tubular epithelial cells into sites of injured urothelial mucosa.[82] The differential diagnosis may vary depending on location (urinary bladder, urethra, prostatic urethra, and so forth).

## Gross Features

Grossly, nephrogenic adenomas are papillary, sessile, or polypoid structures that generally are small (less than 1 cm). A papillary nephrogenic adenoma can mimic urothelial carcinoma at cystoscopy, whereas tubular proliferations may be biopsied as an indeterminate mucosal abnormality or raised lesion, sometimes at a previous biopsy site.

## Microscopic Features

Nephrogenic adenoma can have varying composition including tubular (**Fig. 13**A), cystic, polypoid, papillary (see **Fig. 13**B), fibromyxoid, and flat patterns.[83] These structures are lined by a single layer of flattened, cuboidal, low columnar, or hobnail cells with generally scant eosinophilic or amphophilic cytoplasm and bland nuclei.[73,84] Cystic dilatation of the tubules, containing eosinophilic or basophilic secretions, can occur and some tubular structures are surrounded by a prominent layer of basement membrane (see **Fig. 13**C). Very small tubules may have a signet ring cell-like appearance, if only 1 nucleus and the tubular lumen are visualized in the plane of section (see **Fig. 13**D).

## Differential Diagnosis

Differential diagnosis varies depending on the predominant histologic pattern and site of involvement. Papillary lesions often raise consideration of a urothelial tumor; however, the monolayered cuboidal lining is the most valuable clue to the diagnosis in such cases. Prostatic adenocarcinoma may also be a consideration when there is a predominantly tubular proliferation, especially because alpha-methylacyl-CoA racemase (AMACR) immunohistochemistry can be positive

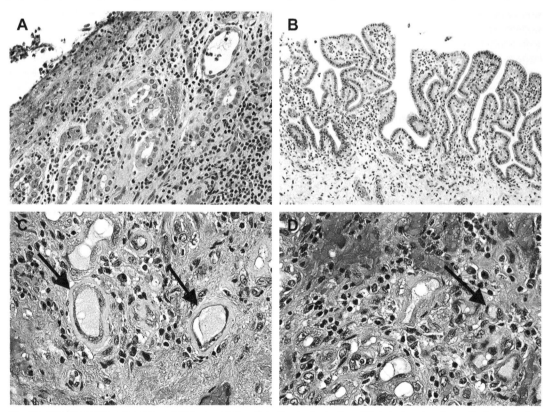

**Fig. 13.** Nephrogenic adenoma exhibits a variety of patterns, including (*A*) tubular structures that may mimic prostate cancer (H&E stain, original magnification ×20) and (*B*) papillary structures that may mimic a urothelial neoplasm (H&E stain, original magnification ×10). The lining by a single, cuboidal cell layer is a clue to the renal origin of this proliferation. (*C*) In some cases, tubular structures are surrounded by a thick layer of basement membrane (*arrows*) (H&E stain, original magnification ×40). (*D*) Occasionally tubular structures may be very small (*arrow*), mimicking signet ring cells (H&E stain, original magnification ×40).

in nephrogenic adenoma and no basal cells are identified using p63.[73] PAX2 and PAX8, renal-specific transcription factors, are useful in confirming the renal tubular origin of these cells, because prostate and urothelial cancers are typically negative with these antibodies.[85,86] The hobnail appearance of the tubules and slight cytologic atypia may bring clear cell adenocarcinoma into the differential diagnosis.[87] Clear cell adenocarcinoma has a predominance of cells with clear cytoplasm, more marked cytologic atypia, and usually recognizable mitotic activity. In contrast, nephrogenic adenoma usually has minimal cytologic atypia, infrequent mitosis, male predominance, small to microscopic size, and infrequent abundant clear cytoplasm.[87] High MIB-1 proliferative rate, positive carcinoembryonic antigen, and p53 have been proposed as adjunctive tools to identifying clear cell adenocarcinoma, although in a given case differences in these staining patterns may not be sufficient to entirely resolve the differential diagnosis.[84] PAX8 is not useful because it is positive in both nephrogenic adenoma and clear cell adenocarcinoma of the bladder.[86] Fibromyxoid nephrogenic adenoma is an unusual variant that contains fibromyxoid stroma, often associated with history of treatment of prior prostate or bladder carcinoma. These lesions may mimic infiltrating mucinous adenocarcinoma and awareness of the unique appearance, combined with the typical nephrogenic adenoma histologic and immunohistochemical features, as well as clinical information, should prevent misdiagnosis.[88]

## Diagnosis

The diagnosis of nephrogenic adenoma is based mainly on morphology, but immunohistochemistry plays a role in difficult cases by excluding a papillary urothelial neoplasm or a prostatic adenocarcinoma. Distinction from clear cell adenocarcinoma can be more challenging and requires integration of the entire constellation of clinicopathologic features.

**Pitfalls**

! Positivity for AMACR and negative staining for p63 may mimic prostate cancer.

! Papillary configuration may mimic urothelial neoplasia.

! Hobnail arrangement of cells overlaps with clear cell adenocarcinoma of the urinary tract; both are positive for PAX8.

## Prognosis

Nephrogenic adenoma is a benign lesion that occasionally may recur. It is not currently regarded as precancerous; however, the morphologic similarity to clear cell adenocarcinoma has led some investigators to question whether it is sometimes capable of progression to clear cell adenocarcinoma.[86]

## PAPILLARY CYSTITIS AND POLYPOID CYSTITIS

Papillary cystitis and polypoid cystitis are nonspecific reactive processes secondary to an inflammatory insult, such as indwelling catheter, colovesical fistula, calculi, urinary tract obstruction, and prior radiation. Clinically and pathologically, these lesions can mimic urothelial neoplasms.

### Gross Features

Grossly, papillary cystitis and polypoid cystitis forms a friable mucosal irregularity or a broad-based, edematous polyp or papillary lesion. These foci may be single or multifocal, raising cystoscopic suspicion for a urothelial tumor.

### Microscopic Features

Microscopically, polypoid cystitis and papillary cystitis are composed of broad (polypoid) or narrow-based (papillary) projections of the lamina propria with edema (**Fig. 14A**) and inflammatory cell infiltrates (see **Fig. 14B**).[89] The lining urothelium lacks the cytologic atypia or architectural disorganization of urothelial carcinoma, and complex branching is absent. Reactive epithelial changes, similar to those seen in flat reactive urothelial atypia, however, may be present.[89]

### Differential Diagnosis

The differential diagnosis includes papillary urothelial neoplasm of low malignant potential (PUNLMP) and papillary urothelial carcinoma. Helpful clues to this distinction include the broad base of the edematous fibrovascular cores seen in polypoid cystitis, in contrast to the narrowed neck, thin, and delicate fibrovascular cores seen in urothelial carcinoma. In papillary cystitis, the fronds are of narrower diameter, and they do not branch into smaller papillae as seen in papillary urothelial carcinoma. Awareness of the clinicopathologic context may also provide helpful insight, especially if the submitting urologist suspects an inflammatory process rather than a neoplastic lesion.[89]

### Diagnosis

Diagnosis of papillary cystitis and polypoid cystitis relies mainly on recognition of the edematous and

*Fig. 14.* Papillary cystitis and polypoid cystitis are composed of edematous (*A*) or inflamed (H&E stain, original magnification ×10) (*B*) projections of urothelial mucosa, lined by urothelium without significant cytologic atypia or branching papillae, arguing against a diagnosis of urothelial neoplasia (H&E stain, original magnification ×10).

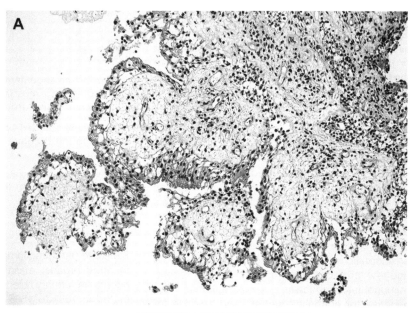

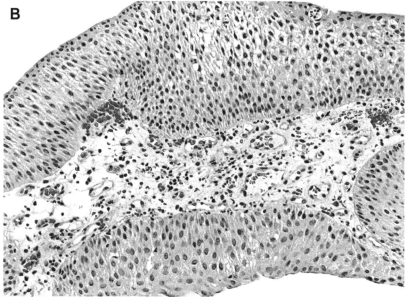

inflammatory background in which the polypoid or papillary structures develop, integrated with clinical history of any inflammatory or irritative processes and absence of cytologic atypia and complex branching architecture.

### Prognosis

Papillary cystitis and polypoid cystitis are benign, reactive conditions that have no known precursor status. With long-standing irritation, these changes may occur more diffusely throughout the urinary bladder.

## PARAGANGLIOMA

Paraganglioma, or extra-adrenal pheochromocytomas, uncommonly occurs as a primary urinary bladder tumor,[90] thought to be derived from paraganglion cells in the bladder wall. Clinical clues to the diagnosis include sustained or paroxysmal hypertension, intermittent gross hematuria, or micturition attacks, characterized by pheochromocytoma or paraganglioma-type symptoms related to bladder filling or micturition.

## Gross Features

Grossly, urinary bladder paragangliomas are well circumscribed or multinodular, with variably intact or ulcerated overlying mucosa.[90,91] Presence of the tumor in the muscularis propria may be a major differential diagnostic pitfall with urothelial carcinoma.

## Microscopic Features

Similar to paragangliomas of other sites, urinary bladder tumors show the so-called Zellballen, or nested, pattern separated by a network of fine collagenous septa containing blood vessels and sustentacular cells. Other less common patterns include diffuse and ribbon-like growth patterns. Cells are round with clear, amphophilic, or eosinophilic cytoplasm. The nuclei are ovoid and few large or bizarre nuclei may be present. Immunohistochemically, paragangliomas are negative for epithelial markers and positive for neuroendocrine markers, such as chromogranin and synaptophysin. S-100 protein highlights the sustentacular cells in the periphery of the nests.[90,92,93]

## Differential Diagnosis

The most critical step in recognizing a primary urinary bladder paraganglioma is considering it in the list of differential diagnoses. Due to the extension into muscularis propria, nested configuration, cytologic atypia, and cautery artifact, a substantial fraction of cases, in particular those encountered in fragmented transurethral resection specimens, may be misdiagnosed as muscle-invasive urothelial carcinoma (**Fig. 15**).[90,92,93] Once the possibility of a nonurothelial tumor is entertained, application of immunohistochemistry for neuroendocrine markers, S-100, and epithelial markers can resolve this problem. A recently recognized diagnostic pitfall, however, is that paragangliomas may show positive nuclear staining for GATA3,[91] a novel transcription factor that has recently emerged as helpful in confirming the urothelial origin of tumors. Therefore, awareness of this staining pattern is also crucial to avoid falsely interpreting GATA3 positivity as confirming a diagnosis of urothelial carcinoma.[91]

## Diagnosis

The diagnosis of bladder paraganglioma can be achieved based on morphology and immunohistochemical stains. A high index of suspicion is necessary in transurethral resection specimens with cautery artifact, in which the overall morphology might be distorted.[90]

### Pitfalls

! Nested arrangement of epithelioid cells extending into muscularis propria may mimic muscle-invasive urothelial carcinoma.

! Positivity for GATA3 in paragangliomas can compound the false impression of urothelial origin.

! Architecture may be concealed in transurethral resection specimens.

## Prognosis

Similar to paraganglioma and pheochromocytoma of other organs, malignant behavior sometimes occurs in urinary bladder paraganglioma, estimated in 10% to 15% of cases, although in the absence of known metastasis, optimal criteria for predicting malignant behavior are elusive.[91] Recently, a fraction of bladder paragangliomas have been recognized as related to germline mutation of SDH subunit genes, similar to paragangliomas elsewhere (see also Pinto and Barletta. Adrenal Tumors in Adults. Surgical Pathology Clinics, 2015, Volume 8, Issue 4).[94]

## PROSTATE

### BASAL CELL HYPERPLASIA

Basal cell hyperplasia is 1 manifestation of prostatic nodular hyperplasia. Usually, basal cell hyperplasia is focally encountered in transurethral resection specimens and causes no diagnostic problems; however, florid and unusual patterns of basal cell hyperplasia can mimic malignancies.

## Gross Features

Grossly, prostate glands with nodular hyperplasia have apparent periurethral nodularity in the transition zone, including cystic and solid nodules. Basal cell hyperplasia in particular does not necessarily confer any specific gross appearance.

## Microscopic Features

Microscopically, the identification of discrete, circumscribed nodules is the most important diagnostic clue to the presence of nodular hyperplasia and basal cell hyperplasia. Nodules contain stromal and glandular elements in different proportions, ranging from pure stromal proliferation to predominantly glandular proliferation. Basal cell hyperplasia is 1 such manifestation,

*Fig. 15.* (*A*) Paraganglioma in the urinary bladder may be a major diagnostic pitfall, as transurethral resection specimens may contain tight nests of cells with cautery artifact that mimic an invasive urothelial carcinoma. Paraganglioma also often intermingles with the muscularis propria, which could be misinterpreted as muscle-invasive urothelial carcinoma (H&E stain, original magnification ×4). (*B*) In areas with preserved morphology, the typical nested pattern with amphophilic cytoplasm may be more readily appreciable. Consideration of this diagnosis when encountering a monomorphic tumor with nested configuration in the urinary bladder helps to avoid this pitfall (H&E stain, original magnification ×20).

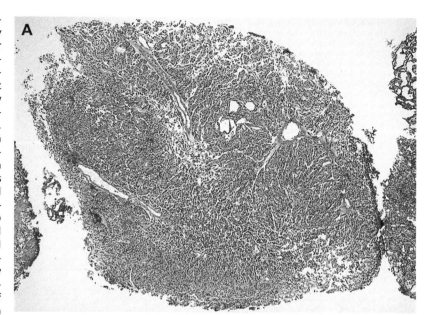

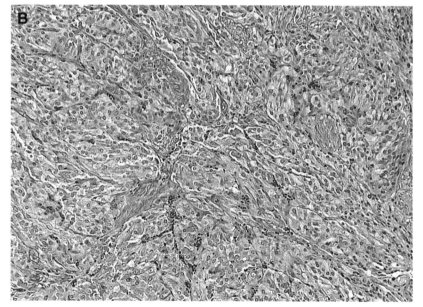

characterized by multilayering of basal cells that may impart a small gland appearance with high cellularity. Heaping of basal cells is often so prominent that the secretory cell layer is inconspicuous and a lumen may appear entirely absent.[95–97]

## Differential Diagnosis

Basal cell hyperplasia, which can be found focally within nodular hyperplasia, consists of tubules or glands with multilayering of the basal cell layer and, when florid, may be confused with prostate cancer, particularly if basal cell hyperplasia focally involves a hyperplastic nodule and, therefore, appears infiltrative (Fig. 16), or if nucleoli are conspicuous. Features useful in distinguishing basal cell hyperplasia from cancer includes multilayering of basal cell nuclei with scant cytoplasm, forming solid nests with scant luminal cytoplasm, pseudocribriform glands, intracytoplasmic eosinophilic globules, and well-formed lamellar calcifications.[95–97] In difficult cases, immunohistochemistry can confirm the presence of numerous basal cells, which are positive for high-molecular-weight cytokeratin and p63.[96,98] Although it is not infrequent for the glands to

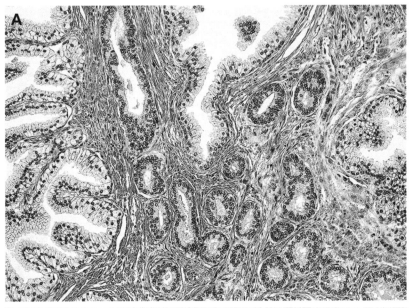

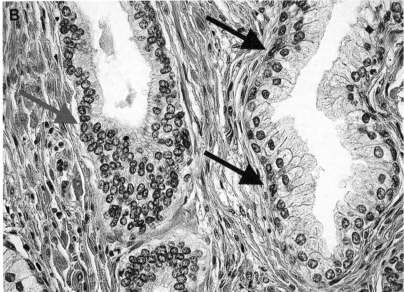

*Fig. 16.* (*A*) Basal cell hyperplasia in the prostate may mimic invasive prostate cancer, particularly if basal cell hyperplasia only partially makes up a hyperplastic nodule (H&E stain, original magnification ×20). (*B*) Higher magnification reveals multiple layers of cells (*red arrow*), with similar cytologic features to the basal cells of the adjacent benign glands (*black arrows*). Although basal cells may contain recognizable nucleoli, large prominent nucleoli and other cytologic features of prostate cancer are lacking (H&E stain, original magnification ×40).

appear entirely filled with basal cells, surprisingly the immunohistochemical labeling may be preferentially located in only some of the layers, often greater in the outer layers (**Fig. 17**). Some foci of basal cell hyperplasia resemble adenoid cystic carcinoma of the salivary glands (**Fig. 18A**), composed of cribriform-appearing glands with multiple lumina and nodules of collagenous material. In the past, a variety of names have been used for this pattern, such as florid basal cell hyperplasia, basal cell adenoma, adenoid basal cell tumor, and adenoid cystic-like tumor.[97] For lesions that are circumscribed and contained within hyperplastic nodules, however, clinical outcomes appear similar to those of usual basal cell hyperplasia, suggesting that all these entities can be diagnosed together under the umbrella of basal cell hyperplasia (see **Fig. 18B**).[97] In contrast, features, such as location in the peripheral zone or extension into the peripheral zone, infiltrative growth pattern, interconnecting glands, desmoplastic or myxoid stromal response, perineural invasion, and absence of concurrent nodular hyperplasia, have been suggested as helpful clues to the diagnosis of true basal cell carcinoma or adenoid cystic carcinoma of the prostate.[97,99]

*Fig. 17.* In this example of basal cell hyperplasia that partially involves a hyperplastic nodule, numerous basal cells are evident using p63 immumohistochemistry in the pseudoinfiltrative glands. Although morphologically the small glands contained multiple cell layers with similar cytologic features, only a subset of the cells (peripherally) label for p63, a known occurrence in prostatic basal cell proliferations (p63 IHC stain, original magnification ×10).

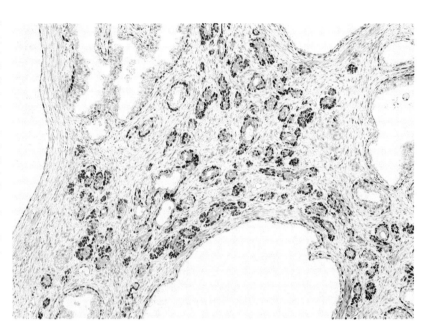

## Diagnosis

In most cases, diagnosis of basal cell hyperplasia is readily apparent based on the circumscription of the lesion and containment within hyperplastic nodules; however, for lesions that mimic acinar adenocarcinoma, immunohistochemical staining for basal cell markers may be helpful in confirming the presence of numerous basal cells. For lesions that raise concern for basal cell carcinoma, attention to infiltrative growth and other features of malignancy (discussed previously) can aid in resolving this question.

### Pitfalls

! Basal cell hyperplasia may falsely appear infiltrative due to focal or partial involvement of a hyperplastic nodule.

! Small glands with basal cell hyperplasia may contain recognizable nucleoli, mimicking acinar adenocarcinoma.

! Cribriform structures may mimic higher-grade adenocarcinoma.

## Prognosis

Even when florid, basal cell hyperplasia pursues a benign clinical course similar to that of usual nodular hyperplasia, as long as features of basal cell carcinoma (discussed previously) are absent.

## ATYPICAL ADENOMATOUS HYPERPLASIA (ADENOSIS) AND SCLEROSING ADENOSIS

Atypical adenomatous hyperplasia, also known as adenosis, is a benign transition zone proliferation that may be confused with acinar adenocarcinoma due to several overlapping morphologic and immunohistochemical features, including composition by small, round glands, incomplete basal cell layer, and positivity for AMACR.[100] Based on these overlapping characteristics, the status of atypical adenomatous hyperplasia as a precursor to adenocarcinoma is debated,[101–103] although it is currently not regarded as precancerous. Similarly, sclerosing adenosis is another transition zone proliferation composed of small glands with increased stromal cellularity that is unique among prostate lesions for the presence of myoepithelial differentiation of the basal cells.[100,104]

### Gross Features

Grossly, atypical adenomatous hyperplasia and sclerosing adenosis are not recognizable, because they typically are focal microscopic lesions within nodular hyperplasia.

### Microscopic Features

Microscopically, both atypical adenomatous hyperplasia and sclerosing adenosis are lobular glandular proliferations, composed of some large glands with a branching configuration, similar to the usual benign glands that comprise hyperplastic nodules. Both lesions, however,

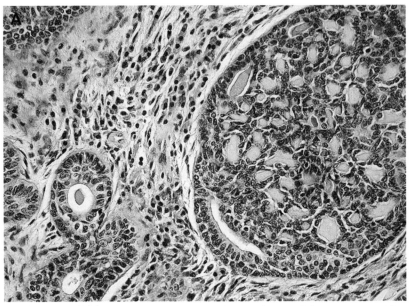

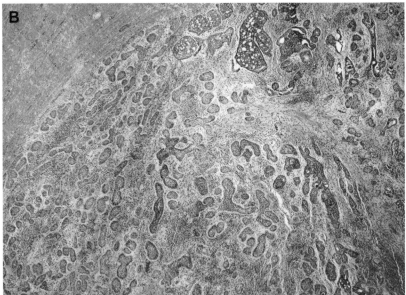

*Fig. 18.* (*A*) Basal cell hyperplasia of the prostate rarely exhibits multiple cribriform-like lumina and eosinophilic material within the nests, similar to salivary gland adenoid cystic carcinoma (H&E stain, original magnification ×40). (*B*) If such a proliferation is localized to a hyperplastic nodule without an infiltrative growth pattern, however, outcomes seem similar to those of nodular hyperplasia rather than basal cell carcinoma/adenoid cystic carcinoma of the prostate (H&E stain, original magnification ×4).

contain a proliferation of smaller glands that generally have similar cytologic features to the larger glands, typically located at the periphery of the nodule (Fig. 19A). Proceeding to the outermost aspect of the nodule, basal cells typically become less conspicuous in the smaller glands (see Fig. 19B), and, in sclerosing adenosis, the combination of minute glands and stromal cellularity may mimic Gleason pattern 4 or 5 cancer glands (poorly formed glands or single cells [Fig. 20A, B]).[100] In sclerosing adenosis, a prominent layer of basement membrane may partly surround the glands.[100] Usually both lesions are well circumscribed, although there may be a focal suggestion of infiltrative growth at the periphery of the nodule. Luminal crystalloids or blue mucin is sometimes present in atypical adenomatous hyperplasia, which may compound the differential diagnostic challenge with low-grade acinar adenocarcinoma.[100,105] Rarely, sclerosing adenosis may also show some cytologic atypia.[106]

## Key Features

- Atypical adenomatous hyperplasia and sclerosing adenosis are circumscribed proliferations of small glands within hyperplastic nodules

- A partial basal cell layer is present in many of the glands

- Morphology of glands lacking basal cells is similar to those with a partial basal cell layer.

- Crystalloids, blue mucin, and small glands can mimic adenocarcinoma.

- Myoepithelial differentiation is present in sclerosing adenosis

### Differential Diagnosis

The most important consideration in attempting to distinguish foci of atypical adenomatous hyperplasia and sclerosis adenosis from adenocarcinoma is to evaluate the entire lesion as a whole. Although some of the small round glands resemble those of an adenocarcinoma and some contain no basal cells as detected by immunohistochemistry (p63 or high-molecular-weight keratin), other glands with similar cytologic features consistently contain at least a partial layer of basal cells, arguing in favor of interpretation of the lesion as a whole as benign. In cases of sclerosing adenosis, immunohistochemistry also reveals positivity for myoepithelial markers, contrasting to normal prostate basal cells, which do not exhibit a myoepithelial phenotype, including actin HHF-35 or S-100 (Fig. 20C, D).[100,104]

### Diagnosis

Diagnosis of atypical adenomatous hyperplasia (adenosis) and sclerosing adenosis requires assessment of the constellation of pathologic features in the entire visualized lesion. If there are no appreciable morphologic differences between glands that contain basal cells and those that do not, this argues strongly against diagnosis of adenocarcinoma.

### Prognosis

Although the precursor status of atypical adenomatous hyperplasia is debated, there is currently no compelling evidence to suggest that its presence indicates an increased risk of developing cancer. Likewise, sclerosing adenosis is also a benign lesion.

## TESTIS

### ADENOMATOID TUMOR

Adenomatoid tumor is a benign mesothelial proliferation and the most common tumor of the paratesticular region, typically occurring near the head of the epididymis but occasionally also involving other sites, such as the rete testis or rarely the testis itself.[107,108] Due to a variety of morphologic patterns, adenomatoid tumors may cause diagnostic difficulty with a spectrum of other testicular and paratesticular tumors.

### Gross Features

Grossly, adenomatoid tumor usually forms a 3-cm to 5-cm circumscribed gross mass in the paratesticular region or less commonly appearing to involve the testis itself, with a white-tan, firm cut surface.[108] A subset of tumors has been recognized to contain necrosis,[109] which may obscure the benign nature of these tumors.

### Microscopic Features

Microscopically, adenomatoid tumors are composed variably of tubular structures, nests, and cords of cells (Fig. 21A), characteristically showing cytoplasmic vacuoles and often at least focally, strands of cytoplasm bridging the gland-like lumina or bridging between cells (see Fig. 21B).[108,110] In some cases, prominent muscle bundles are admixed with the proliferation.

### Differential Diagnosis

Given the heterogeneity in morphology of adenomatoid tumors, the presence of signet ringlike cells, vacuolated cells, glandlike structures, cords of cells, or apparent solid nests may raise a differential diagnosis with metastatic carcinoma, a primary vascular tumor, yolk sac tumor, or sex cord–stromal tumors.[108] Clues to resolving this differential diagnosis include the primarily paratesticular location, circumscription of the lesion, strands of cytoplasm bridging the lumina of the glandlike structures,[110] and reactivity for markers of mesothelial origin, including cytokeratin, calretinin, podoplanin (D2-40), keratin 5/6, thrombomodulin, and WT1. Negative staining for vascular markers (CD31, CD34, and FLI-1) and adenocarcinoma markers (carcinoembryonic antigen, MOC-31, and BER-EP4) facilitates excluding other considerations from the differential diagnosis.[107,108] Despite that some adenomatoid tumors contain necrosis (infarct) with granulation tissue, fibrosis, and/or a fibroblastic proliferation (Fig. 22),[109] an accurate diagnosis can be made when careful

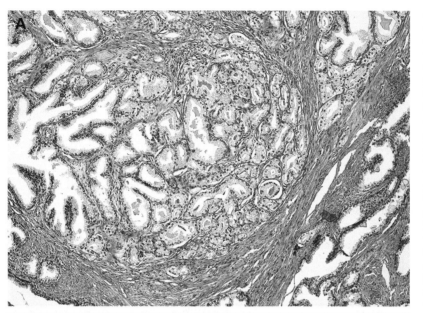

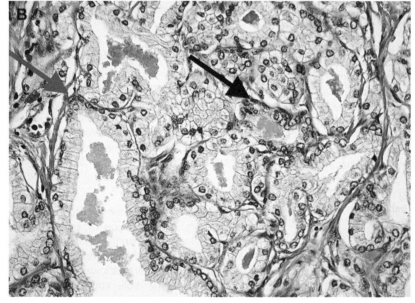

Fig. 19. (*A*) Atypical adenomatous hyperplasia or adenosis is composed of hyperplastic nodules with smaller glands at the periphery of the nodules, mimicking prostate cancer (H&E stain, original magnification ×10). (*B*) At high magnification, however, basal cells can be recognized in both the benign-appearing glands (*red arrow*) and the smaller, atypical glands (*black arrow*), including via immunohistochemistry. Although some of the small glands often lack appreciable basal cells (morphologically or with immunohistochemistry), if their morphology is otherwise the same as that of the benign glands, this argues strongly against diagnosis of adenocarcinoma (H&E stain, original magnification ×40).

attention is paid to the gross and histologic features. In particular, the changes associated with infarct may raise the possibility of malignant mesothelioma; however, the presence of a single circumscribed lesion in the paratesticular region rather than multifocal studding of the tunica vaginalis and usual absence of a papillary component argue against malignant mesothelioma.[109] Positivity for calretinin and WT1 is a shared feature with some sex cord–stromal tumors; however, the location usually outside of the testicular parenchyma is a clue to the diagnosis.

**Key Features**

- Adenomatoid tumor is a paratesticular proliferation of small glandlike structures that may mimic signet ring cells, adenocarcinoma, vascular proliferation, or sex cord–stromal tumor

- Positivity for mesothelial markers and circumscribed configuration confirms the diagnosis.

## Diagnosis

Although adenomatoid tumor is the most common paratesticular tumor, its heterogeneity of morphologic patterns may make diagnosis more challenging. Awareness of its occurrence in this location, its spectrum of morphologies, and the positivity for mesothelial markers facilitates diagnosis and discrimination for the wide array of other tumor types that can be morphologically mimicked by adenomatoid tumor.

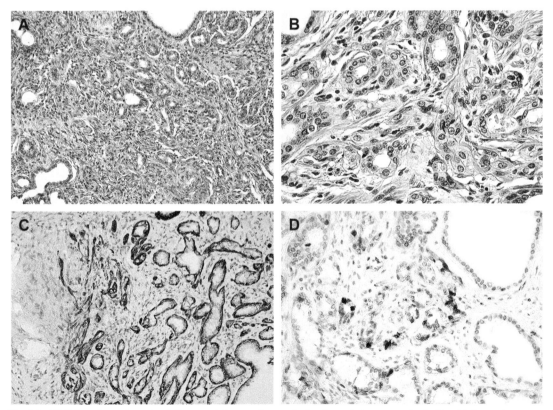

*Fig. 20.* (*A*) Sclerosing adenosis of the prostate may be a mimic of prostate cancer, including high-grade cancer, due to its composition by numerous small glands, sometimes without appreciable lumina (H&E stain, original magnification ×20). (*B*) Small glands without discrete lumina may resemble Gleason pattern 4 or 5 adenocarcinoma glands. The increased stromal cellularity and lack of overtly malignant cytologic features, however, are clues to the benign nature of this proliferation (H&E stain, original magnification ×40). (*C*) Immunohistochemistry for basal cells reveals an intact basal cell layer (High molecular weight cytokeratin IHC stain, original magnification ×20). (*D*) In contrast to normal prostate glands, myoepithelial differentiation is present in sclerosing adenosis, such as detected by S-100 immunohistochemistry in this case (S100 IHC stain, original magnification ×40).

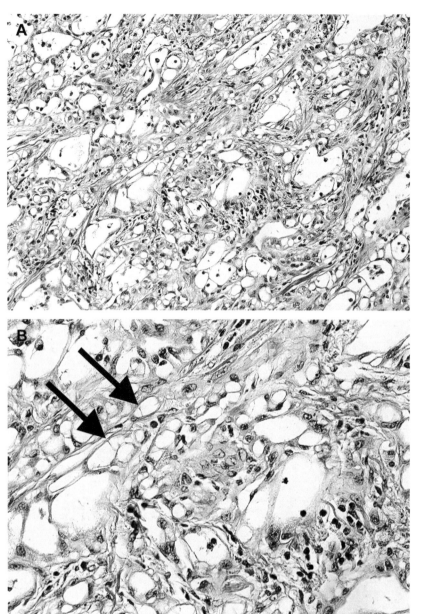

*Fig. 21.* Adenomatoid tumor is the most common tumor of the paratesticular region, composed of (*A*) small glandlike structures formed by mesothelial proliferation (H&E stain, original magnification ×20). (*B*) High magnification reveals variably sized, glandlike structures and single cells. Threadlike bridging strands of cytoplasm across lumina (*arrows*) have been described as a helpful diagnostic clue to the diagnosis (H&E stain, original magnification ×40).

*Fig. 22.* Necrosis and infarct have been described in a small subset of adenomatoid tumors, which may obscure the diagnosis. (*A*) In this case, adenomatoid tumor at left is juxtaposed to a zone of necrosis at right (H&E stain, original magnification ×10). (*B*) Higher magnification reveals glandlike structures with threadlike bridging strands (*arrows*), adjacent to the neutrophilic infiltrate and karryorhectic debris of the necrotic area (*right*) (H&E stain, original magnification ×40).

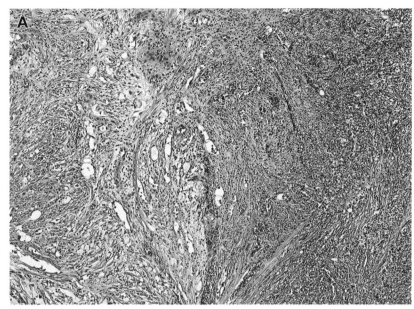

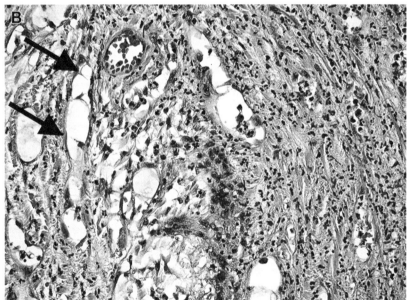

## Prognosis

Adenomatoid tumor is benign. Despite that it morphologically intermingles with paratesticular tissue, lesions are usually circumscribed and lack the recurrent behavior of malignant mesothelioma.

## REFERENCES

1. Adsay NV, Eble JN, Srigley JR, et al. Mixed epithelial and stromal tumor of the kidney. Am J Surg Pathol 2000;24:958–70.
2. Michal M, Hes O, Bisceglia M, et al. Mixed epithelial and stromal tumors of the kidney. A report of 22 cases. Virchows Arch 2004;445:359–67.
3. Antic T, Perry KT, Harrison K, et al. Mixed epithelial and stromal tumor of the kidney and cystic nephroma share overlapping features: reappraisal of 15 lesions. Arch Pathol Lab Med 2006;130:80–5.
4. Jevremovic D, Lager DJ, Lewin M. Cystic nephroma (multilocular cyst) and mixed epithelial and stromal tumor of the kidney: a spectrum of the same entity? Ann Diagn Pathol 2006;10:77–82.

5. Moch H. Cystic renal tumors: new entities and novel concepts. Adv Anat Pathol 2010;17:209–14.

6. Zhou M, Kort E, Hoekstra P, et al. Adult cystic nephroma and mixed epithelial and stromal tumor of the kidney are the same disease entity: molecular and histologic evidence. Am J Surg Pathol 2009;33: 72–80.

7. Turbiner J, Amin MB, Humphrey PA, et al. Cystic nephroma and mixed epithelial and stromal tumor of kidney: a detailed clinicopathologic analysis of 34 cases and proposal for renal epithelial and stromal tumor (REST) as a unifying term. Am J Surg Pathol 2007;31:489–500.

8. Srigley JR, Delahunt B, Eble JN, et al. The International Society of Urological Pathology (ISUP) vancouver classification of renal neoplasia. Am J Surg Pathol 2013;37:1469–89.

9. Tickoo SK, Gopalan A, Tu JJ, et al. Estrogen and progesterone-receptor-positive stroma as a nontumorous proliferation in kidneys: a possible metaplastic response to obstruction. Mod Pathol 2008; 21:60–5.

10. Karafin M, Parwani AV, Netto GJ, et al. Diffuse expression of PAX2 and PAX8 in the cystic epithelium of mixed epithelial stromal tumor, angiomyolipoma with epithelial cysts, and primary renal synovial sarcoma: evidence supporting renal tubular differentiation. Am J Surg Pathol 2011;35: 1264–73.

11. Kum JB, Grignon DJ, Wang M, et al. Mixed epithelial and stromal tumors of the kidney: evidence for a single cell of origin with capacity for epithelial and stromal differentiation. Am J Surg Pathol 2011;35: 1114–22.

12. Eble JN. Multilocular cystic renal cell carcinoma. In: Eble JN, Sauter G, Epstein JI, et al, editors. World Health Organization classification of tumours: pathology and genetics of tumours of the urinary system and male genital organs. Lyon (France): IARC Press; 2004. p. 26.

13. Halat S, Eble JN, Grignon DJ, et al. Multilocular cystic renal cell carcinoma is a subtype of clear cell renal cell carcinoma. Mod Pathol 2010;23: 931–6.

14. von Teichman A, Comperat E, Behnke S, et al. VHL mutations and dysregulation of pVHL- and PTEN-controlled pathways in multilocular cystic renal cell carcinoma. Mod Pathol 2011;24:571–8.

15. Williamson SR, Halat S, Eble JN, et al. Multilocular cystic renal cell carcinoma: similarities and differences in immunoprofile compared with clear cell renal cell carcinoma. Am J Surg Pathol 2012;36: 1425–33.

16. Fine SW, Reuter VE, Epstein JI, et al. Angiomyolipoma with epithelial cysts (AMLEC): a distinct cystic variant of angiomyolipoma. Am J Surg Pathol 2006;30:593–9.

17. Davis CJ, Barton JH, Sesterhenn IA. Cystic angiomyolipoma of the kidney: a clinicopathologic description of 11 cases. Mod Pathol 2006;19: 669–74.

18. Argani P, Faria PA, Epstein JI, et al. Primary renal synovial sarcoma: molecular and morphologic delineation of an entity previously included among embryonal sarcomas of the kidney. Am J Surg Pathol 2000;24:1087–96.

19. Schoolmeester JK, Cheville JC, Folpe AL. Synovial sarcoma of the kidney: a clinicopathologic, immunohistochemical, and molecular genetic study of 16 cases. Am J Surg Pathol 2014;38:60–5.

20. Sukov WR, Cheville JC, Lager DJ, et al. Malignant mixed epithelial and stromal tumor of the kidney with rhabdoid features: report of a case including immunohistochemical, molecular genetic studies and comparison to morphologically similar renal tumors. Hum Pathol 2007;38: 1432–7.

21. Suzuki T, Hiragata S, Hosaka K, et al. Malignant mixed epithelial and stromal tumor of the kidney: Report of the first male case. Int J Urol 2013; 20(4):448–50.

22. Kuroda N, Sakaida N, Kinoshita H, et al. Carcinosarcoma arising in mixed epithelial and stromal tumor of the kidney. APMIS 2008;116:1013–5.

23. Jung SJ, Shen SS, Tran T, et al. Mixed epithelial and stromal tumor of kidney with malignant transformation: report of two cases and review of literature. Hum Pathol 2008;39:463–8.

24. Cheng L, Gu J, Eble JN, et al. Molecular genetic evidence for different clonal origin of components of human renal angiomyolipomas. Am J Surg Pathol 2001;25:1231–6.

25. Martignoni G, Pea M, Reghellin D, et al. PEComas: the past, the present and the future. Virchows Arch 2008;452:119–32.

26. Hornick JL, Fletcher CD. PEComa: what do we know so far? Histopathology 2006;48:75–82.

27. Folpe AL, Kwiatkowski DJ. Perivascular epithelioid cell neoplasms: pathology and pathogenesis. Hum Pathol 2010;41:1–15.

28. Patil PA, McKenney JK, Trpkov K, et al. Renal leiomyoma: a contemporary multi-institution study of an infrequent and frequently misclassified neoplasm. Am J Surg Pathol 2015;39:349–56.

29. Bonsib SM. HMB-45 reactivity in renal leiomyomas and leiomyosarcomas. Mod Pathol 1996;9:664–9.

30. Zheng G, Martignoni G, Antonescu C, et al. A broad survey of cathepsin K immunoreactivity in human neoplasms. Am J Clin Pathol 2013;139: 151–9.

31. Martignoni G, Bonetti F, Chilosi M, et al. Cathepsin K expression in the spectrum of perivascular epithelioid cell (PEC) lesions of the kidney. Mod Pathol 2012;25:100–11.

32. Chilosi M, Pea M, Martignoni G, et al. Cathepsin-k expression in pulmonary lymphangioleiomyomatosis. Mod Pathol 2009;22:161–6.

33. Bonsib SM. Leiomyosarcoma. In: Eble JN, Sauter G, Epstein JI, et al, editors. World Health Organization classification of tumours: pathology and genetics of tumours of the urinary system and male genital organs. Lyon: IARC Press; 2004. p. 63.

34. Nese N, Martignoni G, Fletcher CD, et al. Pure epithelioid PEComas (so-called epithelioid angiomyolipoma) of the kidney: A clinicopathologic study of 41 cases: detailed assessment of morphology and risk stratification. Am J Surg Pathol 2011;35:161–76.

35. He W, Cheville JC, Sadow PM, et al. Epithelioid angiomyolipoma of the kidney: pathological features and clinical outcome in a series of consecutively resected tumors. Mod Pathol 2013;26:1355–64.

36. Eble JN, Amin MB, Young RH. Epithelioid angiomyolipoma of the kidney: a report of five cases with a prominent and diagnostically confusing epithelioid smooth muscle component. Am J Surg Pathol 1997;21:1123–30.

37. Brimo F, Robinson B, Guo C, et al. Renal epithelioid angiomyolipoma with atypia: a series of 40 cases with emphasis on clinicopathologic prognostic indicators of malignancy. Am J Surg Pathol 2010;34:715–22.

38. Aydin H, Magi-Galluzzi C, Lane BR, et al. Renal angiomyolipoma: clinicopathologic study of 194 cases with emphasis on the epithelioid histology and tuberous sclerosis association. Am J Surg Pathol 2009;33:289–97.

39. Klein MJ, Valensi QJ. Proximal tubular adenomas of kidney with so-called oncocytic features. A clinicopathologic study of 13 cases of a rarely reported neoplasm. Cancer 1976;38:906–14.

40. Ng KL, Rajandram R, Morais C, et al. Differentiation of oncocytoma from chromophobe renal cell carcinoma (RCC): can novel molecular biomarkers help solve an old problem? J Clin Pathol 2014;67:97–104.

41. Kryvenko ON, Jorda M, Argani P, et al. Diagnostic approach to eosinophilic renal neoplasms. Arch Pathol Lab Med 2014;138:1531–41.

42. Amin MB, Crotty TB, Tickoo SK, et al. Renal oncocytoma: a reappraisal of morphologic features with clinicopathologic findings in 80 cases. Am J Surg Pathol 1997;21:1–12.

43. Trpkov K, Yilmaz A, Uzer D, et al. Renal oncocytoma revisited: a clinicopathological study of 109 cases with emphasis on problematic diagnostic features. Histopathology 2010;57:893–906.

44. Hes O, Michal M, Sima R, et al. Renal oncocytoma with and without intravascular extension into the branches of renal vein have the same morphological, immunohistochemical, and genetic features. Virchows Arch 2008;452:193–200.

45. Tickoo SK, Amin MB, Zarbo RJ. Colloidal iron staining in renal epithelial neoplasms, including chromophobe renal cell carcinoma: emphasis on technique and patterns of staining. Am J Surg Pathol 1998;22:419–24.

46. Tan PH, Cheng L, Rioux-Leclercq N, et al. Renal tumors: diagnostic and prognostic biomarkers. Am J Surg Pathol 2013;37:1518–31.

47. Brunelli M, Eble JN, Zhang S, et al. Eosinophilic and classic chromophobe renal cell carcinomas have similar frequent losses of multiple chromosomes from among chromosomes 1, 2, 6, 10, and 17, and this pattern of genetic abnormality is not present in renal oncocytoma. Mod Pathol 2005;18:161–9.

48. Cheng L, Williamson SR, Zhang S, et al. Understanding the molecular genetics of renal cell neoplasia: implications for diagnosis, prognosis and therapy. Expert Rev Anticancer Ther 2010;10:843–64.

49. Sperga M, Martinek P, Vanecek T, et al. Chromophobe renal cell carcinoma–chromosomal aberration variability and its relation to Paner grading system: an array CGH and FISH analysis of 37 cases. Virchows Arch 2013;463:563–73.

50. Liu L, Qian J, Singh H, et al. Immunohistochemical analysis of chromophobe renal cell carcinoma, renal oncocytoma, and clear cell carcinoma: an optimal and practical panel for differential diagnosis. Arch Pathol Lab Med 2007;131:1290–7.

51. Hes O, Michal M, Kuroda N, et al. Vimentin reactivity in renal oncocytoma: immunohistochemical study of 234 cases. Arch Pathol Lab Med 2007;131:1782–8.

52. Williamson SR, Eble JN, Amin MB, et al. Succinate dehydrogenase-deficient renal cell carcinoma: detailed characterization of 11 tumors defining a unique subtype of renal cell carcinoma. Mod Pathol 2015;28(1):80–94.

53. Housley SL, Lindsay RS, Young B, et al. Renal carcinoma with giant mitochondria associated with germ-line mutation and somatic loss of the succinate dehydrogenase B gene. Histopathology 2010;56:405–8.

54. Gill AJ, Pachter NS, Chou A, et al. Renal tumors associated with germline SDHB mutation show distinctive morphology. Am J Surg Pathol 2011;35:1578–85.

55. Gill AJ, Hes O, Papathomas T, et al. Succinate Dehydrogenase (SDH)-deficient Renal Carcinoma: a morphologically distinct entity: a clinicopathologic series of 36 tumors from 27 patients. Am J Surg Pathol 2014;38(12):1588–602.

56. Ricketts CJ, Shuch B, Vocke CD, et al. Succinate dehydrogenase kidney cancer: an aggressive

example of the Warburg effect in cancer. J Urol 2012;188:2063–71.

57. Martignoni G, Pea M, Bonetti F, et al. Oncocytoma-like angiomyolipoma. A clinicopathologic and immunohistochemical study of 2 cases. Arch Pathol Lab Med 2002;126:610–2.

58. Montgomery E, Epstein JI. Anastomosing hemangioma of the genitourinary tract: a lesion mimicking angiosarcoma. Am J Surg Pathol 2009;33:1364–9.

59. Mehta V, Ananthanarayanan V, Antic T, et al. Primary benign vascular tumors and tumorlike lesions of the kidney: a clinicopathologic analysis of 15 cases. Virchows Arch 2012;461:669–76.

60. Lin J, Bigge J, Ulbright TM, et al. Anastomosing hemangioma of the liver and gastrointestinal tract: an unusual variant histologically mimicking angiosarcoma. Am J Surg Pathol 2013;37:1761–5.

61. Kryvenko ON, Haley SL, Smith SC, et al. Haemangiomas in kidneys with end-stage renal disease: a novel clinicopathological association. Histopathology 2014;65:309–18.

62. Kryvenko ON, Gupta NS, Meier FA, et al. Anastomosing hemangioma of the genitourinary system: eight cases in the kidney and ovary with immunohistochemical and ultrastructural analysis. Am J Clin Pathol 2011;136:450–7.

63. Brown JG, Folpe AL, Rao P, et al. Primary vascular tumors and tumor-like lesions of the kidney: a clinicopathologic analysis of 25 cases. Am J Surg Pathol 2010;34:942–9.

64. Buttner M, Kufer V, Brunner K, et al. Benign mesenchymal tumours and tumour-like lesions in end-stage renal disease. Histopathology 2013;62:229–36.

65. Pelosi G, Sonzogni A, Viale G. Intravascular papillary endothelial hyperplasia of the renal vein. Int J Surg Pathol 2011;19:518–20.

66. Akhtar M, Aslam M, Al-Mana H, et al. Intravascular papillary endothelial hyperplasia of renal vein: report of 2 cases. Arch Pathol Lab Med 2005;129:516–9.

67. Kryvenko ON, Roquero L, Gupta NS, et al. Low-grade clear cell renal cell carcinoma mimicking hemangioma of the kidney: a series of 4 cases. Arch Pathol Lab Med 2013;137:251–4.

68. Verine J. Differential diagnosis of primary benign vascular tumors and/or tumor-like lesions of the kidney: immunohistochemical stains should not be restricted to vascular and pan cytokeratin markers. Virchows Arch 2013;462:365–7.

69. Williamson SR, MacLennan GT, Lopez-Beltran A, et al. Cystic partially regressed clear cell renal cell carcinoma: a potential mimic of multilocular cystic renal cell carcinoma. Histopathology 2013;63:767–79.

70. Zhao M, Williamson SR, Yu J, et al. PAX8 expression in sporadic hemangioblastoma of the kidney supports a primary renal cell lineage: implications for differential diagnosis. Hum Pathol 2013;44:2247–55.

71. Doyle LA, Fletcher CD. Peripheral hemangioblastoma: clinicopathologic characterization in a series of 22 cases. Am J Surg Pathol 2014;38:119–27.

72. Lopez-Beltran A, Cheng L. Histologic variants of urothelial carcinoma: differential diagnosis and clinical implications. Hum Pathol 2006;37:1371–88.

73. Williamson SR, Lopez-Beltran A, Montironi R, et al. Glandular lesions of the urinary bladder:clinical significance and differential diagnosis. Histopathology 2011;58:811–34.

74. Volmar KE, Chan TY, De Marzo AM, et al. Florid von Brunn nests mimicking urothelial carcinoma: a morphologic and immunohistochemical comparison to the nested variant of urothelial carcinoma. Am J Surg Pathol 2003;27:1243–52.

75. Wasco MJ, Daignault S, Bradley D, et al. Nested variant of urothelial carcinoma: a clinicopathologic and immunohistochemical study of 30 pure and mixed cases. Hum Pathol 2010;41:163–71.

76. Holmang S, Johansson SL. The nested variant of transitional cell carcinoma–a rare neoplasm with poor prognosis. Scand J Urol Nephrol 2001;35:102–5.

77. Lopez Beltran A, Montironi R, Cheng L. Microcystic urothelial carcinoma: morphology, immunohistochemistry and clinical behaviour. Histopathology 2014;64:872–9.

78. Morton MJ, Zhang S, Lopez-Beltran A, et al. Telomere shortening and chromosomal abnormalities in intestinal metaplasia of the urinary bladder. Clin Cancer Res 2007;13:6232–6.

79. Rahemtullah A, Oliva E. Nephrogenic adenoma: an update on an innocuous but troublesome entity. Adv Anat Pathol 2006;13:247–55.

80. Gupta A, Wang HL, Policarpio-Nicolas ML, et al. Expression of alpha-methylacyl-coenzyme A racemase in nephrogenic adenoma. Am J Surg Pathol 2004;28:1224–9.

81. Young RH, Scully RE. Nephrogenic adenoma. A report of 15 cases, review of the literature, and comparison with clear cell adenocarcinoma of the urinary tract. Am J Surg Pathol 1986;10:268–75.

82. Mazal PR, Schaufler R, Altenhuber-Muller R, et al. Derivation of nephrogenic adenomas from renal tubular cells in kidney-transplant recipients. N Engl J Med 2002;347:653–9.

83. Pina-Oviedo S, Shen SS, Truong LD, et al. Flat pattern of nephrogenic adenoma: previously unrecognized pattern unveiled using PAX2 and PAX8 immunohistochemistry. Mod Pathol 2013;26:792–8.

84. Adeniran AJ, Tamboli P. Clear cell adenocarcinoma of the urinary bladder: a short review. Arch Pathol Lab Med 2009;133:987–91.

85. Tong GX, Melamed J, Mansukhani M, et al. PAX2: a reliable marker for nephrogenic adenoma. Mod Pathol 2006;19:356–63.

86. Tong GX, Weeden EM, Hamele-Bena D, et al. Expression of PAX8 in nephrogenic adenoma and clear cell adenocarcinoma of the lower urinary tract: evidence of related histogenesis? Am J Surg Pathol 2008;32:1380–7.

87. Cheng L, Cheville JC, Sebo TJ, et al. Atypical nephrogenic metaplasia of the urinary tract: a precursor lesion? Cancer 2000;88:853–61.

88. Hansel DE, Nadasdy T, Epstein JI. Fibromyxoid nephrogenic adenoma: a newly recognized variant mimicking mucinous adenocarcinoma. Am J Surg Pathol 2007;31:1231–7.

89. Lane Z, Epstein JI. Polypoid/papillary cystitis: a series of 41 cases misdiagnosed as papillary urothelial neoplasia. Am J Surg Pathol 2008;32:758–64.

90. Zhou M, Epstein JI, Young RH. Paraganglioma of the urinary bladder: a lesion that may be misdiagnosed as urothelial carcinoma in transurethral resection specimens. Am J Surg Pathol 2004;28:94–100.

91. So JS, Epstein JI. GATA3 expression in paragangliomas: a pitfall potentially leading to misdiagnosis of urothelial carcinoma. Mod Pathol 2013;26:1365–70.

92. Menon S, Goyal P, Suryawanshi P, et al. Paraganglioma of the urinary bladder: a clinicopathologic spectrum of a series of 14 cases emphasizing diagnostic dilemmas. Indian J Pathol Microbiol 2014;57:19–23.

93. Cheng L, Leibovich BC, Cheville JC, et al. Paraganglioma of the urinary bladder: can biologic potential be predicted? Cancer 2000;88:844–52.

94. Mason EF, Sadow PM, Wagner AJ, et al. Identification of succinate dehydrogenase-deficient bladder paragangliomas. Am J Surg Pathol 2013;37:1612–8.

95. Rioux-Leclercq NC, Epstein JI. Unusual morphologic patterns of basal cell hyperplasia of the prostate. Am J Surg Pathol 2002;26:237–43.

96. Hosler GA, Epstein JI. Basal cell hyperplasia: an unusual diagnostic dilemma on prostate needle biopsies. Hum Pathol 2005;36:480–5.

97. McKenney JK, Amin MB, Srigley JR, et al. Basal cell proliferations of the prostate other than usual basal cell hyperplasia: a clinicopathologic study of 23 cases, including four carcinomas, with a proposed classification. Am J Surg Pathol 2004;28:1289–98.

98. Yang XJ, Tretiakova MS, Sengupta E, et al. Florid basal cell hyperplasia of the prostate: a histological, ultrastructural, and immunohistochemical analysis. Hum Pathol 2003;34:462–70.

99. Ali TZ, Epstein JI. Basal cell carcinoma of the prostate: a clinicopathologic study of 29 cases. Am J Surg Pathol 2007;31:697–705.

100. Srigley JR. Benign mimickers of prostatic adenocarcinoma. Mod Pathol 2004;17:328–48.

101. Green WM, Hicks JL, De Marzo A, et al. Immunohistochemical evaluation of TMPRSS2-ERG gene fusion in adenosis of the prostate. Hum Pathol 2013;44:1895–901.

102. Cheng L, Davidson DD, Maclennan GT, et al. Atypical adenomatous hyperplasia of prostate lacks TMPRSS2-ERG gene fusion. Am J Surg Pathol 2013;37:1550–4.

103. Zhang C, Montironi R, MacLennan GT, et al. Is atypical adenomatous hyperplasia of the prostate a precursor lesion? Prostate 2011;71:1746–51.

104. Grignon DJ, Ro JY, Srigley JR, et al. Sclerosing adenosis of the prostate gland. A lesion showing myoepithelial differentiation. Am J Surg Pathol 1992;16:383–91.

105. Yang XJ, Wu CL, Woda BA, et al. Expression of alpha-Methylacyl-CoA racemase (P504S) in atypical adenomatous hyperplasia of the prostate. Am J Surg Pathol 2002;26:921–5.

106. Cheng L, Bostwick DG. Atypical sclerosing adenosis of the prostate: a rare mimic of adenocarcinoma. Histopathology 2010;56:627–31.

107. Delahunt B, Eble JN, King D, et al. Immunohistochemical evidence for mesothelial origin of paratesticular adenomatoid tumour. Histopathology 2000;36:109–15.

108. Amin MB. Selected other problematic testicular and paratesticular lesions: rete testis neoplasms and pseudotumors, mesothelial lesions and secondary tumors. Mod Pathol 2005;18(Suppl 2):S131–45.

109. Skinnider BF, Young RH. Infarcted adenomatoid tumor: a report of five cases of a facet of a benign neoplasm that may cause diagnostic difficulty. Am J Surg Pathol 2004;28:77–83.

110. Hes O, Perez-Montiel DM, Alvarado Cabrero I, et al. Thread-like bridging strands: a morphologic feature present in all adenomatoid tumors. Ann Diagn Pathol 2003;7:273–7.

# United States Postal Service

## Statement of Ownership, Management, and Circulation
### (All Periodicals Publications Except Requestor Publications)

| 1. Publication Title | 2. Publication Number | 3. Filing Date |
|---|---|---|
| Surgical Pathology Clinics | 0 2 5 - 4 7 8 | 9/18/15 |

| 4. Issue Frequency | 5. Number of Issues Published Annually | 6. Annual Subscription Price |
|---|---|---|
| Mar, Jun, Sep, Dec | 4 | $200.00 |

7. Complete Mailing Address of Known Office of Publication (Not printer) (Street, city, county, state, and ZIP+4®)

Elsevier Inc
360 Park Avenue South
New York, NY 10010-1710

Contact Person
Stephen R. Bushing

Telephone (Include area code)
215-239-3688

8. Complete Mailing Address of Headquarters or General Business Office of Publisher (Not printer)

Elsevier Inc., 360 Park Avenue South, New York, NY 10010-1710

9. Full Names and Complete Mailing Addresses of Publisher, Editor, and Managing Editor (Do not leave blank)

Publisher (Name and complete mailing address)

Linda Belfus, Elsevier Inc., 1600 John F. Kennedy Blvd., Suite 1800, Philadelphia, PA 19103

Editor (Name and complete mailing address)

Lauren Boyle, Elsevier Inc., 1600 John F. Kennedy Blvd., Suite 1800, Philadelphia, PA 19103-2899

Managing Editor (Name and complete mailing address)

Adrianne Brigido, Elsevier Inc., 1600 John F. Kennedy Blvd., Suite 1800, Philadelphia, PA 19103-2899

10. Owner (Do not leave blank. If the publication is owned by a corporation, give the name and address of the corporation immediately followed by the names and addresses of all stockholders owning or holding 1 percent or more of the total amount of stock. If not owned by a corporation, give the names and addresses of the individual owners. If owned by a partnership or other unincorporated firm, give its name and address as well as those of each individual owner. If the publication is published by a nonprofit organization, give its name and address.)

| Full Name | Complete Mailing Address |
|---|---|
| Wholly owned subsidiary of | 1600 John F. Kennedy Blvd. Ste 1800 |
| Reed/Elsevier, US holdings | Philadelphia PA 19103-2899 |

11. Known Bondholders, Mortgagees, and Other Security Holders Owning or Holding 1 Percent or More of Total Amount of Bonds, Mortgages, or Other Securities. If none, check box ☐ None

| Full Name | Complete Mailing Address |
|---|---|
| N/A | |

12. Tax Status (For completion by nonprofit organizations authorized to mail at nonprofit rates) (Check one)
The purpose, function, and nonprofit status of this organization and the exempt status for federal income tax purposes:
☑ Has Not Changed During Preceding 12 Months
☐ Has Changed During Preceding 12 Months (Publisher must submit explanation of change with this statement)

| 13. Publication Title | 14. Issue Date for Circulation Data Below |
|---|---|
| Surgical Pathology Clinics | September 2015 |

PS Form 3526, July 2014 (Page 1 of 3 (Instructions Page 3)) PSN 7530-01-000-9931 PRIVACY NOTICE: See our Privacy policy in www.usps.com

| 15. Extent and Nature of Circulation | | | Average No. Copies Each Issue During Preceding 12 Months | No. Copies of Single Issue Published Nearest to Filing Date |
|---|---|---|---|---|
| a. Total Number of Copies (Net press run) | | | 802 | 631 |
| b. Legitimate Paid and/Or Requested Distribution (By Mail and Outside the Mail) | (1) | Mailed Outside-County Paid Requested Mail Subscriptions stated on PS Form 3541. (Include paid distribution above nominal rate, advertiser's proof copies and exchange copies) | 388 | 317 |
| | (2) | Mailed In-County Paid/Requested Mail Subscriptions stated on PS Form 3541. (Include paid distribution above nominal rate, advertiser's proof copies and exchange copies) | | |
| | (3) | Paid Distribution Outside the Mails Including Sales Through Dealers And Carriers, Street Vendors, Counter Sales, and Other Paid Distribution Outside USPS® | 72 | 75 |
| | (4) | Paid Distribution by Other Classes of Mail Through the USPS (e.g First-Class Mail®) | | |
| c. Total Paid and/or Requested Circulation (Sum of 15b (1), (2), (3), and (4)) | | | 460 | 392 |
| d. Free or Nominal Rate Distribution (By Mail and Outside the Mail) | (1) | Free or Nominal Rate Outside-County Copies included on PS Form 3541 | 3 | 4 |
| | (2) | Free or Nominal Rate In-County Copies included on PS Form 3541 | | |
| | (3) | Free or Nominal Rate Copies mailed at Other classes Through the USPS (e.g. First-Class Mail) | | |
| | (4) | Free or Nominal Rate Distribution Outside the Mail (Carriers or Other means) | | |
| e. Total Nonrequested Distribution (Sum of 15d (1), (2), (3) and (4)) | | | 3 | 4 |
| f. Total Distribution (Sum of 15c and 15e) | | | 463 | 396 |
| g. Copies not Distributed (See instructions to publishers #4 (page #3)) | | | 339 | 235 |
| h. Total (Sum of 15f and g) | | | 802 | 631 |
| i. Percent Paid and/or Requested Circulation (15c divided by 15f times 100) | | | 99.35% | 98.99% |

* If you are claiming electronic copies go to line 16 on page 3. If you are not claiming Electronic copies skip to line 17 on page 3.

| 16. Electronic Copy Circulation | Average No. Copies Each Issue During Preceding 12 Months | No. Copies of Single Issue Published Nearest to Filing Date |
|---|---|---|
| a. Paid Electronic Copies | | |
| b. Total Paid Print Copies (Line 15c) + Paid Electronic copies (Line 16a) | | |
| c. Total Print Distribution (Line 15f) + Paid Electronic Copies (Line 16a) | | |
| d. Percent Paid (Both Print & Electronic copies) (16b divided by 16c X 100) | | |

☐ I certify that 50% of all my distributed copies (electronic and print) are paid above a nominal price.

17. Publication of Statement of Ownership
☑ If the publication is a general publication, publication of this statement is required. Will be printed in the December 2015 issue of this publication.

| 18. Signature and Title of Editor, Publisher, Business Manager, or Owner | Date |
|---|---|
| *Stephen R. Bushing* | September 18, 2015 |

Stephen R. Bushing – Inventory Distribution Coordinator

I certify that all information furnished on this form is true and complete. I understand that anyone who furnishes false or misleading information on this form or who omits material or information requested on the form may be subject to criminal sanctions (including fines and imprisonment) and/or civil sanctions (including civil penalties).

PS Form 3526, July 2014 (Page 3 of 3)

Printed and bound by CPI Group (UK) Ltd, Croydon, CR0 4YY

03/10/2024

01040379-0002